EAT
FOR BEAUTY

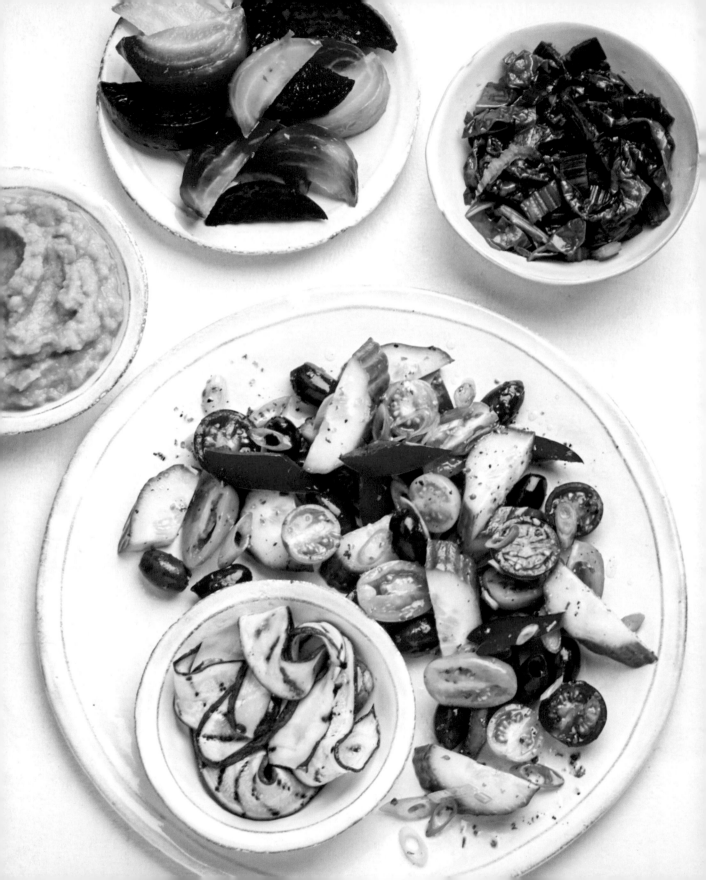

EAT
FOR BEAUTY

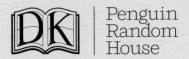

Penguin
Random
House

Editor Kayla Dugger
Americanizer Christy Lusiak
Project Editor Claire Cross
Senior Art Editors Emma Forge, Tom Forge,
Karen Constanti, Alison Gardner
Editorial Assistant Alice Horne
Managing Editor Dawn Henderson
Managing Art Editor Marianne Markham
Jackets Co-ordinator Libby Brown
Jackets Designers Amy Keast, Harriet Yeomans
Pre-Production Producer Catherine Williams
Producer Luca Bazzoli
Art Director Maxine Pedliham
Publisher Mary-Clare Jerram

First American Edition, 2017
Published in the United States by DK Publishing
345 Hudson Street, New York, New York 10014

Copyright © 2017 Dorling Kindersley Limited
DK, a Division of Penguin Random House LLC
17 18 19 20 21 10 9 8 7 6 5 4 3 2 1
001–293591–March/2017

A catalog record for this book is available from the Library of
Congress.
ISBN 978-1-4654-5684-7

DISCLAIMER See page 256.

DK books are available at special discounts when purchased
in bulk for sales promotions, premiums, fund-raising, or
educational use. For details, contact: DK Publishing Special
Markets, 345 Hudson Street, New York, New York 10014
SpecialSales@dk.com

Printed and bound in China

All images © Dorling Kindersley Limited
For further information see: www.dkimages.com

A WORLD OF IDEAS:
SEE ALL THERE IS TO KNOW
www.dk.com

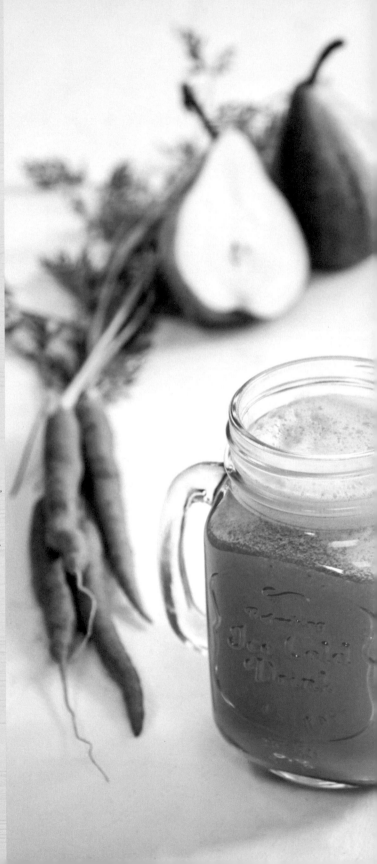

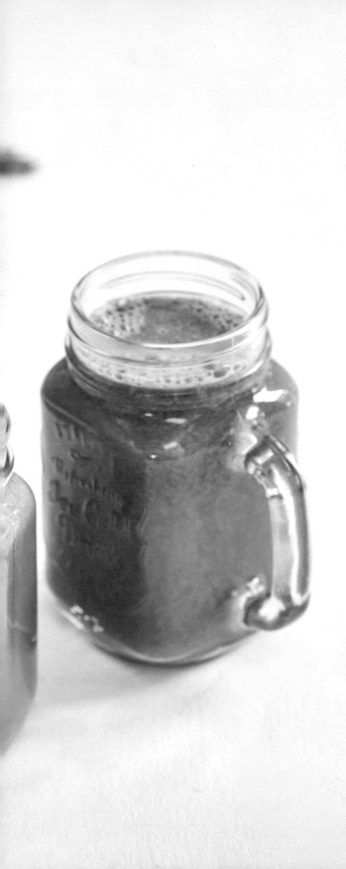

The Authors

Fiona Waring is a qualified nutritional therapist with over 25 years' experience in the health and fitness industry. While running a busy nutrition clinic and nutrition consultancy, she is also working towards a Master's degree in public health nutrition. Passionate about her chosen profession, Fiona believes in making nutrition understandable, enjoyable, practical, and adaptable to each individual's lifestyle and needs.

Tipper Lewis is Head of Training for Neal's Yard Remedies and a qualified naturopathic herbalist. She is passionate about helping spread the word about how natural remedies can help with wellness. Outside of work, she loves being outdoors in nature: on her allotment, gardening, or taking her dog on long country walks.

Susan Curtis is a qualified homeopath and naturopath and is the Director of Natural Health for Neal's Yard Remedies. She is the author of several books, including *Looking Good and Feeling Younger* and *Essential Oils,* and co-author of *Natural Healing for Women.* Susan has two grown-up children and is passionate about helping people live a more natural and healthy lifestyle.

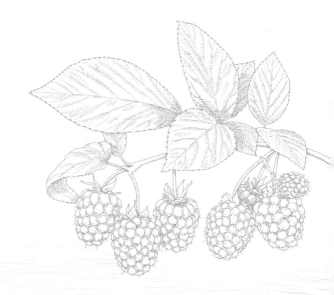

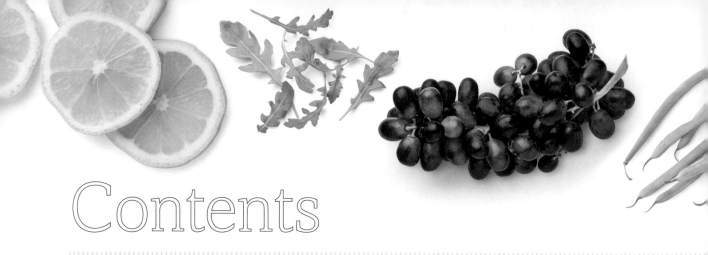

Contents

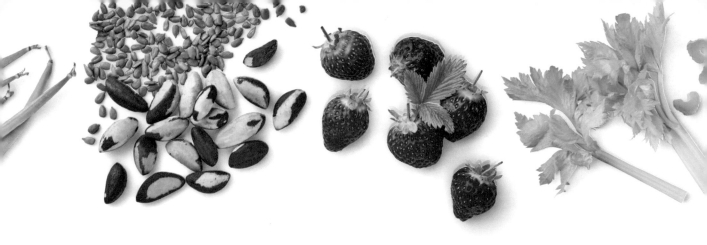

Introduction

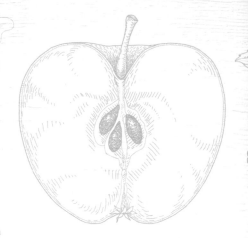

What do we think of when we think of **beauty**? For some, it could be a certain way of looking, and for others, a feeling or quality. Society often links beauty with **health** and **vitality**, so perhaps we should think of beauty as a combination of factors, and of how we look as a reflection of what is going on inside us.

While different cultures have their own ideals of what makes someone beautiful, most people recognize that real beauty isn't simply a collection of well-placed features, it is who a person is and how they feel, and how these things are radiated on the outside.

Modern-day living

In today's society we face many challenges and expectations as to how we look. The media bombards us with airbrushed images of models with perfect complexions and bodies, and there is unspoken pressure to aim for this level of perfection, even though, realistically, this is unachievable. There are also many factors that affect how we look, from pollution to poor food and lifestyle choices, to stress and increasingly busy lives that don't leave time for relaxation. All of these make looking and feeling beautiful a challenge.

There are encouraging signs that certain parts of the media are starting to change the narrative about beauty, and with it our perception of beauty. One of the effects of the growth of social media is that health and food bloggers have been gaining more attention, increasingly promoting the idea that health equals beauty—that if you look after what you eat and how you live, you will radiate wellness and desirability.

Research from the business magazine *Forbes* shows that a relatively minor group of health and wellness consumers are increasingly influential in redefining our food culture: focusing on "real" whole foods and drinks, with the emphasis on fresh and unprocessed, and showing us that eating this way can be fun, not a chore. They are sharing their enthusiasm and knowledge with mainstream consumers who are hungry for guidance, inspiration, and direction.

Along with this global interest in food and wellness is a growing body of information and research on how what we eat affects how we look, feel, and manage our lives. Some of this information is very new, and much of it backs up our traditional understanding about what a healthy diet should be. In this book we

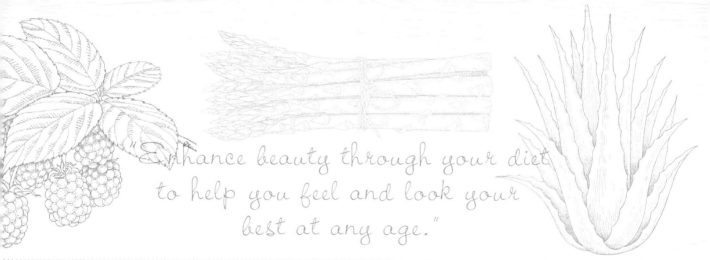

"Enhance beauty through your diet to help you feel and look your best at any age."

draw on a wealth of knowledge to help you find your way through the sometimes confusing messages around what you should and shouldn't eat, so that you can confidently choose the best foods to enhance your beauty and well-being, while also enjoying your food to the utmost, knowing it is doing you good.

Eating for beauty

Your skin is one of the first things you notice in the morning: how healthy does it look, do you look tired or stressed, or do you have spots? This check in the mirror can have a huge impact on how you feel during the day and how you face the world, and if you're not always happy with what you see, this can be difficult.

Naturopaths and holistic practitioners have long been aware that for us to enjoy healthy skin, it's also vital to pay attention to the health of our minds, as a healthy outlook can help you to make the positive lifestyle choices that will enhance your appearance. These good choices in turn impact on the health of our digestive systems, and when we digest foods well and absorb healthy nutrients, this is reflected in our skin. In this book we look at how to choose foods to enhance your face, body, hair, mouth, and hands and feet. For each of these areas we look at specific beauty concerns and show you which foods have a positive

impact. You will notice that certain foods crop up frequently, and these "star performers" provide a foundation of nutrients that will ensure you have the perfect platform to nurture how you look and feel.

A selection of delicious, nutrient-dense recipes helps you put this theory into practice, with meals formulated to address specific beauty concerns, and nutritionally balanced meal plans draw on these recipes, showing you how to plan your meals across the week to tackle a particular beauty concern.

A cleansing detox is the perfect start to your healthy eating regime, clearing your body of built-up toxins so that it can fully absorb beauty nutrients. A dedicated detox chapter maps out an easy-to-follow, two-week detox to set you off on your beauty food regime. And a range of topics, such as how to eat seasonally, how to cook for nutrients, and how to choose the healthiest foods, give you knowledge and confidence to make the right choices and get the most out of your beauty foods.

Enjoy exploring the foods and recipes throughout this book, eat beautiful, and experience more luminous, radiant skin and a greater sense of well-being.

***Susan Curtis**, Director of Natural Health, Neal's Yard Remedies, **Tipper Lewis**, Head of Training, Neal's Yard Remedies, and **Fiona Waring**, Nutritional Therapist*

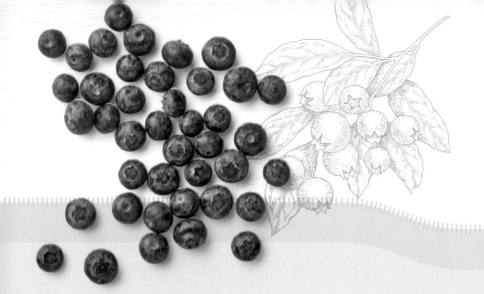

Beauty detox
kickstart

Start your beauty-food plan with this cleansing and rejuvenating two-week detox program. Replace beauty-zapping foods with the top skin-protecting, antioxidant-rich ingredients to help you flush out accumulated toxins and restore a healthy outer glow.

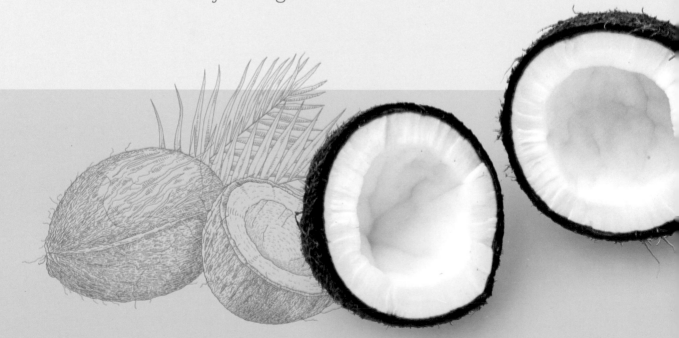

Why detox?

Our skin is a **reflection** of our inner health. Nutritional deficiencies and environmental toxins can lead to dull, dry, itchy skin, lackluster hair, and an untoned body. A cleansing detox will remove built-up toxins and start to restore nutrients, optimizing your body's ability to absorb the beauty-boosting nutrients recommended in this book.

The benefits of detox

Our bodies are under constant assault from toxins, which can come from unhealthy diet and lifestyle choices, the environment, and stress. Too many toxins mean our bodies struggle to get rid of them fast enough, which can make us feel bloated and impact on our skin. Our skin can be affected because when the main organs of detoxification, the liver and kidneys, are unable to cope, the skin takes over, which can result in skin problems as toxins are flushed out.

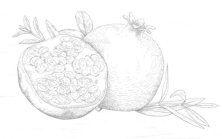

A cleansing detox gives your body a chance to recover, resetting the digestive system and leaving you feeling rejuvenated and revitalized.

The two-week beauty-renewing detox outlined in this chapter is designed to start you off on your beauty food regime, cleansing the body so that it is prepped to best utilize the healthy nutrients recommended in this book for specific beauty concerns. At first it may feel challenging to make the necessary dietary changes, but over time your body will crave the nutrients in these skin-enhancing foods. Once your body is working efficiently inside, healthy-looking skin and hair and a more toned body will start to reveal themselves on the outside. You are likely to find detox such a positive experience for your body, mind, and well-being that you'll make it a yearly ritual!

Common concerns

 How do I know if I need to detox?

Mood swings, headaches, insomnia, worsening menstrual symptoms, skin problems, joint and muscle pains, bloating, gas, bad breath, lowered energy levels, a lack of mental clarity, and lowered immunity can all suggest that your body is under stress. If you're experiencing one or several of these symptoms, a cleansing detox may be beneficial. A qualified naturopath can help you assess your need to detox. Before you detox, consult your doctor about any symptoms that may need further investigation.

 How long should I detox for?

It's best to detox over an extended period of time so that your body—especially your liver and excretory organs—isn't placed under stress. Gradually eliminating foods makes the experience more enjoyable and you'll be more likely to continue your healthy lifestyle

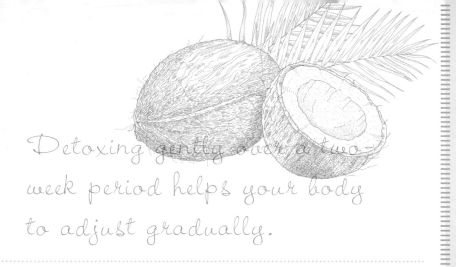

Detoxing gently over a two-week period helps your body to adjust gradually.

afterward. This detox is split into two weeks, each of which focuses on different areas.

 Am I likely to experience detox symptoms?

By detoxing over two weeks you should avoid, or have limited, symptoms because your excretory organs won't be overburdened. If you have symptoms, these should last for a few days only and could include headaches, mood swings, nausea, digestive upsets, lethargy, colds, poor concentration, and irritability. Occasionally, skin can worsen before it improves.

 Are there times when I should avoid detoxing?

Avoid detoxing when you're pregnant or breastfeeding. If you're on medication, talk to your doctor and a qualified naturopath first.

 Is it true that you shouldn't detox in winter?

The ideal time to detox is spring, when the body feels a renewal of energy. A winter detox is also

possible, but you will simply need to adapt and build your detox around broths, soups, and smoothies and juices with warming aromatic herbs.

 Can I work while I'm detoxing?

Yes, you should be able to live life as normal. Any symptoms should be short-lived, and you may find that you have even more energy. Follow the guidelines outlined in this chapter, and make sure that for every food you eliminate you introduce a nutrient-dense food to ensure you have sufficient energy. On this detox you will eat plenty of delicious, healthy foods so you have a wide variety of nutrients and you won't feel you're on a restricted diet.

 Can I exercise when I detox?

Yes, this is helpful, because exercise stimulates the lymphatic and circulatory systems, helping the body to eliminate toxins. Moderate exercise, such as yoga, walking, or Pilates, is ideal.

Detox language

Some of the language around detox can be confusing. Understanding what terms mean demystifies the process:

Free radicals, free oxidizing radicals, oxidants These are all the same thing: unstable chemicals that cause damage to healthy cells, breaking down the skin proteins collagen and elastin, causing skin to sag and wrinkle. They are unavoidable since they're produced by breathing and eating, but are increased by poor diet and lifestyle choices, medications, pollution, and the sun.

Antioxidants These are substances that prevent free-radical damage. We get antioxidants from brightly colored foods, spices, and herbs. The best known are vitamins C and E.

Oxidative stress This is when the number of free radicals outweighs the neutralizing ability of antioxidants. As we age, our ability to fight free radicals slows, so we need more antioxidants.

Dietary toxins These come from the foods we eat. They may be synthetic, such as pesticide residues, or microbial toxins from fungi and bacteria. Burnt, smoked, and fried foods have an increased number of toxins.

Phytonutrients Also called phytochemicals, these compounds in plants protect the plant's vitality and provide us with health-promoting properties when we eat them.

How to detox

Easing into and coming out of detox gently, following the steps below, will make your detox an enjoyable process, reducing the likelihood of side effects, such as cravings, headaches, nausea, and irritability, and making you more likely to continue a healthy eating regime afterward.

1 Prepare

Taking some time to prepare your body before starting your two-week detox program (see pp.20–23) will ensure you get the most out of the process. Detoxing requires both a physical and a mental adjustment. Starting off the cleansing process slowly means your body will be less likely to be overwhelmed by toxins once you begin your main two-week detox, and will also boost your nutritional status, ensuring that your body is able to cleanse most efficiently.

Before you start to detox, try keeping a food diary for a week. Record every food you eat each day, then look back to see which foods you eat excessively and think how you feel about giving up these foods. If you think you can't live without them, they are probably the first foods you should cut back on or eliminate altogether. As more research is being carried out into our gut microbiomes—the good and bad organisms that inhabit our guts—it's becoming increasingly clear that the type of bacteria we have in our guts can often dictate what types of food we choose to eat, causing cravings for certain foods. An imbalance of good and bad gut bacteria is reflected in our food choices—and we may find that we are eating too many sugary, refined, and processed foods rather than healthier whole-food, high-nutrient options.

Once you begin to explore different food options, your body and gut will start to adapt and you are likely to be more inclined to make healthy dietary choices and to avoid the latest diet fad.

2 Ease in

Once you've completed your food diary, ease yourself into detox. Take one to two weeks predetox to eliminate problem foods. If your diet is quite healthy, you could take just one week to prepare, but if you have several foods to eliminate, take two weeks. Foods often eliminated pre- and during detox are sugar, dairy, caffeine, wheat, alcohol, meat, processed and fast foods, and any foods you think you may have an intolerance to. The following tips will help you prepare. When you feel ready, start your detox.

• **Eliminate several foods at once**, or if that feels too daunting, choose the worst offender and cut this out first. You can do this in stages. For example, if you drink eight cups of coffee a day, cutting coffee out completely could lead to headaches and irritability. Instead, cut back to four cups a day in the first week, then eliminate it completely in the second week.

• **Each time you eliminate a food, it's essential to replace** it with a nutrient-dense food. The

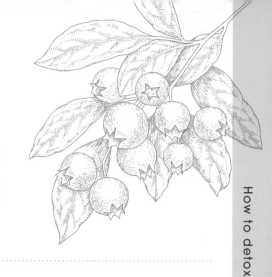

ALKALINES

To function at its best, the pH balance of the body should be mildly **alkaline**. Green leafy veggies are abundant in alkalizing minerals such as sodium, calcium, and potassium.

body needs nutrients to "bind" and neutralize toxins. This is a chance to try new, healthy foods. Increase your intake of foods with essential fatty acids, such as avocados, colorful vegetables and fruit, salad greens, whole grains, oats, legumes, sprouted seeds, and nuts and seeds.

• **Take a multivitamin and mineral supplement**, as well as an antioxidant supplement to neutralize free radicals, and an organic, cold-pressed blend of essential fatty acids to replace bad fats. Take these throughout your detox and afterward if you wish.

• **Review your cooking methods**. Steaming, casseroles, broths, and roasts help preserve nutrients. Don't eat too many raw foods at this point, as they are strong detoxifiers that are helpful later, once your body has adapted to the detox.

• **Drink at least 2 liters of water daily** to hydrate the body and help the lymphatic system and kidneys to eliminate toxins. Start each day with a glass of warm water and a squeeze of lemon juice to flush out impurities processed overnight. Then sip water throughout the day.

③ Ease off

Once you've finished detoxing, ease yourself off it. Resist returning to unhealthy habits, which can be a shock to your newly cleansed body. Enjoy the benefits you've gained: improved energy, concentration, and sleep; clearer skin; healthier digestion; and balanced emotions.

Eat similar foods to when you prepared to detox, and address beauty concerns by focusing on the foods in this book. A probiotic complex supports good gut bacteria, promoting skin health, immunity, and possibly reducing allergic responses. Fermented foods, such as kefir and sauerkraut, will also promote healthy gut bacteria.

Detox your pantry!

It's helpful to remove any temptation lurking in your pantry before you start to detox and restock with healthy options.

Remove any foods that are processed and refined. Look for foods that have artificial sweeteners, food colorings, and additives, such as sugary snacks and fizzy drinks, foods containing hydrogenated fats, and convenience foods such as instant coffee.

Replace each unhealthy food with a healthy option. Visit your local health food store to see if there are new foods you could try. Look at healthy recipes and make a note of ingredients you don't know or are intrigued by before your visit. Invest in superfoods that you can keep a supply of to add to meals and drinks, such as spirulina, baobab, and seaweed. And make some simple swaps, such as short-grain brown rice for white rice and honey for sugar.

Foods to exclude

Certain foods should be avoided when detoxing because they put stress on the digestive and excretory systems, making these less efficient and affecting the uptake of nutrients. Other foods are helpful later when the focus is on cleansing, but should be avoided in week 1. Find out which foods to cut out when before following the detox on pp.20–23.

Detox week 1

During this first week of detox, the main focus is on removing toxins from the bowels. Over time, poor dietary choices and lifestyle factors increase toxin levels, and the digestive organs constantly need to process a high number of toxins. This places the organs under pressure and can compromise their efficiency, making digestion sluggish and leading to problems such as constipation. For bright, vibrant skin we need regular bowel movements to ensure that we are eliminating waste efficiently.

To facilitate the removal of toxins in this first week, you need to eliminate foods that have a slow transit time through the bowels and are difficult to process. You also need to cut out inflammatory foods, which can hamper digestion and exacerbate skin problems.

Some foods are aggressive cleansers, and while these are beneficial later in your detox (see pp.18-19), they should be avoided in this first week because they flush out toxins too quickly, putting undue pressure on the liver and kidneys.

In the first week you will also need to cut out foods that lead to spikes in blood-sugar levels, foods that can affect the balance of good and bad bacteria in the gut, and foods high in salt, which can exacerbate fluid retention.

Detox week 2

In the second half of your detox, you will continue to avoid inflammatory foods, foods that slow down digestion, and high-sugar and high-salt foods.

All types of sugar

Avoid all sugars, including syrup, molasses, honey, fructose, lactose, maltose, and dextrose. **Sugar** is aging as it attaches to **collagen,** the connective tissue that keeps the skin elastic, causing inflammation and breaking it down. Sugar also exacerbates acne, creates insulin surges that disrupt hormone levels, and can imbalance bacteria in our guts.

Yeast products

Foods containing yeast, such as bread, pizza, buns, breadcrumbs, spreads, and gravy should be avoided during detox. These products are often high in additives and in salt, which causes the body to hold onto fluids to balance sodium and fluid levels, leading to puffiness and bloating.

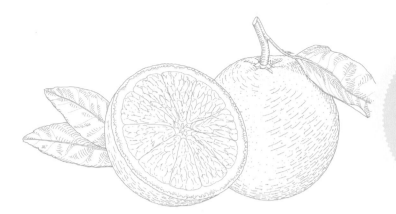

CALORIES

For every food you exclude you need to ensure that you replace it with a nutritious alternative to supply the calories you have lost and meet your energy needs.

Milk and dairy products

Dairy can be slow to pass through the gut, hampering digestion. Also, hormones given to cows to increase milk production end up in our milk and studies suggest these can aggravate acne. Eliminating dairy over these two-weeks allows you to monitor skin improvements. The exception, in week 1, is natural live yogurt and kefir, which support gut bacteria. Avoid all dairy in week 2.

Refined grains

Refined grains and white flour products, such as cakes, cookies, pasta, and cereals, should be cut out during your detox. Gluten from wheat and other grains contains sticky proteins, which are difficult to digest, and that can lead to skin inflammation and skin breakouts. Cereals made from amaranth grain cereal or custom cereals without sugar and salt can still be enjoyed.

Red meats and cured and smoked products

Red meats, in particular beef and pork, should be avoided now. Red meat can be inflammatory and also has a slow transit time through the bowels. While lamb is more easily broken down by the body, this can also be removed. Cut out processed meats and cured and smoked products, such as bacon and hot dogs, which contain toxins.

Citric acid

Avoid all artifically flavored foods, such as chips and other foods that contain artifical sources of citric acid, such as stock cubes, preserves, soft drinks, and canned fruit. Citric acid can lead to sensitivites in some people and aggravate conditions such as acid reflux, which can interfere with the digestive process.

Citrus fruits

Cut out citrus fruits, apart from a small amount of lemon juice, during the first week. Citrus is a strong cleanser, so it should be kept back until the excretory organs are under less pressure. Too much fruit of any sort should be avoided because the sugars in fruits feed unhealthy bacteria in the gut.

Caffeine and alcohol

Food and drinks containing caffeine can increase the levels of the stress hormone cortisol, which increases inflammation in the body, exacerbating skin conditions such as acne and increasing signs of premature aging. During detox cut out caffeine-containing foods and drinks such as coffee, tea, carbonated drinks, and chocolate. Cut out or reduce alcohol, too. This can impair the absorption of nutrients, and is high in aging sugars.

Foods to include

During your two-week detox cleanse (see pp.20–23) you'll include plenty of fresh, antioxidant-rich foods and healthy fats and proteins. As well as detoxifying the body, these foods calm and rehydrate skin, support healthy gut flora, and increase the production of the skin proteins collagen and elastin, essential for supple, healthy skin.

Detox week 1

During your first week, when you are focusing on removing a build-up of toxins from your bowels, you need to include foods that support your body and bowels. It's essential that for each food that is removed, you replace this with a nutrient-dense food so your body receives the fuel it needs to function properly.

Healthy fats, proteins, and complex carbohydrates will provide the calories you need to meet your energy requirements. Foods with a high water content will help to keep you hydrated while your body flushes out toxins, and antioxidant-rich wholefoods with skin-supporting vitamin C, which promotes collagen production, and vitamin E will nourish and revitalize skin during the detox process. Good sources of fiber are essential now to help the bowels work efficiently, as are prebiotic foods that support healthy gut micro-organisms.

Detox week 2

In the second week, the main organs of detoxification are under less pressure since toxins have been gradually removed. The focus now is on giving the bowel and colon a really thorough cleanse, so this is the time to introduce foods that have antiseptic properties or foods that contain chlorophyll, which draws toxins out and is a deep cleanser. Once your digestive tract is clean it will be primed to absorb valuable nutrients.

You should continue to eat foods that help to build collagen to keep skin supple, strong, and toned.

Fresh vegetables and fruit

Eat raw veggies and juices in week 2. Include onions; garlic; chlorophyll-containing cruciferous veggies such as cabbage and kale; fennel; leafy greens; asparagus; bright vegetables such as tomatoes, sweet potatoes, beets, and carrots; seaweeds; and avocados. Include limited fruits to keep sugar intake low, but in the second week, include citrus fruits since these are powerful cleansers.

Beans and legumes

Legumes, or pulses, such as lentils and dried beans, provide complex carbohydrates, healthy proteins, folate, and a range of essential vitamins and minerals to support digestion during detox and promote collagen production for healthy skin, hair, and nails.

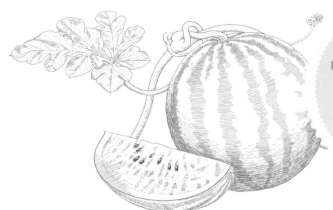

FLUIDS

It's vital to keep your healthy fluid levels up during the detox process (see p.15). As well as water, you can include herbal teas, juices, and smoothies.

Whole grains

Make easily digested whole grains part of your detox diet to provide complex carbohydrates that will supply energy during your detox. Include naturally leavened whole-grain sourdough and rye breads, brown rice, quinoa, millet, buckwheat, rye, barley, and amaranth.

Fermented foods

To promote and support healthy gut microflora, include natural live yogurt, kefir, kombucha, sauerkraut, miso, and tempeh. These fermented foods contain probiotics, which help to repopulate gut bacteria.

Nuts and seeds

These provide healthy proteins and fats as well as vitamins and minerals. Include chia seeds, flaxseeds, walnuts, hazelnuts, Brazil nuts, and almonds.

Healthy oils and fats

Using coconut oil for cooking releases fewer toxins at high heats as well as providing skin-nourishing properties. Use extra-virgin olive oil, flaxseed oil, and sesame oil in salads and to drizzle over foods to provide healthy omega fats.

Oily fish and lean meats

Fresh, oily fish provides protein and healthy fats to help the absorption of nutrients during your detox and to promote collagen production. Aim to eat oily fish two or three times a week. Some lean chicken can also be included in your detox diet if you find it too hard to give up meat.

Herbs and spices

These are a good source of antioxidant nutrients. Flavor foods with spices such as turmeric and ginger, which have cleansing properties, and use aromatic herbs, such as sage, basil, and thyme.

Detox planner week 1

In this first week of detox, the purifying process is underway as your body begins to flush out accumulated toxins. Here we show you the foods you should be concentrating on this week, and give you a day-by-day eating plan to help you incorporate these foods and ensure you are getting a balance of nutrients throughout the week.

How your body adapts

During your first detox week, your body is acclimating to its new diet, processing some new foods and learning how to cope without others. You may find that you feel energized from the outset, or you could experience some minor side effects as your body adapts.

Coldlike aches and pains, headaches, and energy dips are possible symptoms in this first week. Many of the foods you are excluding from your diet now would previously have stimulated your body, and may have been mildly addictive, such as caffeine and, it's increasingly believed, sugar. You may have relied on these foods to pick you up at certain times of the day, and struggle once they are dropped. Be encouraged that these symptoms are temporary, usually lasting a few days at the most. Moreover, it's likely that some of the foods you're excluding now contributed to more chronic symptoms in the past and troughs of low energy, and once your body adjusts to coping without them, you will find that your energy levels are on a more even keel and many symptoms disappear.

Digestive changes

As more bulking, fiber-rich foods are introduced into your diet, you may experience mild constipation. This is quite normal as your body adjusts. Making sure you stay well hydrated will soften and ease bowel movements.

Meal plan

Start each day of your detox with a hot-water drink with a generous squeeze of lemon juice to cleanse the liver. Drinking this on an empty stomach stimulates bile flow and encourages liver detoxification.

Monday

Breakfast

Green smoothie (p.244)

Snack

Handful of nuts and raisins

Lunch

Avocado on toast with mixed-herb pesto (p.180)

Snack

Cup of berries with natural live yogurt

Dinner

Salmon with samphire (p.215) OR Japanese ocean soup (p.201)

Tuesday

Breakfast

Poached egg on a slice of rye bread

Snack

Pineapple smoothie (p.239)

Lunch

Spring veggie salad (p.183)

Snack

Handful of nuts and apricots

Dinner

Summer salad with pomegranate and pistachio (p.202)

Wednesday

Breakfast

Spiced apple oatmeal (p.170)

Snack

Berry nice skin! (p.238)

Lunch

Summer asparagus salad (p.189)

Snack

Cup of berries with natural live yogurt

Dinner

Baked stuffed squash (exclude the optional cheese) (p.203)

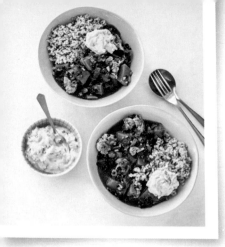

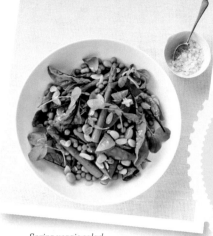

Black lentil and coconut curry (p.204)

Spring veggie salad (p.183)

TOP TIPS

Timing meals while detoxing helps to balance blood sugar. Eat at least every three hours to avoid sugar spikes that raise the stress hormone, cortisol. Aim for smaller, more frequent meals made up of three main meals and two healthy snacks a day.

Useful foods week 1

In your first week include grains such as brown rice, quinoa, millet, and buckwheat; chia and flaxseeds; cruciferous veggies; sprouted seeds; fennel; sweet potato; onion; tomato; carrots; watercress; asparagus; legumes; salad greens; vegetable juices; seaweed; berries; pineapple; pear; apple; cranberry; and aromatic herbs and spices.

• **Whole grains** *are important in this first week of detox to provide fiber to support the digestive system. Vegetables such as squash and legumes are also good sources of fiber.*

• **Light leafy greens** *such as spinach and salad leaves are helpful to include in week 1 of your detox. As well as providing essential vitamins and minerals, these also help to hydrate the body, upping fluid intake to keep the body refreshed and rejuvenated while toxins are being flushed out.*

• **Colorful fruit and vegetables** *are pcked with powerful antioxidants that have numerous benefits for your skin, hair, and body; these are essential throughout your detox.*

• **Seeds** *such as chia and flax are high in healthy essential fats, especially omega-3, which supports and nourishes skin.*

• **Cruciferous vegetables** *support the colon and bowel and have anti-inflammatory properties that help to support the digestive system and calm skin flare-ups that can occur during the detox process.*

Thursday

Breakfast

Berry, seed, and nut granola (p.166)

Snack

Coconut smoothie (p.235) and handful of almonds

Lunch

Sweet potato and mackerel mash (p.219, variation) OR Zucchini noodles (p.186)

Snack

2 oatcakes with hummus

Dinner

Greek vegetable mezze (p.198)

Friday

Breakfast

Overnight oats with superberry compote (p.168)

Snack

Red berry smoothie (p.235)

Lunch

Thai chicken and noodle soup (p.214)

Snack

Handful of fruits with raisins

Dinner

Black lentil and coconut curry (p.204)

Saturday

Breakfast

Oatmeal with apples and dessicated coconut

Snack

Green smoothie (p.244)

Lunch

Salad with crunchy apples and carrots

Snack

Handful of of Hot nuts! (p.194)

Dinner

Garlic salmon with coconut rice (p.215, variation) OR Barley vegetable risotto (p.200)

Sunday

Breakfast

Bluberry and chia pancakes (p.171)

Snack

Hemp seed butter (p.172) on a slice of rye bread

Lunch

Nutty rice salad (p.220)

Snack

Handful of of Hot nuts! (p.194)

Dinner

Japanese ocean soup (p.201)

Detox planner week 2

The focus during your second week of detox is on deep cleansing now that any built-up toxins have been eliminated. Here we have highlighted the foods that are key to your detox this week, and provided a day-by-day planner to help you include these healthy foods and ensure that you are getting all the nutrients you need throughout the week.

Maintaining stamina

During your second week of detox, you may struggle a little to maintain your initial resolve and have moments when you question your stamina and ability to give up certain foods. This is perfectly normal as your body continues to adjust to doing without high-sugar and high-salt quick fixes. As you carry on with your healthy eating this week, your body and gut will start to appreciate the increase in healthy nutrients, and you will find that cravings recede more and you begin to desire the more nutrient-dense, healthier alternatives you're eating now.

If you're feeling fatigued, this can affect your resolve. Check that you're eating sufficient calories for your energy needs and that you're not cutting anything out of the meal plan. It's important not to treat detox as a calorie-restricting diet, and remember that for every food you exclude, you should be replacing this with a nutritious alternative.

Skin changes

One of your main motivations for your beauty detox is likely to be to improve the condition of your skin, so if you suddenly have an acne outbreak you may feel dispirited. This can happen as residual toxins are flushed out through the skin, and is actually a positive sign that the detox is working. The nutrient-dense foods that you're eating now will soon start to have a cleansing effect and result in a more toned, balanced complexion.

Meal plan

Start each day of your detox with a hot-water drink with a generous squeeze of lemon juice to cleanse the liver. Drinking this on an empty stomach stimulates bile flow and encourages liver detoxification.

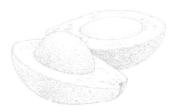

Monday

Breakfast

Fruity quinoa breakfast (p.169) and Vitamin C boost (p.245)

Snack

Handful of berries with natural live yogurt

Lunch

Chile guacamole (p.190) with 2 oatcakes

Snack

Green smoothie (p244)

Dinner

Miso-glazed tofu with quinoa (p.218)

Tuesday

Breakfast

Green smoothie (p.244)

Snack

Handful of nuts and apricots

Lunch

Winter veggie slaw (p.185)

Snack

Pineapple smoothie (p.239)

Dinner

Roasted broccoli and cauliflower with couscous (p.206)

Wednesday

Breakfast

Oatmeal with berry compote

Snacks

Green smoothie (p244)

Lunch

Green salad with cannellini beans

Snack

1 cup of berries with natural live yogurt

Dinner

Greek vegetable mezze (p.198)

TOP TIPS

Add concentrated superfood powders to your detox diet to boost your antioxidant count. You can buy powdered green food complexes such as spirulina and simply add ¼ tsp to a juice, glass of water, or smoothie.

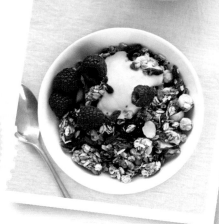

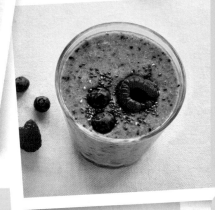

Berry nice skin! (p.238)

Berry, seed, and nut granola (p.166)

Useful foods week 2

Foods to include this week include citrus fruit, especially grapefruit; dark green vegetables, such as broccoli, Brussels sprouts, cabbage, and kale; wheatgrass; salad greens; sprouted seeds; seaweeds; avocado; beets and other bright veggies; turmeric; garlic; ginger; and flax, olive, and sesame oils.

• **Protein is vital** *during detox to ensure sufficient amino acids to bind and detoxify toxins safely. Vegetable proteins are best since these are clean and don't slow down the bowels. You could choose from tofu, tempeh, miso, peas, beans and legumes, or if you don't want to be completely vegetarian include oily fish, unsmoked and unprocessed, and lean chicken.*

• **Raw foods** *are perfect this week because they are potent detoxifiers, bursting with nutrients and enzymes. You could choose to go completely raw for the week, but if that's not for you try to eat some raw foods regularly in the week in juices, smoothies, or salads. When you do cook foods, use gentle steaming or cook foods slowly in a broth.*

• **Dark green foods** *are ideal now. These contain the pigment chlorophyll that plants use to make energy, which has a powerful cleansing effect and is a traditional ingredient for detoxing.*

• **Citrus fruits** *can be reintroduced this week because these have antiseptic and cleansing properties that are especially beneficial now.*

Thursday

Breakfast

Berry, seed, and nut granola (p.166) with coconut yogurt

Snack

Green smoothie (p244) and handful of almonds

Lunch

Fall flavors soup (p.179)

Snack

2 oatcakes with hummus and Berry nice skin! (p238)

Dinner

Japanese ocean soup (p.201)

Friday

Breakfast

2 slices toasted rye bread with almond butter and Vitamin C boost (p.245)

Snack

Green smoothie (p244)

Lunch

Fava bean soup (p.182)

Snack

Handful of nuts and raisins

Dinner

Barley vegetable risotto (p.200)

Saturday

Breakfast

2 slices toasted rye bread with a poached egg

Snack

Green smoothie (p.244)

Lunch

Avocado, kale, and wheatgrass salad

Snack

Handful of Hot nuts! (p.194)

Dinner

Miso-glazed tofu with quinoa (p.218)

Sunday

Breakfast

Green smoothie (p244)

Snack

Fruity chia jam (p.173) on a slice of rye bread with Cucumber and kale juice (p.243)

Lunch

Beet and chickpea soup (p.192)

Snack

Handful of Hot nuts! (p.194)

Dinner

Greek vegetable mezze (p.198)

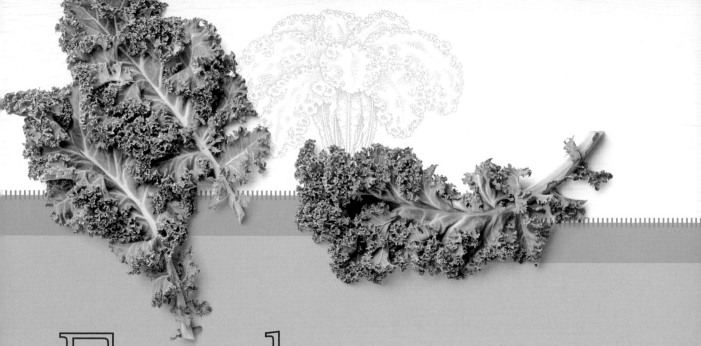

Foods
for the face

Your complexion reflects your lifestyle, and the foods you eat each day influence the way you look. Discover the very best nutrients for boosting your complexion, and follow **nutritionally balanced** meal plans tailored for a range of skin types to help you achieve radiant-looking skin.

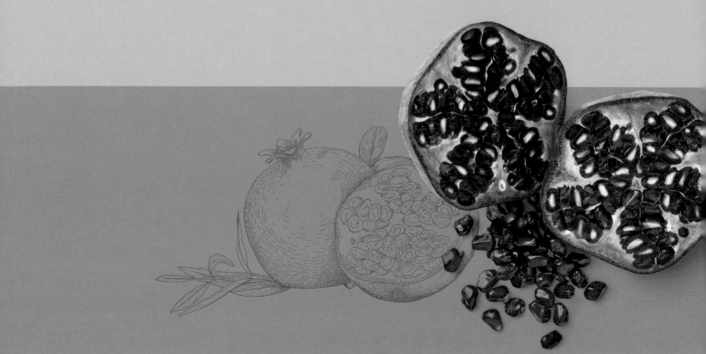

Eat for beauty: face

For skin to look **radiant** and feel smooth and toned, it needs to be nourished by the very best beauty nutrients. Discover the top **skin-nurturing** nutrients that form the foundation for a healthy complexion, helping to keep skin looking **luminous** and beautiful every day.

Nutrients for your face

Before you explore the foods for specific beauty concerns in this chapter, find out why a few key nutrients are fundamental overall for balanced, healthy-looking skin.

Antioxidants These essential compounds, found in many plants, play a critical role in protecting the body against the damaging effect of "free radicals"—the unstable chemicals that result from environmental and dietary toxins that have an aging effect on skin, causing a loss of skin tone and signs of aging such as fine lines and wrinkles. Antioxidants protect collagen and elastin, vital proteins that maintain our skin's elasticity, and boost the circulation to the tiny blood vessels near the skin's surface, enhancing our skin's natural radiance. The main skin antioxidants, such as carotenoids, vitamins C and E, flavonoids, and

resveratrol, are found abundantly in fresh fruit and vegetables. To ensure you're getting enough of these beauty-promoting nutrients, you need to eat a whole "rainbow" of fresh vegetables and fruit from berries and green leafy vegetables, to squash, carrots, sweet potatoes, and beets. One 2015 study found that organically grown fruit and vegetables provided even more antioxidants, and that switching to organic produce was the equivalent of eating one or two extra portions of fruit and vegetables each day.

Vitamin C This essential vitamin, found in many fresh fruits and vegetables, deserves a special mention because it's key to collagen production, the protein that aids the growth of cells and blood vessels, gives skin its firmness and strength, and helps skin to repair itself. An antioxidant, vitamin C reduces the impact of harmful free

radicals on collagen, and research suggests that it protects the skin against the harmful effects of UVB short rays from the sun. Our bodies can't store vitamin C, so it's vital to include it in our diet each day.

Essential fatty acids Healthy skin needs healthy fats, and in particular, a group of polyunsaturated fats called essential fatty acids (EFAs), the two main ones being omega-3 and omega-6. These fats support healthy cell membranes and help maintain the skin's natural oil barrier, critical for keeping skin hydrated, plump, and smooth. Your body can't make EFAs on its own, so you need to obtain them through your diet. It's important, too, to get the right balance of omega-3 and omega-6. Omega-6, found in vegetable oils such as sunflower and corn, helps cells to function, but too much has an inflammatory effect, while omega-3, found in

The healthy nutrients you eat each day will feed your skin from the inside, nourishing and hydrating skin to leave it looking smooth, supple, and radiant.

foods such as oily fish, eggs, nuts, chia, flaxseeds, and hemp seeds, is anti-inflammatory, thereby calming skin. Many of us eat too much omega-6 and not enough omega-3, so try to reverse this balance to optimize health and beauty.

15%

of your diet should be based on healthy proteins.

High-quality proteins Our skin is formed mainly of protein, and a lack of healthy proteins can result in a loss of skin tone and signs of premature aging such as fine lines

and sagging skin. Like EFAs, protein is obtained through the foods you eat daily, and around 15 percent of our diet should be based on protein. Sources of healthy proteins come from fish, lean meat, dairy, and vegetable products, such as hemp seeds, tofu, eggs, quinoa, algae, spinach, nuts, and beans and legumes.

Hyaluronic acid This gel-like, water-holding molecule helps skin cells to retain moisture and also facilitates the passage of nutrients into the skin and the removal of waste products. Studies show that hyaluronic acid (HA), an antioxidant, increases hydration, stimulates collagen production, and improves skin elasticity. The body manufactures HA from certain vegetables, in particular soy foods and sweet potatoes, so increase your intake of organic tofu, miso, and sweet potato.

Sulfur This mineral is one of the most important raw materials for healthy new skin cells. With the help of vitamin C and other key nutrients, it builds and maintains supple, permeable cell walls. It also has detoxifying properties that can help to clear blemishes, and it is thought to help reduce the appearance of acne scars and pigmentation issues such as age spots and sun damage. Sulfur is plentiful in green leafy vegetables such as kale, broccoli, spinach, and arugula.

Hydration Staying hydrated is essential for the health of your skin. Dehydrated skin feels tight and can appear flaky, rough, and finely lined. As well as drinking up to 2 liters of water daily, supplement hydration through your diet by eating foods with a high water content, such as cucumbers, watermelon, and celery.

What affects our skin?

The way we look is dependent on several factors, from what we eat to our genetic inheritance, lifestyle, environment, and stress. Being aware of what can affect your skin will help you to choose foods that support your skin type and help counter the effects of skin stressors.

Hereditary and aging The tendency of skin to be oily, dry, or both is partly down to genetics. While you can't change your skin type, you can adjust your diet to support it. For instance, cleansing foods such as raw vegetables and fruits help to balance oily skin, while dry or sensitive skin benefits from a diet high in omega-3 fats.

As you age, skin loses moisture. Hydrating it with sufficient fluids (see p.42) minimizes signs of aging, and eating high-quality proteins and vitamin C–rich foods supports collagen levels to keep skin supple.

Diet and lifestyle A poor diet and unhealthy lifestyle choices impact negatively on skin. Processed and fast foods are high in sugar and hydrogenated fats, both of which damage collagen. Eat fresh foods to ensure high levels of beneficial nutrients, and choose organic if possible to avoid skin-damaging toxins from pesticide residues. Use good-quality olive or coconut oil; reduce or eliminate sugar, or replace white, nutrient-poor sugar with mineral-rich maple or date syrup (in moderation); and swap highly processed table salt with good-quality sea or Himalayan pink salt that's high in minerals.

Black tea and coffee dehydrate skin. Replace these with herbal teas or hot water and lemon drinks. Avoid, too, sugary, carbonated drinks, which block the absorption of nutrients. Alcohol also dehydrates

Eat for your age

It's a fact that our skin ages, but that doesn't mean we can't keep it looking as fresh and line-free as possible with help from the foods we eat. Over the decades, skin gradually loses elasticity, so from your 30s onward, it's essential to eat foods that support collagen production. You can support your diet and skin with a good multivitamin and mineral supplement. In later decades, omega oil and hyaluronic acid supplements are helpful.

In your 20s

A busy social life can mean a healthy diet is low priority. You may go through a phase of not eating well and overloading your body with toxins that can be prematurely aging for skin. Up until your late 20s you may also still be dealing with outbreaks of acne and other skin problems such as eczema. Many young women are lacking in iron, which leads to pale skin and dark undereye circles.
Eat: Antioxidant-rich fruit and vegetables, especially those high in vitamin C, such as kale, kiwi, and peppers. Eat green leafy vegetables, nuts and seeds, whole grains, and legumes to ensure you have enough iron.

In your 30s

The first signs of aging, such as fine lines, may start to appear now as sebum production slows down. Skin may look dry and dull, and you may have the odd spot still. Pores enlarge, and skin pigment can become patchy, which can be linked to hormonal changes in pregnancy. Skin needs plenty of nourishment now to lay foundations for healthy skin in the future.
Eat: Brightly colored, nutrient-dense foods, such as tomatoes, carrots, and broccoli, with carotenoids that protect skin against aging free radicals. Aid collagen with healthy proteins from oily fish, legumes, nuts, seeds, and lean meats.

35%

of your calories can come from healthy essential omega fatty acids.

skin and aggravates redness or sensitivity. Try to keep alcohol consumption to under 5 drinks a week. And aim to quit smoking. Apart from the health implications, smoking accelerates aging.

Stress Stress can be etched on our faces, causing worry lines and dark undereye circles, as well as aggravating problems such as eczema. We can't avoid all stress, but we can minimize its effects by eating healthy fats from sources such as oily fish, and nutrient-rich fresh vegetables and fruit.

Environment Pollution, harsh winter weather, and overexposure to sun all impact negatively on skin. Irritants in the air from exhaust fumes and other chemicals can inhibit the skin's ability to repair itself. A lack of humidity in colder months dries skin, and too much sun damages skin layers, increasing aging free radicals. Eat antioxidant-rich foods to protect skin, and essential fatty acids to keep skin conditioned and more robust.

In your 40s

Nose-to-mouth lines become more obvious now and skin loses moisture as sebum production continues to drop. Skin can look dry overall and thinner, and skin tone may be uneven. **Eat:** Plenty of good, skin-nourishing oils such as coconut, linseed, and hemp, and fresh, oily fish, such as salmon and mackerel. B vitamins are also crucial to help prevent dry skin. Get B vitamins from grains such as brown rice, whole-grain cereals, and whole-wheat bread. For vitamin B12 you will need to eat fish, poultry, and lean meat or take a supplement if you're vegetarian.

In your 50s

Elastin and collagen levels can drop to unhealthy levels now so this is when we need to work hardest to make sure our diets contain the optimum nutrients to maintain these important skin proteins at healthy levels. Changes in hormones can lead to flushing and rosacea. **Eat:** Essential fatty acids to keep skin supple from olive and coconut oils, avocado, and oily fish. Include healthy proteins from legumes, nuts, eggs, fish, and lean meat. Red foods, such as berries and tomatoes, contain collagen-boosting lycopene, and organic soy products and legumes help to balance hormones.

60s plus

Our collagen levels and ability to manufacture antioxidants decline as we get older, so it's even more important to get an abundance of antioxidants from our diets. The manufacture of hyaluronic acid also declines with age. This acid is vital for healthy collagen and helps skin to retain moisture, keeping it plump and preventing dryness and wrinkles. **Eat:** Healthy proteins and oils from oily fish, coconut, and olive oils, and antioxidant-rich fruit and vegetables, including leafy greens and root veg. Include foods with hyaluronic acid, such as soy products and sweet potatoes.

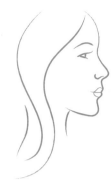

Combination skin

This common skin type is characterized by a shiny forehead, nose, and chin, known as the "T-zone," where sebaceous glands are most active. Processed and fried foods and too much dairy, wheat, and sugar can increase sebum production. Healthy proteins repair and renew skin, while hydrating foods, and foods high in anti-inflammatory essential fatty acids, zinc, and natural pro- and prebiotics help to balance sebum and restore vitality.

Superfood recipe suggestions...Berry, seed, and nut granola p166   Hemp seed butter on whole-wheat bread p172   Spring veggie salad p183   Huevos rancheros p184   Roasted broccoli and cauliflower with couscous p206   Salmon with samphire p215

Chia seeds

These tiny seeds are the richest known source of omega-3 fatty acids. Omega-3s are powerful anti-inflammatories, helping to soothe skin and also to balance sebum production to even skin tone. Flaxseeds, pumpkin, sunflower, and sesame seeds are also great sources of omega-3 fatty acids.
Key nutrients: Omega-3, fiber, manganese.
How to eat: 2–3 tsp daily, sprinkled over meals.

high in omega-3

28%
FIBER RI

high in chlorophyll

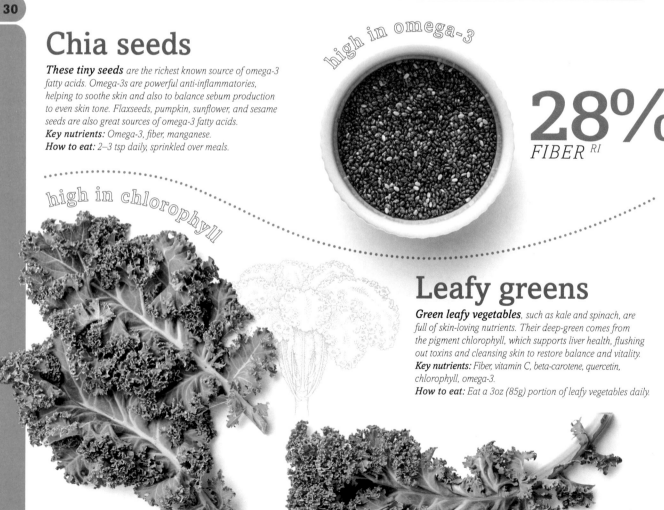

Leafy greens

Green leafy vegetables, such as kale and spinach, are full of skin-loving nutrients. Their deep-green comes from the pigment chlorophyll, which supports liver health, flushing out toxins and cleansing skin to restore balance and vitality.
Key nutrients: Fiber, vitamin C, beta-carotene, quercetin, chlorophyll, omega-3.
How to eat: Eat a 3oz (85g) portion of leafy vegetables daily.

Aloe vera juice

Rich in nutrients, aloe vera juice has antibacterial, antifungal, and antiviral properties that help to balance skin.
Key nutrients: *Vitamins A, C, and E, salicylic acid, polysaccharides, calcium, chromium, selenium, zinc, magnesium, potassium.*
How to eat: *3 tbsp daily; try adding to a smoothie or juice.*

vitamins A, C, and E

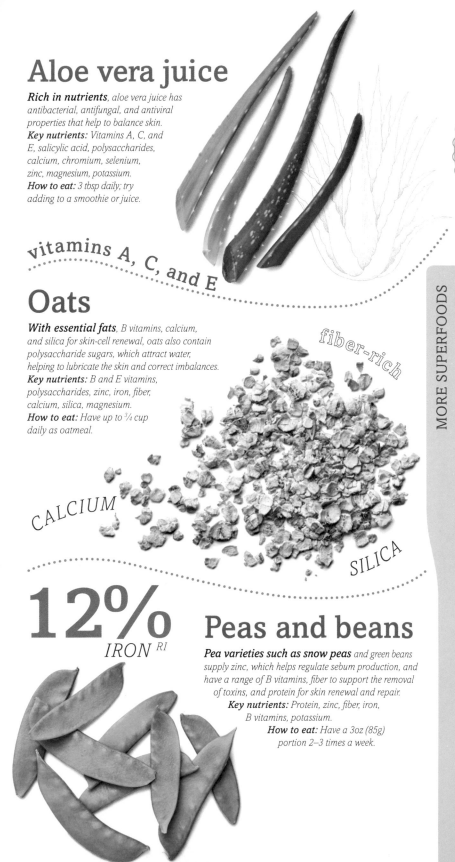

Oats

With essential fats, *B vitamins, calcium, and silica for skin-cell renewal, oats also contain polysaccharide sugars, which attract water, helping to lubricate the skin and correct imbalances.*
Key nutrients: *B and E vitamins, polysaccharides, zinc, iron, fiber, calcium, silica, magnesium.*
How to eat: *Have up to ¾ cup daily as oatmeal.*

fiber-rich

CALCIUM

SILICA

12%
IRON RI

Peas and beans

Pea varieties such as snow peas *and green beans supply zinc, which helps regulate sebum production, and have a range of B vitamins, fiber to support the removal of toxins, and protein for skin renewal and repair.*
Key nutrients: *Protein, zinc, fiber, iron, B vitamins, potassium.*
How to eat: *Have a 3oz (85g) portion 2–3 times a week.*

QUICK FIX

Make a **skin-renewing** smoothie. Mix ⅓ cup oats with 1 cup natural live yogurt and add 3 tbsp aloe vera juice. Add your favorite fruits. Blend and drink immediately.

MORE SUPERFOODS

Nuts
Nuts, such as walnuts and cashews, contain omega-3, -6, and -9, key to controlling sebum overproduction and inflammation.
Key nutrients: *Omega fats, protein, sulfur.*
How to eat: *Up to 2 tbsp daily as snacks.*

Yogurt and kefir
Natural live yogurt and kefir, a fermented milk drink, contain good bacteria for a healthy gut, protein, and minerals.
Key nutrients: *Protein, calcium, B vitamins, potassium.*
How to eat: *Have up to 9oz (250g) daily.*

Seaweed
Full of minerals, sea vegetables help detoxify and hydrate, and in turn balance fluids.
Key nutrients: *Omega-3 and -6, vitamin B6, iodine, calcium, iron, carotenoids.*
How to eat: *Add 1 tsp of dried seaweed daily to food, or use kelp flakes for seasoning.*

Lemon
Astringent and antiseptic, lemon attacks harmful gut bacteria. It aids the absorption of minerals, detoxifies, and supports the liver.
Key nutrients: *Vitamin C, folate.*
How to eat: *Include a squeeze in water, juices, smoothies, dressings, and meals.*

Spirulina
Spirulina, a detoxifier, is up to 70 percent pure, absorbable protein, great for skin repair. It contains a spectrum of enzymes and other skin-balancing nutrients.
Key nutrients: *Protein, antioxidants, essential fatty acids, B vitamins, calcium.*
How to eat: *Start with ¼ tsp daily in a meal or drink and build up to 1 tsp.*

For supplements, see page 249.

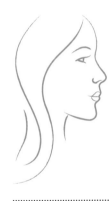

Oily complexion

Overactive sebaceous glands produce a surplus of oil, which combines with dead skin cells, blocking and enlarging pores and causing spots and a "shine." Some people have a genetic tendency to oily skin but processed, fried, and sugary foods can clog pores. Eat foods rich in zinc for skin repair, foods with anti-inflammatory fatty acids to balance sebum, and nutrient-dense antioxidant foods to help keep skin clear.

Superfood recipe suggestions...**Hemp seed butter with rye bread** p172   **Avocado on toast with mixed-herb pesto** p180
Winter veggie slaw p185   **Nutty rice salad** p220   **Miso-glazed tofu with quinoa** p218

Leafy greens

*The **deep green** of vegetables such as Savoy cabbage and spinach indicates chlorophyll, a natural detoxifier. Leafy greens also provide fiber, which supports digestion and waste removal, and are abundant in B vitamins, antioxidants, and healthy fats, all of which help to restore the balance of sebum to keep skin toned.*
Key nutrients: *Fiber, B vitamins, vitamin C, folate, beta-carotene, chlorophyll, folate, quercetin, omega-3.*
How to eat: *Have up to 3½oz (100g) daily.*

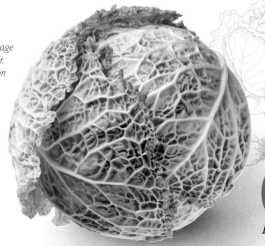

64%
FOLATE RI

HIGH IN VITAMIN C

Lemon juice

*This **simple flavoring** has astringent and antiseptic properties that help to counter the negative effects of a diet high in processed meats and saturated fats, which dull skin. Its purifying properties make it ideal for combating oily skin.*
Key nutrients: *Vitamin C, folate.*
How to eat: *Add a squeeze to water, juices, smoothies, salad dressings, and meals.*

QUICK FIX

Use skin-detoxifying lemons daily. Start the day with a hot water and lemon drink, then add lemon juice and zest to smoothies, dressings, and to flavor meals.

Brightly colored vegetables

Think red, yellow, and orange for the potent skin benefits of the antioxidant beta-carotene. In the body, beta-carotene converts to vitamin A, which helps rejuvenate skin cells.
Key nutrients: Vitamins A, B2, and C.
How to eat: Have a 3oz (85g) portion of bright vegetables daily, raw or lightly steamed.

vitamin A

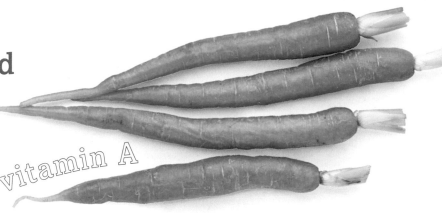

Watercress

This sulfur-rich salad leaf aids protein absorption, supports liver health, and cleanses the blood of impurities. It's especially high in vitamin C and antioxidants, which fight bacterial infections and reduce skin eruptions common to oily skin.
Key nutrients: Sulfur, vitamin C, antioxidants, calcium, iron, folate.
How to eat: Have a large handful as part of your five a day; add to salads or meals.

VITAMIN C–RICH

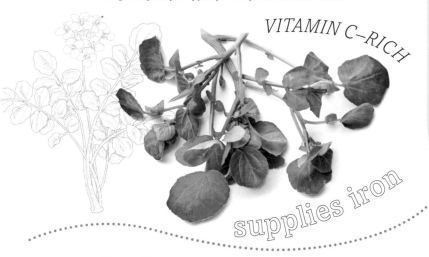

supplies iron

11%
VITAMIN K RI

Sprouted seeds

These are 10–30 times more concentrated in nutrients than vegetables and have easily absorbed nutrients, enzymes, and amino acids. Seeds such as alfalfa aid detoxification, helping to cleanse the skin.
Key nutrients: Vitamins A, B complex, C, E, and K, fiber, iron, sulfur, protein, calcium, selenium, omega-3.
How to eat: Have a large handful of broccoli or alfalfa sprouts daily, sprinkled over salads or main meals.

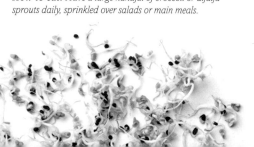

MORE SUPERFOODS

Aloe vera juice
This helps to soothe digestive problems that make the system sluggish. Aloe vera also contains salicylic acid, an anti-inflammatory, and sulfur, which promotes skin repair.
Key nutrients: Vitamins A, C, and E, zinc, salicylic acid, polysaccharides, calcium, chromium, selenium, magnesium, potassium.
How to drink: Have 3 tbsp daily; try adding to smoothies or juices.

Brown rice and legumes
Short-grain brown rice and legumes, such as lentils, are excellent sources of fiber, skin-nourishing healthy fats, B vitamins, and skin-repairing minerals such as zinc. Opt for brown rice as white removes the outer layer of the grain, which is filled with the nutrients.
Key nutrients: Fiber, B vitamins, zinc.
How to eat: Up to 3oz (85g) daily.

Miso paste
Made by fermenting soy, rice, wheat, or barley, miso populates the gut with good bacteria. It has the amino acids needed for skin renewal, and antioxidants to balance and tone skin.
Key nutrients: Kojic acid, vitamin K, zinc, protein, phosphorus, probiotics, omega-3.
How to eat: Up to 2 tbsp 3–4 times a week. Add the paste to dressings or while cooking.

Hemp seeds
These have a healthy balance of oils, with a good ratio of omega-3, -6, and -9, all of which help promote healthy, toned skin.
Key nutrients: Omega fats, protein, sulfur.
How to eat: Up to 2 tbsp daily.

Spirulina
This protein-rich "super" supplement inhibits prostaglandins, which cause inflammation.
Key nutrients: Protein, antioxidants, essential fatty acids, B vitamins, calcium.
How to eat: Start with ¼ tsp daily in a meal or drink and build up to 1 tsp.

Meal planner Skin balancing

Our skin is our biggest organ and works with the kidneys and bowels to excrete toxins. A build-up of toxins can exacerbate problems such as oily skin. The meal planner below, using recipes from this book and additional meal ideas, incorporates foods that help to balance sebum levels and ease skin congestion to promote a balanced, healthy complexion.

34

Your skin-balancing week

This nutritionally balanced one-week meal planner starts you off on your skin-balancing diet. For best results, continue for four weeks, varying meals using the alternatives, opposite. Begin each day with a hot water and lemon drink to aid digestion.

Monday

Breakfast
Green smoothie (p.244)

Snacks
Handful of nuts and raisins

Lunch
Avocado on whole-wheat or spelt toast with sprouted seeds and herb pesto (p.180)

Dinner
Roasted sea bass with tomato salsa (p.212)

Tuesday

Breakfast
Hemp seed butter (p.172) with whole-wheat or spelt toast

Snacks
Sliced carrot and celery with 2 tablespoons of hummus

Lunch
Scrambled tofu (p.181)

Dinner
Thai chicken and noodle soup (p.214)

Wednesday

Breakfast
Fruity quinoa breakfast (p.169)

Snacks
Hot nuts! (p.194)

Lunch
Summer asparagus salad (p.189)

Dinner
Miso-glazed tofu with quinoa (p.218)

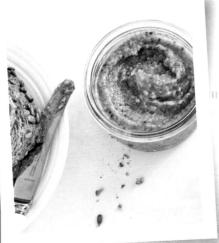

Hemp seed butter (p.172)

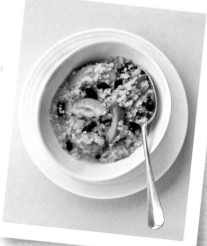

Fruity quinoa breakfast (p.169)

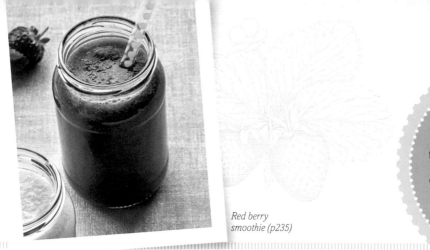

Red berry smoothie (p235)

SPROUTING

Sprouted seeds are a warehouse of **vitamins, minerals, enzymes, fatty acids**, and the largest source of protein of any vegetable, all of which help to promote a balanced complexion. Try growing your own sprouted seeds or simply buy them at the supermarket.

Thursday

Breakfast

Berry, seed, and nut granola (p.166)

Snacks

Red berry smoothie (p.235)

Lunch

Huevos rancheros (p.184) with watercress salad

Dinner

Roasted broccoli and cauliflower with couscous (p.206)

Friday

Breakfast

Rye bread with almond butter

Snacks

Oat cakes with nut butter with raw red bell pepper sticks

Lunch

Cannellini beans with bok choy, arugula, tomatoes, and olive salad

Dinner

Salmon with samphire (p.215)

Saturday

Breakfast

Mixed berry fruit salad with natural live yogurt and ground flaxseeds

Snacks

Sliced apple, spread with almond butter

Lunch

Winter veggie slaw (p.185)

Dinner

Nutty rice salad (p.220)

Sunday

Breakfast

Nutty overnight oats (p.168, variation)

Snacks

Green smoothie (p.244)

Lunch

Dairy-free pesto (p.186, variation) with gluten-free pasta and green salad

Dinner

Baked stuffed squash (p.203)

Sweet treat

Coconut yogurt with baobab and goldenberries (p.226)

Alternatives

To help you on your way, draw on these additional recipe suggestions to vary your meals over the course of four weeks.

Breakfast

Poached egg on rye bread

Sliced banana and cashew butter on rye toast

Snacks

Protein power beauty bites (p.195)

Rye bread with nut butter

Lunch

Spring veggie salad (p.183)

Fava bean soup (p.182)

Dinner

Black lentil and coconut curry (p.204)

Greek vegetable mezze (p.199)

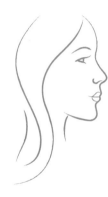

Dry, flaky skin

Skin lacking in sebum can become tight, itchy, red, and flaky. Eating unhealthy fats, smoking, and drinking alcohol and caffeine exacerbate dry skin. Vitamin A– and E–rich foods and brightly colored foods full of beta-carotene repair and replenish damaged skin cells, while healthy fats and essential fatty acids have an anti-inflammatory action that reduces redness and helps to restore sebum.

Superfood recipe suggestions...**Blueberry and chia pancakes** p171 **Fall flavors soup** p179 **Scrambled tofu** p181
Zucchini noodles with basil pesto p186 **Salmon with samphire** p215 **Salted goldenberry chocolate cups** p224

Bananas

A prebiotic, *fructooligosaccharide (FOS), in bananas feeds healthy gut bacteria, supporting the uptake of nutrients and bowel health. Bananas also have the antioxidant lutein, which boosts elasticity and sebum levels, locking in moisture and keeping skin supple.*
Key nutrients: Vitamins B6 and C, manganese, potassium, fiber, biotin, copper, lutein.
How to eat: Snack on a banana daily.

QUICK FIX

Hydrate and nurture skin with this fruity smoothie. Process 1 banana, a handful each of blueberries or redcurrants, and 1¼ cups coconut water. Drink immediately.

Olive oil

A good source of skin-repairing antioxidant *vitamin E, the fat in olive oil is up to 75 percent omega-9 (oleic acid), which aids the absorption of omega-3 fats, enhancing our uptake of nutrients. Cold-pressed, extra-virgin oil is especially good for dry skin as it has anti-inflammatory properties.*
Key nutrients: Vitamins E and K, omega-9, flavonoids, quercetin.
How to eat: Include up to 2 tbsp daily. Use extra-virgin in salads and non-extra-virgin for cooking.

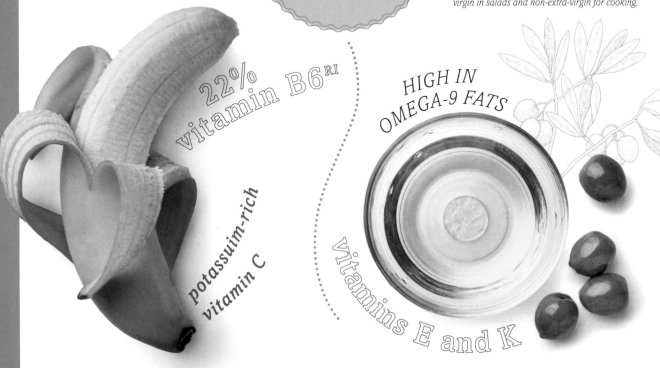

22% vitamin B6 RI

potassuim-rich vitamin C

HIGH IN OMEGA-9 FATS

vitamins E and K

Coconut

Coconut oil is rich in special fats called medium-chain triglycerides (MCTs), which nourish dry skin, while the water is high in electrolyte minerals, which quickly rehydrate the body.
Key nutrients: MCTs, potassium, manganese, fiber, vitamin B6.
How to eat: Use up to 2 tbsp of the oil daily for cooking, or drink up to 1¼ cups of the water.

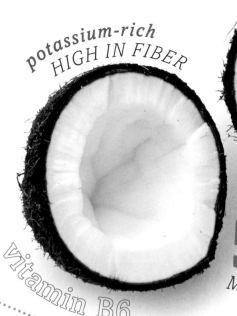
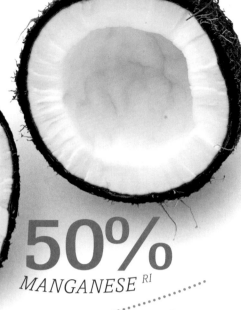

potassium-rich
HIGH IN FIBER

vitamin B6

50%
MANGANESE RI

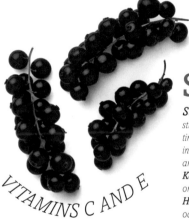

VITAMINS C AND E

Summer berries

Summer berries, such as blueberries and redcurrants, strengthen blood vessel walls, boosting circulation to the tiny blood vessels in the skin. The improved blood supply increases skin nutrition, helping to prevent skin thinning and increase radiance. The seeds are rich in fatty acids.
Key nutrients: Antioxidants, vitamins C and E, omega-3, potassium, magnesium.
How to eat: Add a handful daily to smoothies, oatmeal, or eat as a snack.

MORE SUPERFOODS

Oily fish
These supply anti-inflammatory omega-3, often lacking in dry skin.
Key nutrients: Omega-3, fiber, manganese.
How to eat: Aim to eat 2–3 times a week.

Seeds
Hemp seeds are about 47 percent essential fats. Flaxseeds and chia seeds also supply omega-3.
Key nutrients: Omega-3 and -6, gamma linolenic acid (GLA), protein, sulfur.
How to eat: Snack on 2 tbsp daily.

Avocado
High in healthy fats, omega-3, -6, and -9, and skin-nurturing vitamins.

Key nutrients: Lutein, beta-carotene, omega-3, vitamins A, B6, C, E, and K, folate, copper, potassium.
How to eat: Enjoy 2–4 avocados a week.

Oats
Polysaccharides in oats attract water to moisturize.
Key nutrients: B vitamins, vitamin E, zinc, iron, fiber, calcium, magnesium, polysaccharides.
How to eat: Have ⅓–¾ cups a day.

Eggs
Protein and healthy fats in eggs nourish skin.
Key nutrients: Omega-3, choline, selenium, biotin, vitamins A, B5, 12, and D, protein.
How to eat: Have 2–3 poached eggs a week.

Leafy greens
These are a rich source of vitamins, omega-3, sulfur, and chlorophyll, all of which nourish blood, in turn helping to condition the skin.
Key nutrients: Fiber, vitamin C, beta-carotene, quercetin, omega-3, chlorophyll, sulfur.
How to eat: Have a 3oz (85g) serving of steamed leafy greens up to once a day.

Spirulina
The anti-inflammatory properties of this superfood powder benefit dry skin.
Key nutrients: Protein, antioxidants, essential fatty acids, B vitamins, calcium.
How to eat: Start with ¼ tsp daily in meals and drinks and build up to 1 tsp daily.

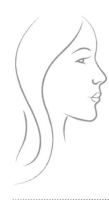

Mature skin

Skin thins as we age, becoming drier as sebum production falls, and less supple, as collagen and elastin production slow. Smoking, alcohol, sugar, sun, and processed foods all accelerate signs of aging. For glowing skin, eat skin-nourishing foods with essential fatty acids; anti-inflammatory foods and easily digested proteins to keep skin supple and firm; and antioxidants to protect skin against UV rays and boost circulation.

Superfood recipe suggestions...**Blueberry and chia pancakes** p171 **Avocado and ground seeds** p180, variation **Salmon pâté** p193 **Beet and chickpea soup** p192 **Miso-glazed tofu with quinoa** p218 **Berry nice skin!** p238

Cold-water fish

Wild salmon, trout, sardines, and herring are protein rich, helping repair skin at a cellular level, and have omega-3 for supple skin. The pink in trout and salmon is a carotenoid, astaxanthin, a powerful anti-inflammatory that increases skin elasticity.
Key nutrients: Omega-3, protein, vitamins B12 and D, selenium, carotenoids.
How to eat: Have an 5½oz (150g) portion 2–3 times a week.

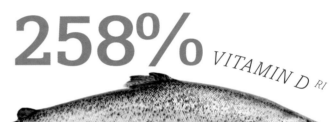

258% VITAMIN D RI

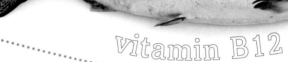

vitamin B12

full of healthy fats

Avocado

The fruit with the highest healthy fat content, including monounsaturated fats, phytosterols, and omega-3, -6, and -9 oils, avocados regenerate and nourish skin. The presence of lutein, a carotenoid, hydrates and boosts elasticity, preserving beneficial skin lipids.
Key nutrients: Lutein, beta-carotene, fatty acids, oleic and pantothenic acid, vitamin K, copper, folate, vitamins B6, C, and E, potassium.
How to eat: Have 1 medium avocado 2–4 times a week.

QUICK FIX

For a **skin-nurturing** snack, quickly rustle up an avocado and vinaigrette. Mix 1 tbsp olive oil, ½ tsp each mustard and honey, and a squeeze of lemon, then drizzle over half an avocado.

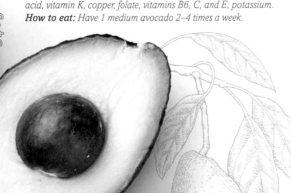

Kiwi fruit

Fiber-rich kiwi *can be yellow or green. Both types are a great source of vitamin C, which aids collagen production, and antioxidants.*
Key nutrients: *Vitamins C, E, and K, copper, fiber, potassium, folate, manganese.*
How to eat: *Have up to 2–3 kiwi daily.*

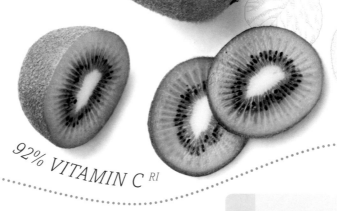

92% VITAMIN C *RI*

Lima beans

Lima beans *help the skin to produce hyaluronic acid; known as nature's moisturizer. As we age, levels of this moisture-packed substance decrease, leading to reduced elasticity and a loss of tone and plumpness.*
Key nutrients: *Fiber, folate, protein, potassium, vitamins B1 and B6, iron, magnesium.*
How to eat: *Have a 1/2-cup portion 2–3 times a week.*

PROTEIN-RICH

high in fiber

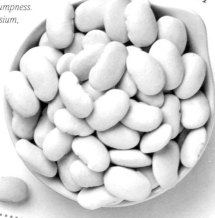
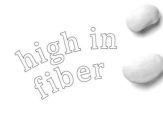

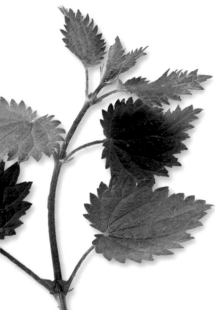

Nettles

These are one of the richest sources *of the beauty mineral silica, crucial for collagen formation, which keeps skin tight and wrinkle-free, and the hydrating molecule hyaluronic acid. Silica deficiency can cause poor elasticity and texture.*
Key nutrients: *Iron, potassium, silica, calcium, vitamins A, D, and K.*
How to eat: *Add a small handful to meals daily.*

48%
CALCIUM *RI*

MORE SUPERFOODS

Summer berries
The intense colors come from antioxidants, which strengthen tiny capillaries near the skin.
Key nutrients: *Flavonoids, anthocyanins, vitamins C and E, omega-3, potassium, magnesium.*
How to eat: *Snack on a handful daily.*

Green tea
Polyphenol in green tea boosts blood flow to the skin and protects against UV damage.
Key nutrients: *Catechins, epigallocatechin gallate (EGCG), L-theanine.*
How to eat: *Drink 1–3 cups daily.*

Sweet potatoes
Rich in beta-carotene, these aid the production of hyaluronic acid for a youthful complexion.
Key nutrients: *Beta-carotene, B vitamins, polysaccharides, vitamin C, potassium.*
How to eat: *A 3oz (85g) portion makes one of your five a day. Steam or bake with the skin on to maximize nutrients.*

Tofu and tempeh
A great source of protein, calcium, and vitamin E, these are thought to firm skin and reduce the appearance of fine lines.
Key nutrients: *Protein, calcium, selenium, omega-3, iron, magnesium, zinc, vitamin E.*
How to eat: *Have up to 2½oz (75g) daily.*

Leafy greens
These are high in anti-inflammatory vitamin E, defending the skin against free radicals.
Key nutrients: *Fiber, vitamins C and E, omega-3, beta-carotene, quercetin.*
How to eat: *Eat a 3oz (85g) portion daily.*

Nuts and seeds
Nuts and seeds provide rejuvenating essential fatty acids and vitamin E.
Key nutrients: *Protein, omega-3, vitamins B and E, calcium, chromium, iron, magnesium, potassium, selenium, zinc.*
How to eat: *A small handful daily.*

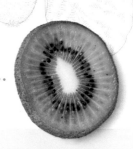
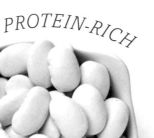
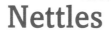

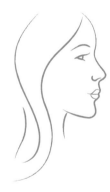

Premature aging

From our late 20s onward, signs of aging begin. The substance hyaluronic acid, which bathes the skin proteins collagen and elastin, keeping them supple, decreases with age. Genes and ethnicity play a role, and eating a poor diet hastens damage. Protective antioxidant-rich foods boost circulation to the skin's tiny blood vessels, and hydration is key: as well as water, foods with essential fatty acids moisturize from within.

Superfood recipe suggestions...Berry, seed, and nut granola p166 Japanese ocean soup p201 Summer salad with pomegranate and pistachio p202 Pineapple with cacao and coconut sauce p228 Matcha beauty shot p237

Super berries

Goji berries and mulberries *are traditionally used in Asia to keep skin moisturized and youthful. Goji berries are the only known food to stimulate human growth hormone (or "youth" hormone), which declines with age. Full of water-attracting polysaccharide sugars, these berries moisturize from the inside out.*
Key nutrients: *Vitamin C, carotenoids, protein, iron, polysaccharides.*
How to eat: *Snack on a handful of dried berries daily, or soak and add to oatmeal or desserts.*

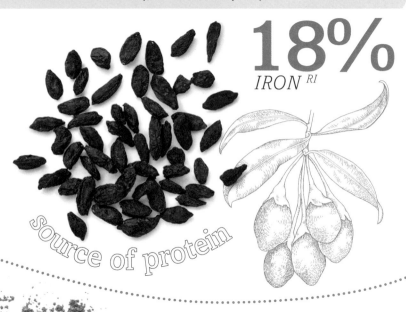

18%
IRON RI

source of protein

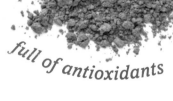

full of antioxidants

Matcha

Matcha has 10 times *the antioxidant value of green tea and the highest antioxidant value of all known foods, making it supremely anti-aging and protective against UV light.*
Key nutrients: *L-theanine, catechins, epigallocatechin gallate (EGCG), vitamin K.*
How to eat: *Add 1 scant tsp daily to drinks or desserts.*

39%
VITAMIN K RI

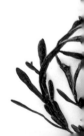

Pomegranate

A symbol of rebirth, fertility, and eternal life, when eaten, natural substances called ellagitannins are broken down by gut bacteria, producing a substance called urolithin A, which has been discovered to be a key rejuvenator, prompting cells to recycle and rebuild themselves.
Key nutrients: Fiber, vitamins C and E, polyphenols, folate.
How to eat: Have a handful of seeds daily.

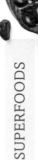

HIGH IN FIBER

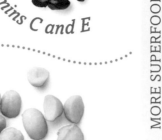

vitamins C and E

QUICK FIX

For a **skin-renewing** smoothie, put 1 cup pomegranate juice, 2 handfuls of blueberries, 1 tbsp chia seeds, 1 tsp coconut oil, and half an avocado in a blender and process until smooth.

Macadamia nuts

These nuts contain up to 80 percent good monounsaturated fats, mainly omega-9 and omega-7, which prevent cell membrane deterioration and hydrate skin.
Key nutrients: Selenium, zinc, essential fatty acids, calcium, iron, magnesium, manganese, zinc.
How to eat: Snack on a handful each day.

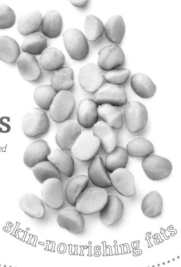

skin-nourishing fats

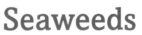

98%
IODINE RI

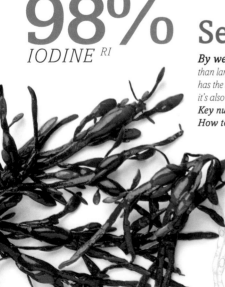

Seaweeds

By weight, seaweed is higher in minerals and vitamins than land vegetables. High in omega-3 fats—a single nori sheet has the same amount as two avocados—to lock in moisture, it's also a great source of the water-holding hyaluronic acid.
Key nutrients: Fatty acids, vitamin B6, iodine, calcium, iron.
How to eat: Add 1 tsp dried seaweed daily to meals.

MORE SUPERFOODS

Baobab
This African fruit stimulates collagen production for healthy skin, hair, and teeth.
Key nutrients: Calcium, vitamins A, B1, B6, and C, potassium, magnesium, zinc, bioflavonoids, fiber.
How to eat: Add 1–2 tsp daily to meals.

Raw cacao
Unlike cocoa, this has no added dairy or sugar and is full of minerals and antioxidants.
Key nutrients: Magnesium, chromium, protein, calcium, carotene, vitamin B1, and B2, sulfur, magnesium, flavonoids, fatty acids.
How to eat: Add 1–6 tsp daily to drinks, oatmeal, or add to baked goods.

Coconut oil
Made up of oxidizing-resistant fats, this has a natural steroidal hormone, pregnenolone, whose manufacture in the body decreases with age, and which promotes skin elasticity.
Key nutrients: Medium-chain triglycerides.
How to eat: Use up to 2 tbsp daily in cooking.

Miso
Made by fermenting soybeans, barley, or rice, this contains linoleic acid to promote supple skin kojic acid, which regulates pigmentation.
Key nutrients: Kojic acid, vitamin K, zinc, protein, phosphorus, probiotics, fatty acids.
How to eat: Up to 2 tbsp 3–4 times a week.

Camu camu
The powder from this Peruvian fruit has 60 times more vitamin C than an orange. An anti-inflammatory, it helps damaged skin.
Key nutrients: Vitamin C, beta-carotene.
How to eat: Add 1 tsp daily to meals.

Chlorella
This microalgae is packed with rejuvenating nutrients that keep skin supple and firm.
Key nutrients: Protein, antioxidants, fatty acids, B vitamins, calcium.
How to eat: Start with ¼ tsp daily in meals and drinks and build up to 1 tsp.

For supplements, see page 249.

10 ways to...
Stay hydrated

Water is necessary for your body to function— it plays a vital role in digestion, blood circulation, and skin health, as well as helping your body absorb nutrients and eliminate toxins. It can be easy not to drink enough—one in five women drinks less than their recommended daily intake—but this can have a negative impact on skin, hair, and nails. Here are some tips to help you keep fluid levels up throughout the day.

1 Consume **your quota**

Fluid requirements vary for each individual and are dependent on your age, gender, and activity level. As a rule of thumb, women should aim to drink around 8 cups of water each day, and men 10 cups. This should come mainly from water and foods (see Did you know?), but herbal teas, tisanes, and milk are other good choices and provide additional skin-friendly nutrients.

2 Prioritize **water**

The only drink that contains no sugar, calories, or additives, water is the best choice to help you stay hydrated. Keep a large bottle with you and sip from it throughout the day to keep you energized and your skin nourished, which in turn helps to reduce the appearance of fine lines.

6 Drink for **exercise**

Drink plenty of liquids before and during exercise in order to stay hydrated and keep your skin glowing. Your body can lose up to 32oz (1l) of water per hour during exercise, through sweating to regulate body temperature and breathing more heavily than usual. Don't drink too much just after you've finished exercising, as this may cause your muscles to cramp.

7 Check your **hunger**

The hormones that trigger hunger and thirst are the same, which means that you can mistake long-lasting thirst for hunger. Next time you feel a hunger pang, try drinking a glass of water instead of reaching for a snack.

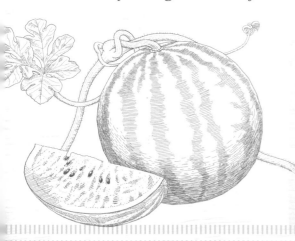

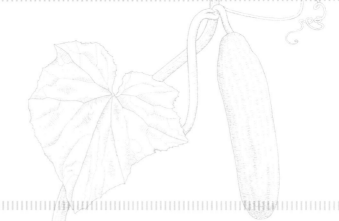

DID YOU KNOW?

We get about 20 percent of our total water intake from the foods that we eat. Fruit and vegetables are particularly good for hydration, as they are made up of around 80 percent water.

3 Drink **first thing**

Your body is mildly dehydrated after sleep, so make sure that you drink a glass of water first thing in the morning. This also helps your body flush out toxins before your first meal, keeps your skin supple and radiant, and boosts your energy for the day ahead, reducing the temptation to snack unnecessarily

4 Limit **tea and coffee**

Caffeinated drinks contain water, so can contribute to your daily fluid intake, but be aware that they have a mild diuretic effect. This means that they cause your body to produce urine, which can lead to dehydration. Tea and coffee also contain tannin, a chemical that blocks the pores of cells and can cause dry skin.

5 Drink **regularly**

If you feel thirsty, it's a sign that your body has been craving water for some time—drink little and often, and don't wait to feel thirsty before drinking. If you urinate infrequently or in small amounts, or if your urine is dark yellow in color, these are other indications that your body is lacking water. When you're adequately hydrated, your urine should be a pale, straw-yellow color.

8 Avoid **alcohol**

Alcohol is a diuretic that causes your kidneys to produce large quantities of urine, depleting the body of skin-nourishing nutrients and drying out skin. Drinking just one alcoholic drink can cause your body to lose a disproportionately large quantity of liquid, and the effects continue even after you've stopped drinking.

9 Drink for **digestion**

Drink a glass of water at least 30 minutes before eating a meal. This will help you avoid overeating and keep your digestive system healthy, maximizing the uptake of beneficial beauty nutrients. Make sure you don't drink just before eating, however, because the water can dilute your digestive juices, hindering the breakdown of food in your digestive tract.

10 Hydrate **before bed**

Make sure you're hydrated before going to sleep to keep skin nourished during the night and reduce the appearance of fine lines. Drink a glass of water shortly before going to bed. The nighttime is usually the longest period your body will go without a drink, so it's important that your hydration levels are topped off beforehand.

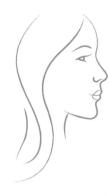

Neck and décolletage

This area often shows signs of neglect with crepey, loose skin, loss of tone, and age spots. It is frequently exposed to harsh sunlight and environmental hazards that damage elastin and collagen, the proteins that allow skin to stretch and contract. Hydrating foods, anti-aging antioxidants, and foods high in healthy proteins and healthy fats that boost collagen and elastin to keep skin firm and toned all offer excellent support.

Superfood recipe suggestions...Spiced apple oatmeal p170   Fall flavors soup p179   Ratatouille p207   Greek vegetable mezze p198   Pineapple with cacao and coconut sauce p228   Sweet green ice cream p229   Pineapple smoothie p239

Cucumber

With a high water content, *the humble cucumber is a top rehydrating beauty food that has collagen-building silica and skin-strengthening sulfur, which tone and firm the fine skin on the neck. A high vitamin count includes A, C, E, and vitamin K, a vitamin that promotes elasticity in blood vessels.*
Key nutrients: *Silica, vitamins A, C, E, and K, sulfur.*
How to eat: *Eat ¼ cucumber daily in salads or snacks.*

95%
WATER

Green tea

The health properties *of the antioxidant polyphenol in green tea are more potent than vitamin C and are thought to offer some protection against aging UV damage.*
Key nutrients: *Antioxidants, L-theanine, catechins, epigallocatechin gallate (EGCG).*
How to eat: *Drink 1–3 cups daily.*

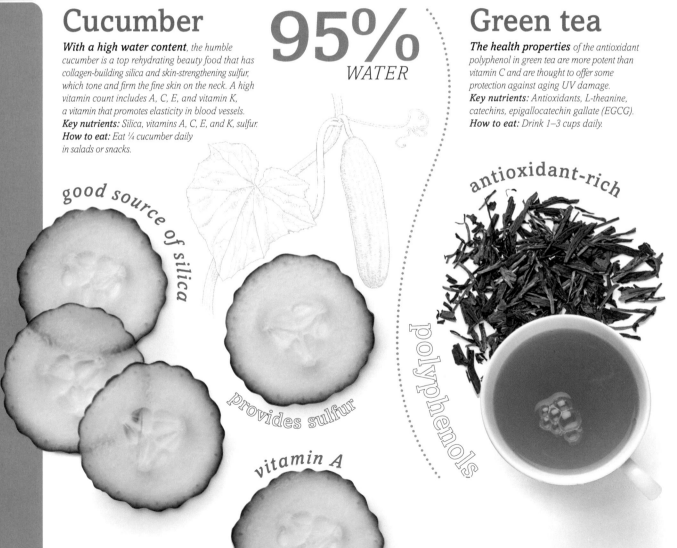

good source of silica

provides sulfur

vitamin A

antioxidant-rich

polyphenols

Pineapple

This is especially high in vitamin C, *which stimulates the production of collagen and elastin and has antioxidant properties that protect the delicate neck skin from damage and breakdown. Other vitamin C–rich fruits include kiwi, papaya, and strawberries.*
Key nutrients: *Vitamin C, manganese, copper, potassium.*
How to eat: *Add vitamin C–rich fruit daily to smoothies or juices, or enjoy as a healthy snack.*

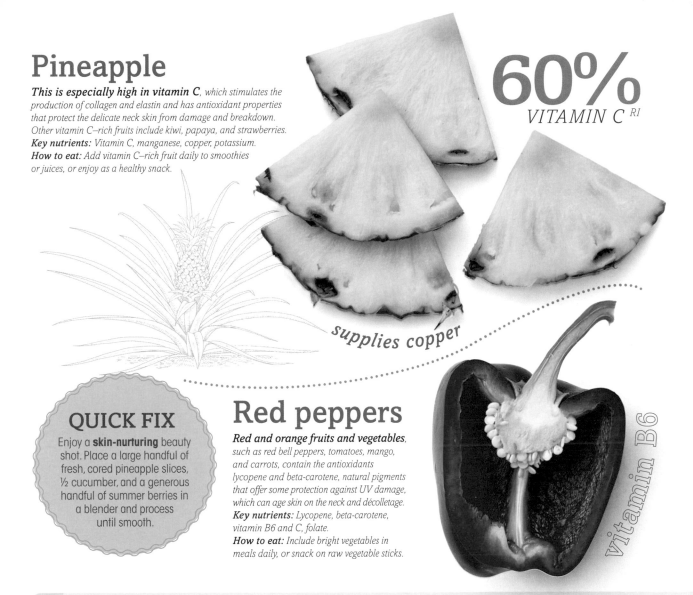

60%
VITAMIN C RI

supplies copper

vitamin B6

QUICK FIX

Enjoy a **skin-nurturing** beauty shot. Place a large handful of fresh, cored pineapple slices, ½ cucumber, and a generous handful of summer berries in a blender and process until smooth.

Red peppers

Red and orange fruits and vegetables, *such as red bell peppers, tomatoes, mango, and carrots, contain the antioxidants lycopene and beta-carotene, natural pigments that offer some protection against UV damage, which can age skin on the neck and décolletage.*
Key nutrients: *Lycopene, beta-carotene, vitamin B6 and C, folate.*
How to eat: *Include bright vegetables in meals daily, or snack on raw vegetable sticks.*

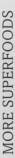

MORE SUPERFOODS

Turmeric
Contains a powerful detoxifying, anti-inflammatory antioxidant called curcumin, which helps to tone skin on the neck to prevent it from sagging.
Key nutrients: *Curcumin, beta-carotene, iron, manganese, vitamin B6.*
How to eat: *Add ½ tsp ground turmeric to smoothies, juices, soups, and cooking grains.*

Oats
These provide essential fatty acids and silica, which aids the manufacture of collagen and elastin for firmer, toned skin and is a component of hyaluronic acid, which bathes collagen and elastin in moisture, keeping the skin hydrated.

Key nutrients: *B vitamins, vitamin E, zinc, iron, fiber, calcium, magnesium.*
How to eat: *Have up to ¾ cup daily.*

Quinoa
This gluten-free seed is high in protein, with all the amino acids needed for skin renewal. It also contains silica for strong, elastic skin.
Key nutrients: *Zinc, l-lysine, protein, silica, quercetin, magnesium.*
How to eat: *Eat up to 60g (3½oz) daily.*

Barley
A great alternative to rice, buy whole rather than pearl barley, as it's less processed, with more nutrients and protein. It has moisture-boosting properties and skin-strengthening silica, both of which protect skin on the neck.
Key nutrients: *Fiber, selenium, vitamin B1 and B3, chromium, phosphorus, magnesium, silica.*
How to eat: *Up to ½ cup six times a week.*

Summer berries
High in antioxidants, summer berries, such as raspberries and blueberries, strengthen blood vessel walls, boosting the microcirculation in tiny vessels near the skin's surface to nurture skin.
Key nutrients: *Vitamin C, carotenoids, protein, polysaccharides.*
How to eat: *Snack on a handful each day.*

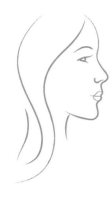

Fine lines

While some skin types have a propensity to develop fine lines, caused by a lack of sebum that can lead to dryness, all skin types can become dehydrated, the loss of moisture leaving skin feeling taut and flaky and prone to fine lines. Super-hydrating foods with minerals that rebalance fluids and electrolytes offer an effective remedy for dry skin, and eat foods that supply nourishing fatty acids to moisturize skin from within.

Superfood recipe suggestions...**Overnight oats with superberry compote** p168 **Zucchini noodles with basil pesto** p186
Gazpacho with watermelon p188 **Japanese ocean soup** p201 **Coconut smoothie** p235

Green beans

French, string, mung, and sprouted beans all provide *hyaluronic acid, a moisture magnet that helps to plump and moisturize skin so that fine lines appear less visible.*
Key nutrients: *Hyaluronic acid, silica, vitamin C and K, fiber, folate, beta-carotene.*
How to eat: *3½oz (100g) as part of your five a day.*

fiber-rich

silica

25% *VITAMIN C* ^RI

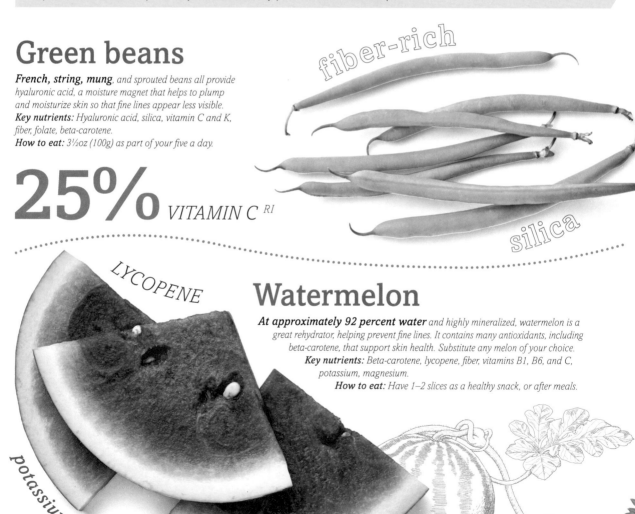

LYCOPENE

Watermelon

At approximately 92 percent water *and highly mineralized, watermelon is a great rehydrator, helping prevent fine lines. It contains many antioxidants, including beta-carotene, that support skin health. Substitute any melon of your choice.*
Key nutrients: *Beta-carotene, lycopene, fiber, vitamins B1, B6, and C, potassium, magnesium.*
How to eat: *Have 1–2 slices as a healthy snack, or after meals.*

potassium

Zucchini

These have a high water content *that refreshes and hydrates skin. Zucchini and squash are also full of antioxidants, such as beta-carotene and vitamin C, for clear, firm skin.*
Key nutrients: *Carotenoids, omega-3, oleic acid, vitamins B6 and C, magnesium, potassium, folate.*
How to eat: *Have ½ lightly steamed squash or zucchini as a side vegetable, or add raw to salads.*

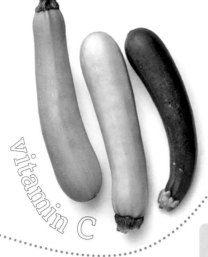

vitamin C

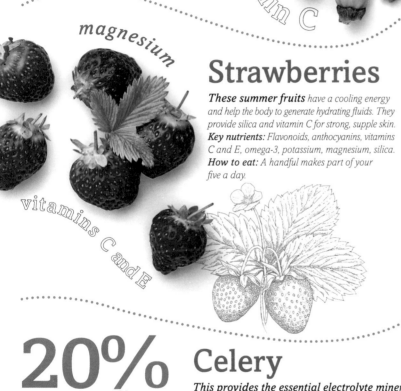

magnesium

vitamins C and E

Strawberries

These summer fruits *have a cooling energy and help the body to generate hydrating fluids. They provide silica and vitamin C for strong, supple skin.*
Key nutrients: *Flavonoids, anthocyanins, vitamins C and E, omega-3, potassium, magnesium, silica.*
How to eat: *A handful makes part of your five a day.*

20%
VITAMIN A ᴿᴵ

Celery

This provides the essential electrolyte minerals *sodium and potassium, which are powerful fluid regulators. Celery is also exceptionally high in silica, which helps to renew connective tissue such as collagen.*
Key nutrients: *Vitamin A, sodium, fiber, potassium, magnesium, quercetin silica.*
How to eat: *Snack on a stick of celery, or add to casseroles or salads.*

PROVIDES SODIUM

MORE SUPERFOODS

Cucumber
This is high in fluid-rebalancing minerals.
Key nutrients: *Silica, vitamins A, C, E, and K, sulfur.*
How to eat: *Snack on cucumber sticks daily.*

Seaweed
Sea vegetables are a top source of detoxifying minerals and improve water metabolism.
Key nutrients: *Fatty acids, vitamin B6, iodine, calcium, iron, carotenoids.*
How to eat: *Add 1 tsp dried daily to meals.*

Chia
The richest known source of omega-3, this seed is a moisture magnet when soaked in water.
Key nutrients: *Protein, omega-3, calcium, magnesium, iron, zinc, vitamins B, D, and E.*
How to eat: *Add up to 2 tbsp daily to meals.*

Lemon
This stimulates the production of fluids in the body to rehydrate skin quickly.
Key nutrients: *Vitamin C, folate.*
How to eat: *Squeeze into drinks and meals.*

Tofu
An easily digested soybean protein, this has a plant hormone that aids collagen production.
Key nutrients: *B vitamins, calcium, selenium, omega-3, iron, magnesium, zinc.*
How to eat: *Up to 2½oz (75g) daily.*

Coconut water
Perfectly balanced with electrolyte minerals, this provides a skin-hydrating drink.
Key nutrients: *Sodium, potassium, B vitamins.*
How to drink: *Up to 1 cup daily.*

Lettuce
High in water and cleansing chlorophyll, this also has skin-firming silica.
Key nutrients: *Vitamins A, C, and K, folate, fiber, potassium, biotin, iron, silica.*
How to eat: *Add a handful to salads.*

Sallow skin

With its yellow tone, sallow skin can be aging as it lacks the brightness and pinky hue of healthy skin. Skin may be dry, uneven, blotchy, and look lifeless and dull. Smoking constricts the tiny capillaries that feed oxygen and nutrients to the skin. Eat iron-rich foods to provide oxygenating red blood cells; B vitamins; anti-inflammatory foods, which help to keep skin smooth; and foods that support the circulation to restore radiance.

Superfood recipe suggestions...**Blueberry and chia pancakes** p171 **Chile guacamole** p190 **Huevos rancheros** p184 **Beet and chickpea soup** p192 **Winter veggie slaw** p185 **Black lentil and coconut curry** p204

QUICK FIX

Boost circulation by making garlic a natural part of your daily diet. Roast whole cloves alongside vegetables, add crushed to salad dressings, and use as a regular flavoring in cooking.

21%
VITAMIN C RI

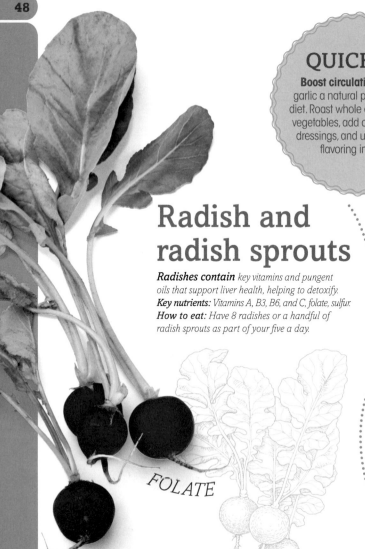

Radish and radish sprouts

Radishes contain *key vitamins and pungent oils that support liver health, helping to detoxify.*
Key nutrients: *Vitamins A, B3, B6, and C, folate, sulfur.*
How to eat: *Have 8 radishes or a handful of radish sprouts as part of your five a day.*

FOLATE

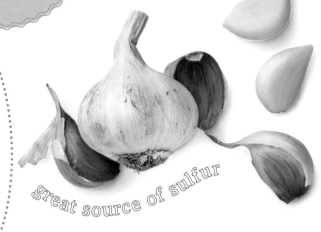

great source of sulfur

Garlic

A natural blood thinner, *garlic is fantastic for improving blood circulation to the extremities, while the sulfur it contains helps to clear the skin and boost the complexion.*
Key nutrients: *Sulfur, selenium, vitamins B6 and C.*
How to eat: *Use 1–2 cloves daily to flavor meals or in dressings.*

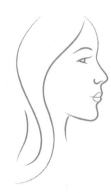

Summer berries

A perfect synergy of vitamin C and blood vessel–supporting flavonoids, berries support conditions associated with poor circulation and lack of radiance. Blackberries in particular boost new blood cell formation and purify blood.
Key nutrients: *Flavonoids, anthoyanins, vitamins C and E, omega-3, potassium, magnesium.*
How to eat: *Snack on a handful of berries daily.*

35%
VITAMIN C [RI]

beta-carotene-rich

potassium

Sweet potato

Full of skin-loving beta-carotene and bursting with vitamin C, these are also a good source of a range of B vitamins for healthy blood that carries skin-boosting nutrients to the skin to help lift the complexion.
Key nutrients: *Beta-carotene, polysaccharides, vitamin C, B vitamins, potassium.*
How to eat: *Steam or bake a 3oz (85g) portion; keep the skins on to maximize nutrients.*

Cayenne pepper

Cayenne has an impressive effect on the circulation, dilating tiny capillaries so blood can reach the extremities and providing blood-thinning agents called salicylates.
Key nutrients: *Capsaicin, beta-carotene, vitamins C and E.*
How to eat: *Use ½–1 tsp dried cayenne pepper daily to flavor meals.*

provides vitamin E

MORE SUPERFOODS

Turmeric
This contains a powerful fat-soluble antioxidant called curcumin that acts as an anti-inflammatory.
Key nutrients: *Curcumin, beta-carotene, iron, manganese, vitamin B6.*
How to eat: *Add ½ tsp ground turmeric to smoothies, juices, soups, and cooking grains.*

Ginger
This contains a natural blood thinner, salicylate. The pungent volatile oils are anti-inflammatory and help boost the body's microcirculation.
Key nutrients: *Gingerols, volatile oils.*
How to eat: *Add ½ tsp ground ginger or 2 tsp freshly grated ginger to drinks and meals.*

Kiwi fruit
High in vitamin C for collagen production, skin texture, and radiance. Flavonoid antioxidants strengthen blood vessels for improved circulation.
Key nutrients: *Vitamins C, E, and K, copper, fiber, potassium, folate, manganese.*
How to eat: *Enjoy 2–3 kiwi fruits daily.*

Legumes, peas, and beans
Protein-rich for skin repair, and high in B vitamins, iron, and fiber for healthy bowels that remove toxins, in turn supporting skin health.
Key nutrients: *Protein, zinc, fiber, iron, B vitamins, potassium.*
How to eat: *Have up to 3oz (85g) daily.*

Leafy greens
Iron-rich, these help red blood cells to transport nutrients, and have chlorophyll to aid the liver.
Key nutrients: *Fiber, B vitamins, vitamin C, beta-carotene, quercetin, omega-3.*
How to eat: *Add to salads or meals daily.*

Avocado
With healthy fats and vitamin E, these can help to thin "sticky blood" to boost circulation.
Key nutrients: *Lutein, beta-carotene, omega-3, vitamins B6, C, E, and K, copper, folate, potassium.*
How to eat: *1 medium avocado 2–4 times a week.*

For supplements, see page 249.

Meal planner Anti-aging

Our skin reflects how our bodies cope with the stresses of life, and we can support it with the right nutrients. This anti-aging meal planner, which draws on the recipes in this book with additional meal ideas, has been devised to provide hydrating, protecting, and moisturizing nutrients to keep skin firm and supple and reduce the appearance of fine lines.

Your anti-aging week
Use this nutritionally balanced one-week meal plan as the starting point for your anti-aging diet. To yield the best results, continue for four weeks, using the alternative meal ideas, opposite, for added variety. Begin each day with a hot water and lemon drink to aid digestion.

Monday

Breakfast
Berry nice skin! (p.238)

Snacks
Handful of macadamia nuts

Lunch
Two-egg omelet with arugula and watercress salad

Dinner
Roasted sea bass with tomato salsa (p.212)

Tuesday

Breakfast
Spiced apple oatmeal (p.170)

Snacks
Matcha fruit shake (p.240)

Lunch
Avocado and ground seeds (p.180, variation) on a rice cake

Dinner
Barley vegetable risotto (p.200)

Wednesday

Breakfast
Blueberry and chia pancakes (p.171)

Snacks
Pineapple smoothie (p.239)

Lunch
Salmon pâté (p.193) with cucumber slices

Dinner
Miso-glazed tofu with quinoa (p.218) with green beans

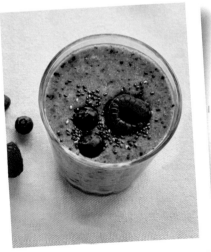

Berry nice smoothie (p.238)

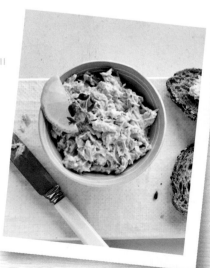

Salmon pâté (p.193)

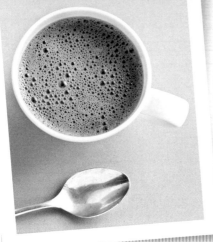

Matcha beauty shot (p.237)

HYDRATION

It is essential to drink at **least 6–7 glasses** of water daily to keep skin hydrated. Pages 42–43 have some good tips to help you reach your full quota. **Herbal teas,** such as nettle, and green tea also contribute to your daily water intake.

Thursday

Breakfast
Jumbo rolled oats with mixed seeds and sliced organic apricots

Snacks
Handful of nuts and raisins and Matcha beauty shot (p.237)

Lunch
Two slices of rye bread toast with hummus and cucumber and green leaf salad

Dinner
Japanese ocean soup (p.201)

Friday

Breakfast
Mixed berry and kiwi fruit salad with natural live yogurt and ground flaxseeds

Snacks
Green smoothie (p.244)

Lunch
Winter salad (p.185, variation)

Dinner
Ratatouille (p.207) with baked potato

Saturday

Breakfast
Berry nice skin! (p.238)

Snacks
Handful of nuts and raisins and a banana

Lunch
2 slices of toasted rye bread with hummus and green salad

Dinner
Summer salad with pomegranate and pistachio (p.202)

Sunday

Breakfast
Poached egg on rye bread

Snacks
Bell pepper and tomato dip (p.190) with celery sticks

Lunch
Fall flavors soup (p.178)

Dinner
Roasted broccoli and cauliflower with couscous (p.206)

Sweet treat
Sweet green ice cream (p.229)

Alternatives

To help you on your way, draw on these additional recipe suggestions to vary your meals over the course of four weeks.

Breakfast
Berry, seed, and nut granola (p.166)

Overnight oats (p.168)

Oatmeal with berries

Snacks
Superfood spread on toast (p.172)

Protein power beauty bites (p.195)

Lunch
Zucchini noodles with basil pesto (p.186)

Gazpacho with watermelon (p.188)

Dinner
Potato mash with veggie mix (p.219)

Ratatouille (p.207) with quinoa

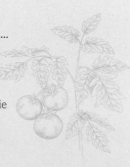

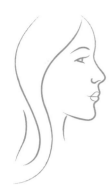

Sensitive skin

Skin that overreacts may develop pustules, bumps, become inflamed, flush, and have weakened capillaries that cause thread veins. Food intolerances, harsh weather, stress, genetics, eczema, and very dry skin can increase sensitivity. The antioxidant quercetin soothes the gut and essential fatty acids strengthen the gut wall, both of which help reduce food sensitivities, and anti-inflammatory foods calm irritated skin.

Superfood recipe suggestions... **Berry, seed, and nut granola** p166   **Fall flavors soup** p179   **Summer asparagus salad** p189
Roasted broccoli and cauliflower with couscous p206   **Green smoothie** p244

Asparagus

This contains anti-inflammatory *compounds called saponins and a starch, inulin, which passes undigested to the large intestine where it supports bacteria associated with nutrient absorption and a lower allergy risk.*
Key nutrients: *Folate, vitamins B1, C, and K, fiber, iron, calcium.*
How to eat: *Add 4–5 raw spears to a salad or eat as a side vegetable.*

86%
FOLATE RI

Red onion

This is a fabulous source *of the antioxidant quercetin, thought to inhibit the release of histamines that leads to allergic reactions. Red onions also provide sulfur, which boosts healthy connective tissue, or collagen.*
Key nutrients: *Inulin, quercetin, flavonoids, sulfur, biotin.*
How to eat: *Add red onions to salads or use as a base for meals.*

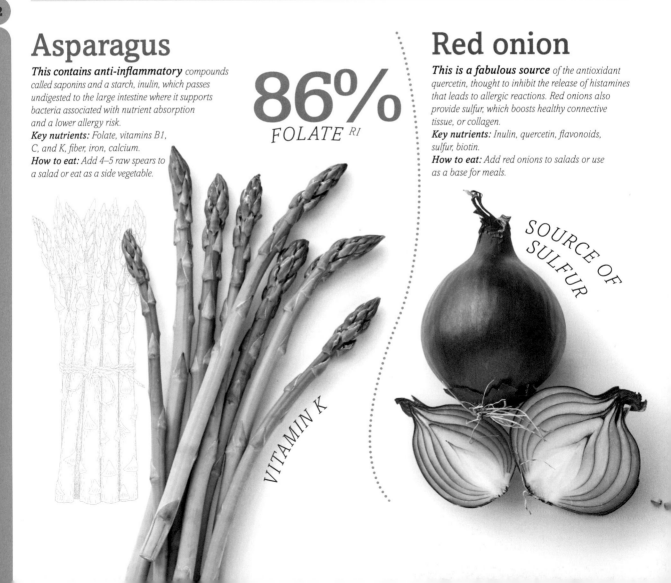

VITAMIN K

SOURCE OF SULFUR

Tomatoes

All colors supply antioxidants: quercetin calms skin, and lycopene and rutin protect and strengthen the blood vessels.
Key nutrients: Lycopene, lutein, beta-carotene, quercetin, vitamin C.
How to eat: Eat up to 7 cherry tomatoes or 1 medium one daily.

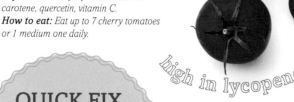

high in lycopene

QUICK FIX

This easy gazpacho recipe is a **soothing treat** for irritated skin. Purée 2 tomatoes, a seeded green bell pepper, a red onion, and a cucumber. Season with freshly ground black pepper to taste.

SOURCE OF IRON

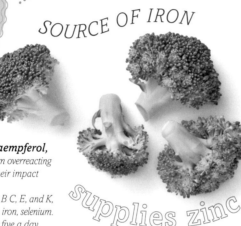

Broccoli

This is high in an antioxidant kaempferol, which helps to stop the immune system from overreacting to allergy-related substances, lessening their impact and lowering the risk of inflammation.
Key nutrients: Sulforaphane, vitamins A, B C, E, and K, chromium, omega-3, protein, zinc, calcium, iron, selenium.
How to eat: 8 florets make part of your five a day.

supplies zinc

55%
MAGNESIUM *RI*

Buckwheat

This is actually a fruit seed related to rhubarb and sorrel, so it's a good grain substitute for those sensitive to wheat or other gluten grains. It also provides the antioxidant rutin, which helps reduce the fragility of blood vessel walls.
Key nutrients: Rutin, quercetin, magnesium, fiber, protein.
How to eat: Have up to 1/3 cup daily.

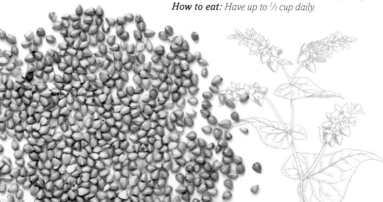

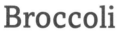

Summer berries

Low in sugar, yet full of antioxidants that protect the skin and blood vessels.
Key nutrients: Flavonoids, anthocyanins, vitamins C and E, omega-3, potassium, magnesium.
How to eat: Snack on a handful daily.

Bell peppers

These have 30 types of carotenoid, flavonoids such as quercetin, and vitamin C. They also contain sulfur, which supports collagen.
Key nutrients: Quercetin, carotenoids, vitamin C, B vitamins.
How to eat: Eat raw in salad or add to meals.

Olive oil

Try to use organic, extra-virgin, cold-pressed oil as this has more anti-inflammatory polyphenols that can calm sensitive skin.
Key nutrients: Quercetin, vitamin E, omega-9.
How to eat: Use up to 2 tbsp daily in salads and for cooking over low heats.

Avocado

Healthy monounsaturated fats in avocado allow 2–6 times more uptake of carotenoids. They contain to help calm skin.
Key nutrients: Lutein, beta-carotene, omega-3, omega-9, vitamins B5, B6, C, E, and K, copper, folate, potassium.
How to eat: 1 medium avocado 2–4 times a week.

Green tea

This has higher levels of antioxidants than black tea, including catechins, which support collagen and elastin.
Key nutrients: L-theanine, catechins, epigallocatechin gallate (EGCG).
How to eat: Drink 1–3 cups daily.

Leafy greens

Rich in vitamins A and C, quercetin, and anti-inflammatory vitamin K.
Key nutrients: Fiber, vitamin C, beta-carotene, quercetin, omega-3.
How to eat: Daily in salads and meals.

Cacao

Just 5 tbsp of cacao contains 314 percent of our daily iron needs. Cacao also has sulfur, supporting collagen production.
Key nutrients: Magnesium, chromium, iron, protein, copper, calcium, carotene, vitamins B1 and B2, magnesium, sulfur, flavonoids, fatty acids.
How to eat: Add 1–6 tsp daily to meals.

For supplements, see page 249.

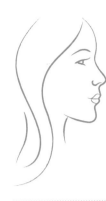

Acne

When hair follicles near sebaceous glands block, this causes pimples, and black- and whiteheads. Linked to hormonal changes, acne can be hereditary but is exacerbated by fried foods, bad fats, and excess salt, sugar, or dairy. Antioxidant-rich foods promote clear skin and healthy proteins, and fiber-rich foods support good gut flora to reduce breakouts, and sulfur and zinc calm skin, speed skin repair, and reduce scarring.

Superfood recipe suggestions...Berry, seed, and nut granola p166   Fruity quinoa breakfast p169
Beet and chickpea soup p192   Japanese ocean soup p201   Baked stuffed squash p203

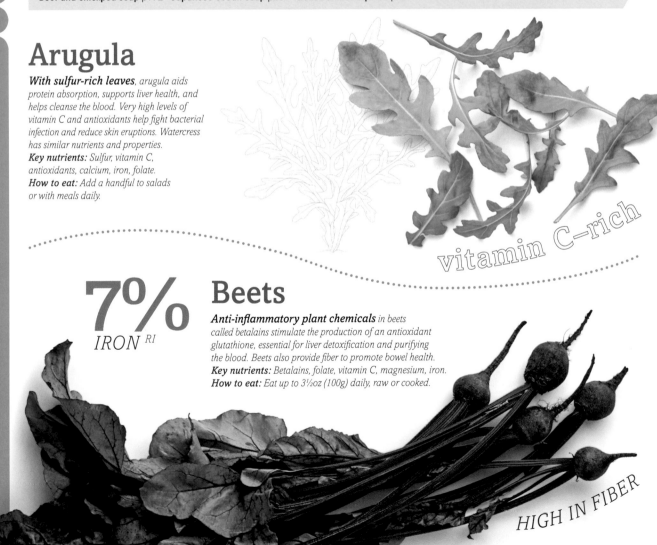

Arugula

With sulfur-rich leaves, *arugula aids protein absorption, supports liver health, and helps cleanse the blood. Very high levels of vitamin C and antioxidants help fight bacterial infection and reduce skin eruptions. Watercress has similar nutrients and properties.*
Key nutrients: *Sulfur, vitamin C, antioxidants, calcium, iron, folate.*
How to eat: *Add a handful to salads or with meals daily.*

vitamin C–rich

7%
IRON RI

Beets

Anti-inflammatory plant chemicals *in beets called betalains stimulate the production of an antioxidant glutathione, essential for liver detoxification and purifying the blood. Beets also provide fiber to promote bowel health.*
Key nutrients: *Betalains, folate, vitamin C, magnesium, iron.*
How to eat: *Eat up to 3½oz (100g) daily, raw or cooked.*

HIGH IN FIBER

Foods for the face

54

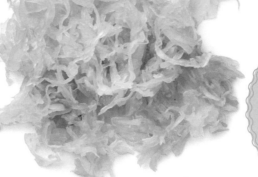

Sauerkraut

Fermented foods *increase healthy gut bacteria, helping promote clear skin. As well as the pickled cabbage sauerkraut, try kimchi, an oriental version of sauerkraut.*
Key nutrients: *Vitamins B, C, and K, prebiotic fiber, calcium.*
How to eat: *Eat up to ½ cup daily as a snack or added to salads.*

NATURAL PREBIOTIC

QUICK FIX

For a simple **sauerkraut**, toss the finely sliced leaves of 1 cabbage, 1 tbsp Himalayan pink salt, and 1 tbsp fennel seeds. Rub the leaves until a juice appears, then transfer them to a sealed jar. Ferment for 3 weeks.

iron source

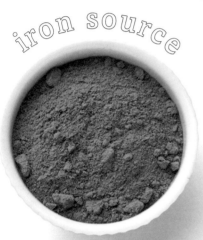

Turmeric

This healing spice *contains a powerful anti-inflammatory antioxidant called curcumin, which in turn increases blood levels of a detoxifying enzyme, glutathione S-transferase. Turmeric is also antibacterial, helping to keep skin clear.*
Key nutrients: *Curcumin, beta-carotene, iron, manganese, vitamin B6.*
How to eat: *Add ½ tsp ground turmeric to smoothies, juices, soups, and while cooking grains.*

5%
COPPER RI

SUPPLIES ZINC

Quinoa

A food of the Incans, *quinoa is rich in protein, including the amino acid lysine that aids tissue repair. It is also plentiful in minerals and anti-inflammatory omega-3, and a good source of zinc, which helps prevent scarring and balances sebum.*
Key nutrients: *Zinc, L-lysine, protein, quercetin, lysine, magnesium.*
How to eat: *Up to ½ cup daily.*

MORE SUPERFOODS

Lentils
They help to balance blood-sugar levels.
Key nutrients: *Protein, zinc, fiber, iron, B vitamins, potassium.*
How to eat: *Eat ½ cup 2–3 times a week.*

Garlic
This contains cleansing volatile oils and inulin, a prebiotic that supports good gut bacteria.
Key nutrients: *Sulfur, inulin, vitamin B6.*
How to eat: *1–2 cloves daily in meals.*

Onion
Like garlic, this has cleansing oils and prebiotics.
Key nutrients: *Inulin, quercetin, biotin.*
How to eat: *Use 1 daily for cooking.*

Sprouted seeds
Sprouted seeds, such as radish, are 10–30 times more concentrated in nutrients than vegetables.
Key nutrients: *Vitamins A, B, C, E, and K, iron, fiber, sulfur, omega-3, protein, calcium.*
How to eat: *Add to salads or meals.*

Pumpkin seeds
These help balance sebum and limit scarring.
Key nutrients: *Fatty acids, fiber, zinc, magnesium, protein, phytosterols.*
How to eat: *Snack on a handful daily.*

Wheatgrass
Wheatgrass is 70 percent cleansing chlorophyll.
Key nutrients: *Chlorophyll, protein, iron, zinc, potassium, fiber, vitamins A, B, C, and E, selenium.*
How to eat: *Have 1oz (25g) twice a week.*

Spirulina
This powder helps to detoxify and repair skin.
Key nutrients: *Protein, antioxidants, fatty acids, B vitamins, calcium.*
How to eat: *Start with ¼ tsp daily in drinks or meals and build up to 1 tsp.*

For supplements, see page 249.

10 ways to... Balance your diet

Focusing on particular foods can help you tackle your beauty concerns, but you should also make sure that you eat a healthy, balanced diet. A diet that encompasses all the major food groups and includes plenty of fresh fruits and vegetables will help your body to function healthily as a whole as well as promote glowing skin and strong, healthy-looking hair and nails.

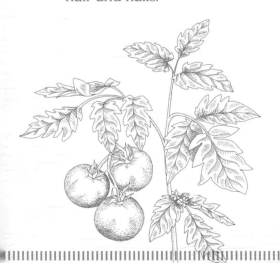

1 Eat good carbs

Choose good-quality, slow-release carbohydrates, and make these the basis of your meals and snacks. Refined carbohydrates, such as sugar and white flour, cause a fast rise in insulin levels, which causes inflammation, so these should be avoided. Good carbohydrates, on the other hand, provide nutrients and slow-release energy—these include whole grains and beans, as well as fresh vegetables and fruit.

2 Add healthy proteins

Make sure you include a protein-containing food, such as nuts, seeds, beans, lentils, lean meat, or fish to each meal. Protein is a vital nutrient because it is the basic building material for cells, so it helps your body form and maintain healthy muscles, bones, hair, skin, and nails. Protein also helps slow down the digestion of carbohydrates, ensuring a gradual release of energy and nutrients.

6 Include minerals

Minerals are vital for your health and beauty—they help build and maintain strong bones and teeth, keep your skin healthy, and help your body transform food into the energy it needs to function. Key minerals include zinc, sulfur, manganese, selenium, potassium, iron, sodium, calcium, phosphorus, and copper. Grains, nuts, seeds, dairy products, eggs, and cruciferous vegetables (including broccoli, cauliflower, cabbage, and watercress) seaweeds, and microalgae are rich sources of these essential minerals.

7 Eat regularly

It's important to maintain your blood sugar levels throughout the day by eating regular, healthy meals. Meals that contain unprocessed, slow-release carbohydrates will keep your physical and mental energy levels stable throughout the day, and won't produce insulin spikes that can cause inflammation and stopping you reaching for a sugar-laden unhealthy snack that will feed bad bacteria in the gut.

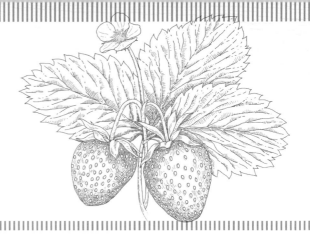

3 Eat plenty of **fiber**

Include fiber-rich foods, such as whole grains, fruit, and vegetables, in your meals throughout the day. Fiber speeds the passage of waste through the digestive tract, preventing constipation and is also a prebiotic, helping to feed good gut bacteria. A healthy digestive system effectively rids your body of toxins, helping protect your skin from breakouts and promote a more radiant complexion.

4 Include **healthy fats**

Your body needs a small amount of certain healthy fats. Healthy fats contain essential fatty acids, such as omega-3 and omega-6. It's important to balance both types of fat in order to maintain healthy skin. Most western diets are deficient in omega-3 fats, which can lead to inflammatory skin conditions, such as acne, eczema, and rosacea. Eat omega-3-rich foods such as sardines, salmon, mackerel, avocado, flaxseeds, chia, and hemp seeds.

5 Eat **colorful** foods

Naturally colorful fresh fruit and vegetables are rich in essential vitamins. Vitamins A, C, and E are antioxidants that help combat free radical damage. The B vitamin biotin may help protect skin against acne, fungal infections, rashes, and dryness. Other B vitamins help your body access the energy in foods. Vitamin D works as an anti-inflammatory agent, while vitamin K helps to keep your blood healthy, in turn ensuring nourishing nutrients reach the skin.

8 Snack **healthily**

Avoid processed, sugary, or fatty snacks. Instead, opt for nutritionally balanced snacks that combine carbohydrates and protein. Oat cakes spread with nut butter, rice cakes with hummus, or a handful of mixed nuts and raisins are all good choices. A simple fruit smoothie can also help maintain your blood sugar levels—try blending quinoa milk with fresh berries, nuts, and seeds for a nutritious, skin-toning smoothie-snack.

9 **Balance** your plate

A simple way to make sure that your meals are well balanced is to check the ratios of each food on your plate. Half of a medium-sized plate (10½in or 27cm in diameter) should be filled with vegetables or salad. A quarter of the plate should be whole grains, such as brown rice, wheat-free pasta, quinoa, millet, or buckwheat. The final quarter should be made up of a healthy protein: a piece of oily fish, eggs, hummus, legumes, such as chickpeas, lentils, beans, or a portion of lean meat.

10 Stay **hydrated**

Your body is made up of nearly two-thirds water, so fluids are a vital component of a balanced diet, and help to hydrate skin and reduce the signs of premature aging, such as fine lines. Healthy fluids can come from water, green tea, herbal teas, or tisanes, and also from foods with a high water content (see pp.42–43). Avoid caffeinated teas, coffee, and alcohol, as these work as a diuretic and can cause dehydration.

Rosacea

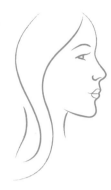

Characterized by redness, flushing, flaking, itchiness, and sometimes small spots and pustules, long-term, rosacea can cause thread veins and, rarely, a bumpy, misshapen nose. Spicy foods, caffeine, and alcohol can cause flare-ups. Eat plenty of antioxidant-rich foods to strengthen blood vessels, skin-repairing zinc-rich foods, pro- and prebiotics to support healthy gut bacteria and in turn soothe skin, and foods with calming B vitamins.

Superfood recipe suggestions...Fruity quinoa breakfast p169   Hot nuts! p194   Japanese ocean soup p201
Miso-glazed tofu with quinoa p218   Cashew and goji berry cheesecake p231   Pineapple smoothie p239

Papaya

This tropical fruit has the digestive enzymes chymonpapain and papain that help the absorption of nutrients, promote healing, and reduce allergies.
Key nutrients: *Vitamins A, C, E, and K, folate, magnesium, potassium, copper.*
How to eat: *Eat up to 1 papaya daily after meals or as a snack.*

75%
VITAMIN C [RI]

A RANGE OF VITAMINS

omega-3

Broccoli sprouts

These are a rich source of the antioxidant kaempferol, which helps to calm the immune system's allergic responses, lowering the risk of inflammation.
Key nutrients: *Sulforaphane, vitamins A, C, E, K, B1, B5, and B6, chromium, omega-3, protein, zinc, calcium, iron, selenium.*
How to eat: *Add a handful to salads or meals daily or simply eat as a snack.*

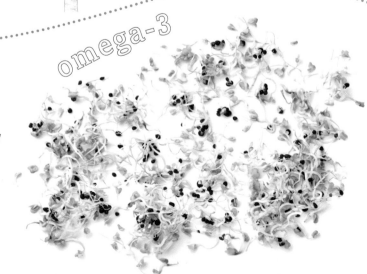

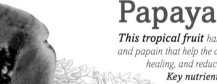

Berries

Summer berries and "super" berries such as goji and mulberry are amazing sources of vitamin C and flavonoids, which strengthen blood vessels, and quercetin, which fights allergic responses.
Key nutrients: *Vitamins C and E, flavonoids, potassium, omega-3, anthocyanins, magnesium, folate.*
How to eat: *Have a handful daily or add to smoothies.*

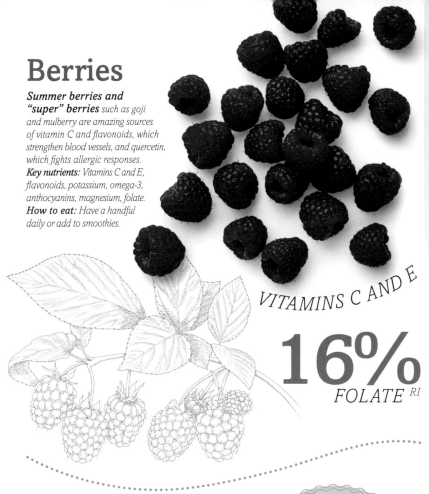

VITAMINS C AND E

16%
FOLATE RI

Nuts and seeds

Brazils, cashews, hazelnuts, and seeds have essential fatty acids, skin-repairing minerals such as zinc, and B vitamins. Star performers are Brazil nuts, with selenium to boost skin elasticity, and hemp seeds for their balance of omega oils that calms inflammation.
Key nutrients: *Protein, omega-3, vitamins B and E, calcium, chromium, iron, magnesium, potassium, selenium, zinc.*
How to eat: *Snack on a small handful daily.*

QUICK FIX
Try this simple pâté for a **fatty acid boost**. Wilt 3oz (85g) spinach leaves. Blend ½ cup cashews until finely ground. Add the spinach, ½ tsp nutmeg, season, and spread on oat cakes or whole-grain bread.

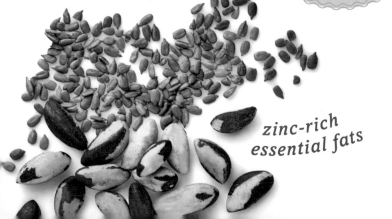

zinc-rich essential fats

Fermented foods
Tempeh, miso, kefir, sauerkraut, and kimchi help support good gut bacteria to promote healthy, calm skin.
Key nutrients: *Vitamins B, C, and K, prebiotic, fiber, calcium.*
How to eat: *Up to 3½ oz (100g) daily.*

Turmeric
An anti-inflammatory in turmeric, curcumin, reduces puffiness, boosts circulation, and aids detoxification.
Key nutrients: *Curcumin, beta-carotene, iron, manganese, vitamin B6.*
How to eat: *Add ½ tsp to smoothies, juices, soups, and while cooking grains.*

Buckwheat
The antioxidant rutin boosts circulation and helps to strengthen blood vessel walls.
Key nutrients: *Rutin, quercetin, magnesium, fiber, protein.*
How to eat: *Up to ⅓ cup daily.*

Red onions
A prebiotic with calming quercetin and sulfur, these promote good gut bacteria.
Key nutrients: *Inulin, quercetin, flavonoids, sulfur, biotin.*
How to eat: *Add to salads and meals.*

Quinoa
The amino acid lysine aids tissue repair.
Key nutrients: *Zinc, L-lysine, protein, quercetin, lysine, magnesium.*
How to eat: *Up to ⅓ cup daily.*

Seaweeds
Full of minerals, these aid immune health, fighting allergies and inflammation.
Key nutrients: *Fatty acids, vitamin B6, iodine, calcium, iron, carotenoids.*
How to eat: *Add 1 tsp dried seaweed daily to meals.*

Leafy greens
With B vitamins and fatty acids, these are key for healthy, calm, clear skin.
Key nutrients: *Fiber, vitamin C, beta-carotene, quercetin, omega-3.*
How to eat: *Add to salads and meals daily.*

Spirulina
This superfood powder has an anti-inflammatory effect that calms skin.
Key nutrients: *Protein, antioxidants, fatty acids, B vitamins, calcium.*
How to eat: *Start with ¼ tsp daily in a meal or drink and build up to 1 tsp.*

For supplements, see page 249.

Meal planner Skin calming

Sensitive skin and conditions such as eczema and rosacea can be affected by the bacteria in our gut. Choosing foods that promote "good" gut bacteria can help to soothe skin. This skin-calming meal planner, using recipes from this book with added meal ideas, provides moisturizing and soothing foods that promote healthy gut bacteria to help relieve irritated skin.

Your skin-calming week
This nutritionally balanced one-week meal planner is a starting point for your skin-calming diet. For optimum results, continue for four weeks, using the alternative meal ideas, opposite, for variety. Start each day with a hot water and lemon drink to aid digestion.

Monday

Breakfast
Hemp seed butter on rye bread (p.172) and Vitamin C boost (p.245)

Snacks
Handful of nuts and raisins

Lunch
Green salad leaves with avocado and red onion

Dinner
Japanese ocean soup (p.201)

Tuesday

Breakfast
Overnight oats with superberry compote (p.168)

Snacks
Matcha fruit shake (p.240)

Lunch
Huevos rancheros (p.184)

Dinner
Sweet potato and mackerel mash (p.219, variation), with a watercress and arugula salad

Wednesday

Breakfast
Spiced apple oatmeal (p.170)

Snacks
Pineapple smoothie (p.239)

Lunch
Chile guacamole (p.190) with crudités

Dinner
Rice salad (p.220, variation)

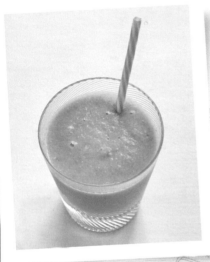

Vitamin C boost (p.245)

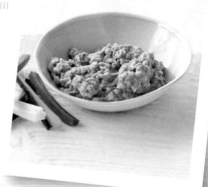

Chile guacamole with crudités (p.190)

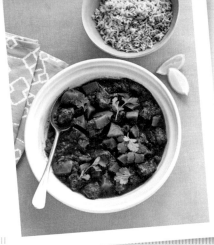

Lamb tagine
(p.208)

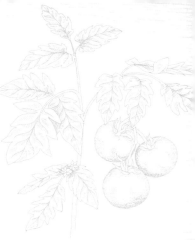

NATURAL PROBIOTICS

Fermented and cultured foods act as probiotics, helping to destroy harmful gut bacteria. Try cultured dairy such as kefir and natural live yogurt, and foods such as miso, sauerkraut, and kimchi, to promote a **healthy gut environment**.

Thursday

Breakfast
Fruity quinoa breakfast (p.169)

Snacks
Homemade oat milk (p.241) with papaya

Lunch
Tomato salsa (p.213)

Dinner
Lamb tagine (p.208)

Friday

Breakfast
Rye bread with almond butter

Snacks
Sliced apple with nut butter

Lunch
Winter veggie slaw (p.185)

Dinner
Salmon with coconut rice (p.215, variation)

Saturday

Breakfast
Mixed berry and kiwi fruit salad with natural live yogurt and ground flaxseeds

Snacks
Handful of nuts and raisins

Lunch
Beet and chickpea soup (p.192)

Dinner
Greek vegetable mezze (p.198)

Sunday

Breakfast
Poached egg on rye bread

Snacks
Bell pepper and tomato dip (p.190) with raw vegetable sticks

Lunch
Mixed tomato salad with avocado

Dinner
Baked stuffed squash (p.203)

Sweet treat
Pineapple with cacao and coconut sauce (p.228)

Alternatives

To help you on your way, draw on these additional recipe suggestions to vary your meals over the course of four weeks.

Breakfasts
Blueberry and chia pancakes (p.171)

Berry nice skin! (p.238)

Snacks
Hot nuts (p.194)

Lunch
Tomato salsa (p.213) with brown rice

Spring veggie salad (p.183)

Dinner
Roasted broccoli and cauliflower (p.206)

Barley vegetable risotto (p.200)

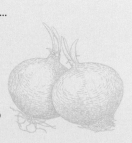

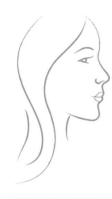

Cold sores

These infectious sores caused by the herpes simplex virus (HSV-1) remain dormant in the nervous system when not active, waiting until conditions are right to recur. Triggers include cold viruses, stress, menstruation, spicy foods, chocolate, beer, and sugary cereals. Eat vitamin C– and zinc-rich foods to boost immunity, foods with antioxidants and the amino acid L-lysine to help suppress the virus, and skin-calming B vitamins.

Superfood recipe suggestions...**Fruity quinoa breakfast** p169 **Scrambled tofu** p181 **Beet and chickpea soup** p192
Protein power beauty bites p195 **Lemon and herb-roasted chicken** p210

Red grapes

Resveratrol, a potent antioxidant *found in grapes, may stop the herpes virus from reactivating. This is a preventative measure, so eat resveratrol-rich foods if you suffer from cold sores. It's also found in blueberries, cranberries, and mulberries.*
Key nutrients: *Resveratrol, vitamins C and K, copper.*
How to eat: *Snack on a handful daily.*

13%
VITAMIN K RI

vitamin C

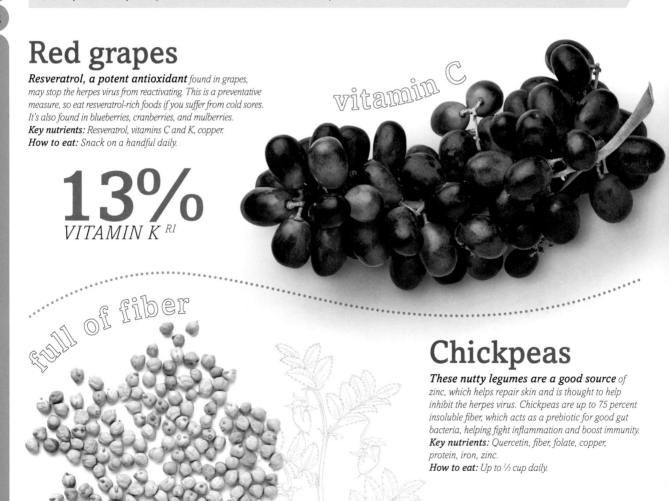

full of fiber

Chickpeas

These nutty legumes are a good source *of zinc, which helps repair skin and is thought to help inhibit the herpes virus. Chickpeas are up to 75 percent insoluble fiber, which acts as a prebiotic for good gut bacteria, helping fight inflammation and boost immunity.*
Key nutrients: *Quercetin, fiber, folate, copper, protein, iron, zinc.*
How to eat: *Up to ⅓ cup daily.*

Oregano

This herb contains two powerful compounds, *carvacrol and thymol, which have antiviral, antibacterial, and antifungal properties. In studies, they deactivated the herpes simplex virus type I by up to 90 percent within an hour.*
Key nutrients: *Volatile oils and antioxidants.*
How to eat: *Add daily to flavor meals.*

antioxidant-rich

Figs

Sweet and delicious *figs are a good source of zinc, which can deactivate the herpes virus that causes cold sores. It also has a range of skin-healing B vitamins.*
Key nutrients: *Fiber, B vitamins, copper, potassium, zinc.*
How to eat: *Makes one of five a day.*

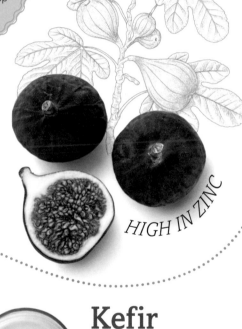

HIGH IN ZINC

20%
CALCIUM RI

protein

omega-3

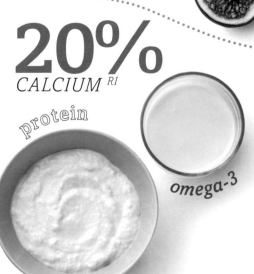

Kefir

Fermented foods *such as kefir milk (left) and kefir yogurt (far left) help balance "good" and "bad" bacteria in the gut to raise immunity and calm inflammation. Try also miso, sauerkraut, kimchi, and tempeh.*
Key nutrients: *Protein, omega-3, calcium, B vitamins, potassium.*
How to eat: *Consume up to 1 cup daily. Add to smoothies or eat with fruit.*

Garlic
A special enzyme called alliinase is made when garlic is crushed or chewed. This in turn produces a sulfur compound called allicin, which, alongside volatile oils, and incredible levels of antioxidants and selenium, makes a natural antibiotic, antiviral, and immune booster, ideal for preventing and fighting cold sores.
Key nutrients: *Sulfur, selenium, vitamin B6.*
How to eat: *Include up to 2 cloves crushed garlic daily in meals and salad dressings.*

Aloe vera juice
Derived from the gel inside the leaf of the aloe vera plant, this juice has a range of antibiotic and antiviral uses that are helpful for cold sores. It has 18 amino acids that help to speed skin repair, as well as salicylic acid, which acts as an anti-inflammatory.
Key nutrients: *Beta-carotene, vitamins C and E, salicylic acid, polysaccharides, calcium, chromium, selenium, magnesium, potassium, zinc.*
How to drink: *Drink up to 3 tbsp daily.*

Turmeric
This has an antioxidant curcumin that has anti-inflammatory and painkilling properties and is thought to help prevent infection by the herpes virus.
Key nutrients: *Curcumin, beta-carotene, iron, manganese, vitamin B6.*
How to eat: *Add ½ tsp ground turmeric to drinks, soups, and while cooking grains.*

Quinoa
The balance of amino acids in quinoa helps to prevent cold sore outbreaks. Quinoa is also rich in protein and zinc, both of which support tissue repair. It also has a range of B vitamins for skin health, and healthy fats to reduce inflammation.
Key nutrients: *Zinc, L-lysine, protein, quercetin, lysine, magnesium.*
How to eat: *Have up to ⅓ cup daily.*

Camu camu
This powder derived from the Peruvian fruit is full of vitamin C, with its antiviral and immunity-boosting effects. It has up to 60 times more vitamin C per serving than an orange. Phytonutrients from the berry makes it more effective than commercial vitamin C.
Key nutrients: *Vitamin C and beta-carotene.*
How to eat: *Add 1 tsp daily to a drink, oatmeal, or a meal.*

For supplements, see page 249.

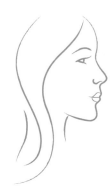

Irregular pigmentation

Darker areas of skin that appear as flat brown marks, most commonly on the face, hands, neck, and décolletage, are caused by an excess of the pigment melanin. Sun damage, pregnancy hormones, acne, genes, alcohol, smoking, and a poor diet can cause dark patches. An antioxidant-rich diet with plenty of raw foods and vitamin C cleanses, tones, and renews skin and helps to protect it from UV damage.

Superfood recipe suggestions...**Overnight oats with superberry compote** p168 **Fall flavors soup** p178
Potato mash with veggie mix p219 **Nutty rice salad** p220 **Pineapple with cacao and coconut sauce** p228

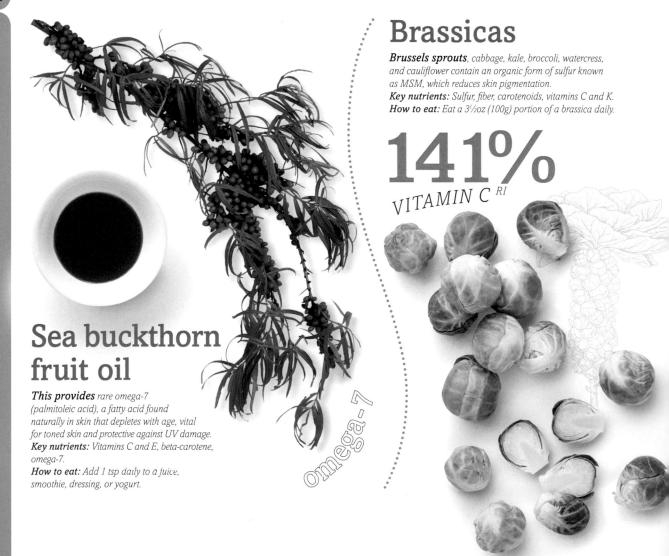

Brassicas

Brussels sprouts, *cabbage, kale, broccoli, watercress, and cauliflower contain an organic form of sulfur known as MSM, which reduces skin pigmentation.*
Key nutrients: *Sulfur, fiber, carotenoids, vitamins C and K.*
How to eat: *Eat a 3½oz (100g) portion of a brassica daily.*

141%
VITAMIN C [RI]

Sea buckthorn fruit oil

This provides *rare omega-7 (palmitoleic acid), a fatty acid found naturally in skin that depletes with age, vital for toned skin and protective against UV damage.*
Key nutrients: *Vitamins C and E, beta-carotene, omega-7.*
How to eat: *Add 1 tsp daily to a juice, smoothie, dressing, or yogurt.*

omega-7

Berries

Cranberries, blackberries, *raspberries, strawberries, goji, and mulberries all provide ellagic acid, a natural chemical that helps even out and brighten skin tone.*
Key nutrients: *Vitamins B6 and C, magnesium.*
How to eat: *Eat a handful of berries daily.*

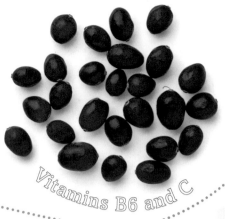

Vitamins B6 and C

QUICK FIX

As well as buying **vitamin C–rich** berries in season, stock frozen berries to enjoy year-round. These defrost quickly, ready to add to desserts, smoothies, or oatmeal.

Miso

A grain or bean paste *fermented from soybeans, this is a good source of kojic acid, which helps to lighten skin by inhibiting the enzyme tyrosinase, in turn reducing the amount of melanin produced.*
Key nutrients: *Kojic acid, vitamin K, protein, zinc, phosphorus, iron, omega-3.*
How to eat: *Add up to 2 tbsp 3–4 times a week to meals.*

13%
IRON RI

protein

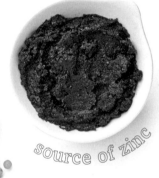

source of zinc

high in antioxidants

Milk thistle

This herbal remedy *contains silymarin, an antioxidant complex that boosts levels of another antioxidant, glutathione. Glutathione regulates melanin, neutralizes damaging free radicals, and is needed for DNA repair.*
Key nutrients: *Vitamins C and E, antioxidants.*
How to eat: *Take a tincture, tea, or capsules daily for several months, take a break, then repeat if you wish.*

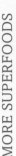

MORE SUPERFOODS

Macadamia nuts or oil
Together with sea buckthorn fruit oil, these also provide omega-7, which protects skin against UV damage. They also contain selenium, which works with the antioxidant glutathione to also protect skin.
Key nutrients: *Omega-7, iron, calcium, vitamin B6, magnesium.*
How to eat: *Eat a small handful daily.*

Carrots
A great source of antioxidant carotenoids: beta-carotene, lutein, and lycopene, which protect and repair UV damage. Carotenoids are also plentiful in other bright vegetables such as sweet potatoes, squash, bell peppers, and tomatoes.
Key nutrients: *Vitamins A, B2, B6, C, and K, iron, magnesium, zinc, phosphorous.*
How to eat: *Include carotenoid-rich foods in your diet daily.*

Beets
A pigment called betalain in beets helps the body detox, neutralizing and removing toxins that can exacerbate skin patches by making them water-soluble for excretion in the urine.
Key nutrients: *Vitamins A, B1, B6, and C, magnesium, folate.*
How to eat: *Eat beets 2–3 times a week.*

Green tea
Catechins, the active antioxidant found in green tea, can help make skin more resistant to UV radiation.
Key nutrients: *Catechins, vitamins A, B1, and B2, potassium, magnesium.*
How to eat: *Drink 1–3 cups daily.*

Camu camu
This is the richest known source of skin-toning vitamin C on the planet, supported by a range of antioxidants, vitamins, and minerals.
Key nutrients: *Vitamin C, manganese, zinc, copper.*
How to eat: *Take ½ to 1 tsp powder daily.*

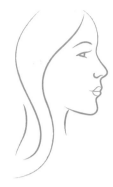

Tired, dull eyes

Too much screen or driving time, close work, poor lighting, and an incorrect prescription can all strain our eyes. As a result, eyes can feel out of focus, sore, either dry or watery, and there may be a dull pain around the eyes that can build to a headache. Foods rich in vitamins A and B, antioxidants, and fatty acids boost circulation around the eye, supporting eye health. If problems persist, consult an optician.

Superfood recipe suggestions...**Berry, seed, and nut granola** p166   **Cacao and chia chocolate "pudding"** p174
Huevos rancheros p184   **Ratatouille** p207   **Salmon with samphire** p215   **Green smoothie** p244

Orange pepper

A study in the British Journal of Ophthalmology found that orange bell peppers had the highest amount of the carotenoid zeaxanthin, which protects the retina, of 33 fruits and vegetables tested.
Key nutrients: Flavonoids, carotenoids, vitamins A, B, and C.
How to eat: Include one as part of your five a day.

70%
VITAMIN A ᴿᴵ

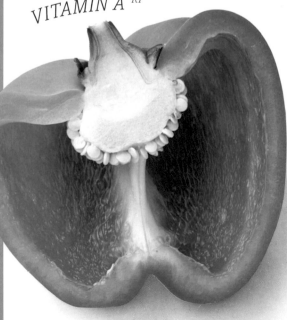

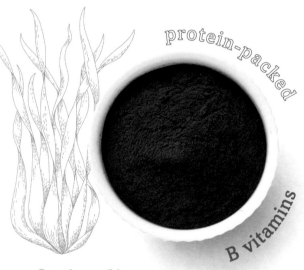

protein-packed

B vitamins

Spirulina

Grown naturally from algae, this superfood powder is extremely nutritious. Rich in highly absorbable protein, spirulina has a spectrum of carotenoid antioxidants that promote eye health.
Key nutrients: Protein, antioxidants, fatty acids, iron, B vitamins, calcium.
How to eat: Add a ¼ tsp daily to a meal or drink, and gradually increase to 1 tbsp.

QUICK FIX

Start the day with a **nutrient boost** for tired eyes. Soak 2 tbsp **chia seeds** with ¾ cup coconut milk overnight. Add a handful of berries, ¼ tsp spirulina, and enjoy.

30%
IRON ᴿᴵ

74%
SELENIUM RI

Wild Alaskan salmon

This is one of the few foods *that contains the super antioxidant astaxanthin: this is fat-soluble, so it passes through cell membranes; it crosses the blood-retinal barrier; and it absorbs UVB, reducing DNA damage to the eyes.*
Key nutrients: *Omega-3, protein, vitamins B12 and D, magnesium, potassium, selenium.*
How to eat: *Eat a 5½oz (150g) portion 2–3 times a week.*

vitamins B12 and D

high in magnesium

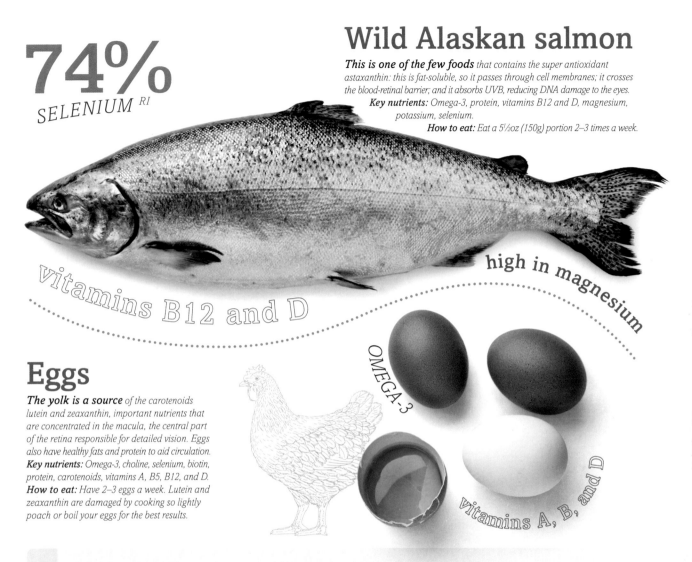

OMEGA-3

Eggs

The yolk is a source *of the carotenoids lutein and zeaxanthin, important nutrients that are concentrated in the macula, the central part of the retina responsible for detailed vision. Eggs also have healthy fats and protein to aid circulation.*
Key nutrients: *Omega-3, choline, selenium, biotin, protein, carotenoids, vitamins A, B5, B12, and D.*
How to eat: *Have 2–3 eggs a week. Lutein and zeaxanthin are damaged by cooking so lightly poach or boil your eggs for the best results.*

vitamins A, B, and D

MORE SUPERFOODS

Berries
These are high in vitamin C, protecting the retina against light. In a Japanese study, blackcurrant extract helped eyes adapt to the dark and relieved tired eyes after two hours of computer work. This is due to the antioxidant anthocyanin, which boosts circulation to the eye area.
Key nutrients: *Flavonoids, vitamins A and C, potassium, copper, iron, magnesium.*
How to eat: *Enjoy a handful each day.*

Cucumber
High in water, antioxidants, and minerals, cucumber helps to hydrate and nourish eyes.
Key nutrients: *Silica, vitamins A,C, E, and K, sulfur.*
How to eat: *Have ¼ cucumber each day.*

Carrots
Beta-carotene in carrots is converted to vitamin A in the body, which is vital for healthy retinas.
Key nutrients: *Beta-carotene, lutein, vitamins B6, C, and K, biotin, fiber, potassium.*
How to eat: *Have up to 1 carrot daily.*

Dark leafy greens
These are a rich source of the carotenoids lutein and zeaxanthin, important nutrients for detailed vision, which also help to protect the eye from UV damage. Kale and spinach are especially high in lutein.
Key nutrients: *Fiber, vitamin C, beta-carotene, quercetin, omega-3.*
How to eat: *Eat a 3½oz (100g) portion a day.*

Chia seeds
These are rich in omega-3, which protects against macular degeneration.
Key nutrients: *Protein, omega-3, calcium, magnesium, iron, zinc, vitamins B, D, and E.*
How to eat: *Sprinkle up to 2 tbsp daily on meals.*

Bee pollen
This contains the antioxidant rutin, which boosts blood vessel walls to improve microcirculation.
Key nutrients: *18 vitamins, all amino acids, fatty acids, protein.*
How to eat: *Eat up to 1 tsp daily. Do not give bee pollen to young children, or take it if you have an allergy to honey or bee stings or if you're pregnant or breastfeeding.*

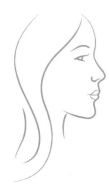

Eye bags and dark circles

The skin around the eyes is the most delicate of the body. When we are dehydrated it thins and blood vessels become prominent, creating dark circles, while excess fluid can cause puffiness. Contributory factors include genetics, lack of sleep, aging, caffeine, alcohol, and sugar. Hydrating foods and circulation-boosting antioxidants make a noticeable difference, as do mineral-rich foods that help to balance fluids.

Superfood recipe suggestions...**Berry, seed, and nut granola** p166 **Huevos rancheros** p184
Gazpacho with watermelon p188 **Greek vegetable mezze** p198 **Ratatouille** p207 **Berry nice skin!** p238

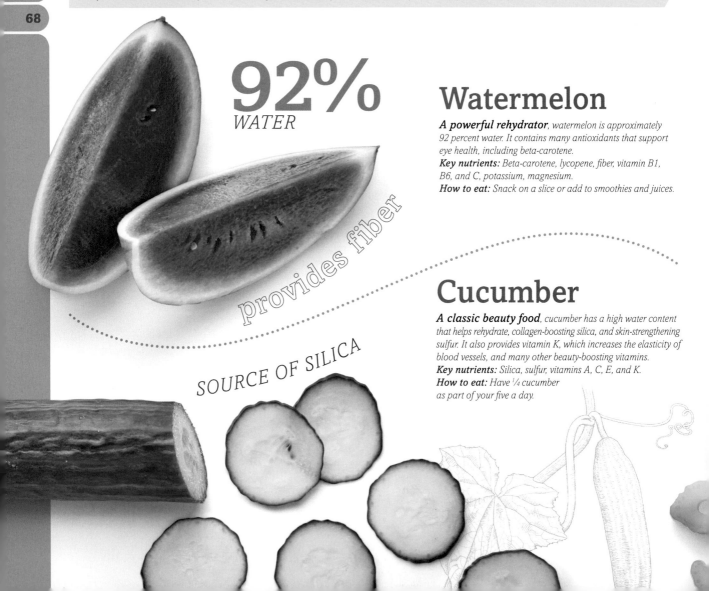

92%
WATER

provides fiber

SOURCE OF SILICA

Watermelon

A powerful rehydrator, *watermelon is approximately 92 percent water. It contains many antioxidants that support eye health, including beta-carotene.*
Key nutrients: *Beta-carotene, lycopene, fiber, vitamin B1, B6, and C, potassium, magnesium.*
How to eat: *Snack on a slice or add to smoothies and juices.*

Cucumber

A classic beauty food, *cucumber has a high water content that helps rehydrate, collagen-boosting silica, and skin-strengthening sulfur. It also provides vitamin K, which increases the elasticity of blood vessels, and many other beauty-boosting vitamins.*
Key nutrients: *Silica, sulfur, vitamins A, C, E, and K.*
How to eat: *Have ¼ cucumber as part of your five a day.*

Blueberries

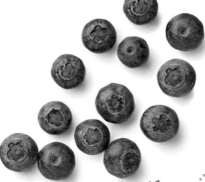

Renowned for their benefits to eye health, blueberries are a prime source of the antioxidants lutein and anthocyanins, which protect the delicate blood vessels, improving the circulation to the eyes.
Key nutrients: Lutein, quercetin, anthocyanins, omega-3, vitamin C and K, manganese.
How to eat: Snack on a handful each day.

provide antioxidants

QUICK FIX

For a quick-to-assemble, **hydrating**, and **circulation-boosting** appetizer, simply skewer some cherry tomatoes, cucumber slices, and basil leaves on toothpicks.

Tomatoes

The bright, dense red pigment in tomatoes indicates powerful antioxidants, in particular lycopene that helps to protect the delicate blood vessels and improve circulation to the eyes.
Key nutrients: Lycopene, lutein, beta-carotene, quercetin, vitamin C.
How to eat: Have 1 medium or 7 cherry tomatoes daily.

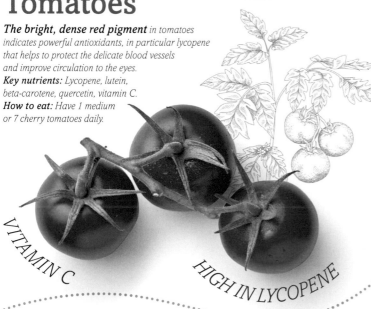

VITAMIN C

HIGH IN LYCOPENE

7%
POTASSIUM ᴿᴵ

Celery

This is a rich source of the electrolyte minerals sodium and potassium, powerful fluid regulators that can help to reduce puffiness. The sodium in celery is very different than white table salt as it promotes the uptake of other nutrients.
Key nutrients: Sodium, potassium, magnesium, quercetin, fiber.
How to eat: Snack on a stick or add to meals or salads.

POTASSIUM

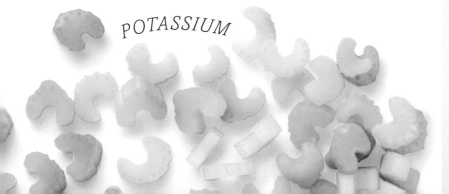

MORE SUPERFOODS

Mulberries

These contain resveratrol, an age-defying antioxidant, iron, and hydrating sugars.
Key nutrients: Vitamins A, B1, B2, and C, protein, anthocyanins, resveratrol.
How to eat: Eat a few dried mulberries daily.

Beets

The red pigment is from the detoxifying antioxidants betalain, useful for eye health.
Key nutrients: Betalains, folate, vitamin C, magnesium.
How to eat: Up to 3oz (85g) a day.

Goji berries

The hydrating carotenoid zeaxanthin in goji berries boosts the skin around the eyes.
Key nutrients: Vitamins B and C, beta-carotene, zeaxanthin, polysaccharides, amino acids, iron, copper, selenium, calcium, zinc.
How to eat: Eat a small handful daily.

Baobab

Nutrient-dense, this has low sodium levels, balancing fluids and preventing puffy eyes.
Key nutrients: Fiber, calcium, vitamins A, B1, B6, and C, potassium, magnesium, zinc, bioflavonoids.
How to eat: Add 1–2 tsp a day to meals.

Bee pollen

The antioxidant rutin aids circulation, and protein renews collagen and elastin.
Key nutrients: 18 vitamins, all amino acids, fatty acids, protein.
How to eat: Eat up to 1 tsp daily. Do not give to children, or take if you have a bee sting allergy, are pregnant, or breastfeeding.

Spirulina

Nutrient-dense, this has protein for tissue renewal and sulfur to strengthen skin.
Key nutrients: Protein, antioxidants, fatty acids, B vitamins, calcium.
How to eat: Start with ¼ tsp daily in a meal or drink and build up to 1 tsp.

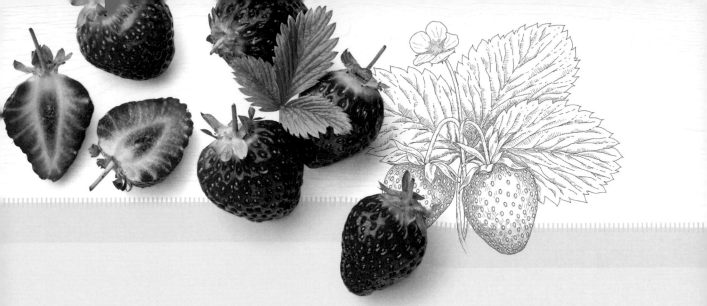

Foods
for the body

Diet and lifestyle inevitably impact how your body looks and feels. Find out how to tailor your diet to include foods that tone your body and leave skin silky smooth, and try nutritionally balanced meal plans designed to ensure you eat the most beneficial foods to keep you looking your very best.

Eat for beauty: body

For your body to look and feel fabulous, it's essential that it's **fueled** by a range of the **top beauty nutrients** to nourish from within and keep it **supple** and toned. Discover the key nutrients to help you hone your physique and keep you looking and feeling at your very best.

Nutrients for your body
Before you address the specific beauty concerns in this chapter, find out how certain nutrients are key to a toned, beautiful body.

Essential fatty acids Your body needs a regular supply of omega-3 and omega-6 fatty acids for the growth and repair of cell membranes. These vital fats have an impressive range of beauty benefits for your body. As well as maintaining the skin's oil barrier to keep skin hydrated, they have an anti-inflammatory action that helps to soothe conditions such as eczema and rough skin. The moisture they provide lubricates skin, keeping it supple and firm, which in turn helps to prevent premature sagging and reduces the appearance of stretch marks. In addition, omega-3 and omega-6 help to balance hormones and reduce premenstrual symptoms

such as bloating. These essential fats cannot be manufactured by the body so you need to obtain them through your diet. And while both omega-3 and omega-6 are important, our bodies need more omega-3 than omega-6 since too much omega-6 can have an inflammatory effect. Eating oily fish at least three times a week will boost your levels of omega-3, and other good sources of this fat are found in flaxseeds and hemp seed oils, nuts, avocados, and dark-green leafy vegetables. Omega-6 sources include meats, cereal grains, flaxseeds, hemp, and grapeseed oils, and nuts and seeds.

High-quality proteins These are essential for collagen, the strong cementlike material that binds the cells of the body together. This structural tissue, made of fibrous protein, comprises 30 percent of the total protein in the body and is

one of the most valuable proteins. Collagen contains the fiber elastin that helps to form the connective tissues throughout our bodies, strengthening the skin, blood vessels, and bones. Supple skin with good elasticity is a sign that the body has ample collagen. As collagen is replaced very slowly, it's important to include sources of healthy protein consistently in your diet. Make sure you have good-quality proteins in every meal from foods such as eggs, fish, chicken, and legumes.

Vitamins A, C, and E The unstable chemicals known as free radicals, whose development is hastened by toxins and unhealthy lifestyle choices, have a damaging effect on our bodies and are a key factor in the aging process. This damage can result in dry skin and poor skin tone, which in turn exacerbates problems such as

Providing your body with all the nutrients it needs to thrive will help your body to feel energized and look supple and toned, and for you to feel fantastic.

cellulite and slows the healing of scars and bruises. The best way to protect your body against these harmful substances is to boost your daily intake of antioxidant vitamins, found most abundantly in fresh fruit and vegetables. The

27%
of our daily vitamin E needs are met by a medium-sized avocado.

most beneficial antioxidants for your body are vitamins A, C, and E. Vitamin A is obtained from foods that have betacarotene, which converts to vitamin A

in the body. Good sources of betacarotene include carrots, sweet potatoes, kale, and spinach. As well as being a powerful antioxidant, vitamin C is also important for the formation of collagen, so it's a particularly crucial nutrient for healthy, firm, supple skin. Good sources of vitamin C include berries, broccoli, kiwi, and sweet potatoes. Vitamin E helps to protect the skin against damaging UV rays and is found in foods such as nuts, seeds, vegetables oils, avocados, and tomatoes.

Zinc This essential trace mineral is found in every single cell in the body and is needed by more than 100 different enzymes to help them function properly. Surface skin cells are especially dependent on zinc, and the top layer of skin contains up to six times more of the mineral than the lower skin

layers. Zinc acts as an antioxidant, helping to slow the aging process, and also has an anti-inflammatory action and healing properties that help to repair skin, reducing the appearance of scars and sun damage and calming conditions such as eczema and skin bumps. Good sources of zinc include nuts and seeds, asparagus, quinoa, oats, spinach, lentils, and whole grains.

Hydration Our bodies need to be well hydrated to function properly. Staying hydrated also helps to lubricate skin and flush out toxins, which in turn stops us feeling bloated and controls problems such as cellulite. Drinking up to 2 liters of water each day (around 6–8 glasses) helps to hydrate us, and we can supplement fluids by eating fresh fruit and vegetables with a high water content, such as leafy greens, cucumbers, celery, and watermelons.

What affects our bodies?

How your body looks is affected by a whole range of factors, including diet and lifestyle, life events such as pregnancy, and the effects of long-term stress. Understanding how foods support your body with nutrients and energy will help you to make the right food choices to look and feel your very best.

Diet and lifestyle Just as a balanced, nutritious diet supports the body and helps us maintain a healthy weight, a poor diet can deplete our bodies of nutrients. Saturated fats and processed oils and foods can produce aging free radicals, while a strict fat-free diet starves the skin of moisture. Refined carbohydrates, such as processed sugars and white flour, can lead to rapid spikes in blood-sugar and insulin levels, which triggers the kidneys to retain sodium. This, together with the high levels of refined salt in processed foods, can cause fluid retention and bloating. Alcohol and caffeine act as diuretics, and although these reduce excess fluids, their addictive nature can mean that too much fluid is lost and the body is stripped of essential nutrients.

Aim for a diet full of healthy fats and protein from fish, lean meat, nuts, and legumes, and complex carbohydrates from wholegrains and colorful fruits and vegetables.

Pregnancy and breastfeeding If you are pregnant or breastfeeding, your body's demand for nutritious foods is greater because you need to nourish both yourself and your growing baby. Many pregnant women and breastfeeding mothers are low in omega-3 fats and other vital nutrients, leaving the body lacking moisture and exacerbating pregnancy concerns such as stretch

Eat for your age

As we age, our body goes through significant changes, some dramatic (for example, in pregnancy), others slower and more subtle (for example, the gradual loss of muscle tone from our 30s). Collagen-boosting proteins and omega fats and a range of vegetables and fruit that provide a full spectrum of nutrients support these changes. A multivitamin with vitamin D as well as a fish oil supplement can help to keep skin supple.

In your 20s

In our 20s we have optimal muscle mass, and collagen and elastin are at their peak, keeping skin firm and supple and ensuring good muscle definition. However, poor dietary choices, too much alcohol, and hectic lifestyles can place stress on our bodies, and your body may be depleted of key healthy nutrients.
Eat: To ensure you are getting a good range of nutrients, eat plenty of good-quality protein from sources such as fish, chicken, and legumes; whole grains to support digestion; and dark greens and colorful vegetables and fruits to supply a whole range of antioxidants.

In your 30s

The rate of new cells being produced slows down in this decade, and collagen production also starts to slow, which means that skin begins to get thinner gradually and loses some plumpness, and muscles start to lose tone. Sebum production starts to slow, making skin drier overall and more susceptible to inflammation, and metabolism slows, so you may gain a few pounds.
Eat: Antioxidant-rich fruit and vegetables help to nourish skin now, and foods high in vitamin C, such as citrus fruits, dark leafy greens, and bell peppers, will help to boost collagen production and elasticity.

12%

of our daily protein needs are met by just ¼ cup pistachio nuts.

Stress and illness Periods of illness can affect weight, leaving us with an unhealthy body mass index (BMI) and depleting the body of nutrients, which need building up again. It's important to focus on a high-nutrient diet to help the body recover. When stressed, we may pay less attention to our diet, often eating insufficient healthy fats and too many refined carbohydrates. Stress also leads to insomnia, and when sleep deprived we may be tempted into unhealthy food choices. Finding coping strategies for dealing with stress can help you to avoid dietary pitfalls.

marks and uneven skin tone. Being well hydrated and eating a balanced diet with healthy proteins, fats, and complex carbohydrates can help avoid unnecessary weight gain and reduce problems such as swelling.

Menopause As we approach menopause it's common to put on weight as our bodies adapt to fluctuating hormones. Eating healthy fats and nutrient-dense foods will help control weight gain.

In your 40s

Collagen production continues to slow now, and skin elasticity decreases. The lymphatic system loses efficiency, making it harder to eliminate toxins and causing bloating. Estrogen levels also start to fall, which can make skin drier and less firm. The effects of accumulated sun damage may start to show with areas of patchy skin and discoloration.
Eat: Eat antioxidant-rich fresh vegetables to detoxify and hydrate. Essential fats from oily fish, nuts, and seeds also hydrate the body. Foods with phytoestrogens, such as tempeh, lentils, chickpeas, and flaxseeds, can help to balance hormones.

In your 50s

Patches of pigmentation and age spots may appear on the body, in particular on the arms and hands. Skin cells have 30 percent less natural moisture now, so sagging is a main concern, and skin is noticeably drier, thinner, tighter, and flakier. For women, a major shift in hormones can disrupt skin function and lead to a loss of elasticity.
Eat: Healthy proteins and brightly colored fruit and vegetables help to balance blood sugar and hormones. In particular, betacarotene-rich yellow and red vegetables also support the growth of new skin cells.

60s plus

The material that attaches to skin called fascia deteriorates, which means that skin continues to lose tone and can become saggier around the underarm area and the tops of the thighs, and overall muscle mass declines. Circulation has slowed down significantly now, which means skin can look dull in appearance and lose its sheen.
Eat: Continue to eat healthy proteins and include foods that are sources of vitamin D, such as legumes, eggs, and oily fish. Fresh fruit and vegetables provide antioxidants, which are increasingly important to keep the body healthy.

Cellulite

Skin with cellulite has a dimpled, lumpy appearance, most noticeably on the buttocks and thighs. Unhealthy fats, excess carbohydrates, salt, caffeine, too little fluid and fiber, and smoking all increase toxin levels. To promote smooth, supple skin, eat fresh foods with a high water content to help flush out toxins and boost circulation. Healthy proteins and antioxidants support collagen production, keeping skin toned and firm.

Superfood recipe suggestions...**Spiced apple oatmeal** p170 **Superfood spread** p172 **Cacao and chia chocolate "pudding"** p174 **Protein power beauty bites** p195 **Black lentil and coconut curry** p204 **Homemade oat milk** p241

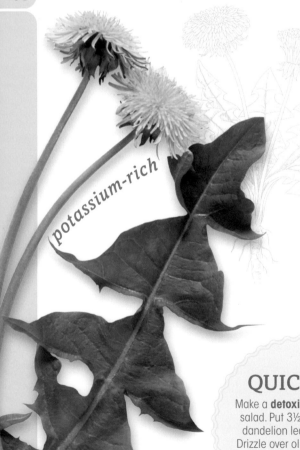

potassium-rich

Dandelions

A diuretic, dandelion helps to release toxins *trapped under the skin and flush waste products out of the liver. It is also high in antioxidants and potassium, which helps to combat fluid retention, keeping skin smooth.*
Key nutrients: *Potassium, calcium, manganese, iron, magnesium, vitamins C and A.*
How to eat: *Add dandelion leaves to salads or drink 1 cup of herbal tea daily.*

Unrefined salt

Swap refined table salt *for Himalayan pink salt or Celtic sea salt. Refined salt is extremely acidic, leaching minerals from the body. It is also highly dehydrating, exacerbating cellulite. Crystal and sea salt are alkaline, packed full of beneficial minerals, and have a fuller flavor.*
Key nutrients: *Calcium, iron, potassium, magnesium.*
How to eat: *Use a small amount to season food.*

QUICK FIX

Make a **detoxifying** dandelion salad. Put 3½oz (100g) torn dandelion leaves in a bowl. Drizzle over olive oil, then add a squeeze of lemon and a pinch of Himalayan pink salt.

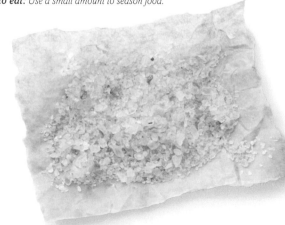

Cinnamon

This sweet spice stimulates the regenerative ability of cells, which boosts circulation, improving the supply of nutrients to the skin and helping to prevent a build-up of toxins that can result in bumpy cellulite.
Key nutrients: *Calcium, manganese, iron.*
How to eat: *Sprinkle ½ tsp of cinnamon on your breakfast or oatmeal each morning.*

MANGANESE CALCIUM

contains saponins

15%
IRON RI

Gotu kola tea

This Asian herb, *a member of the parsley family and commonly used in traditional Chinese and Ayurvedic medicine, has chemical compounds called triterpene saponins that help to boost collagen production and improve blood circulation, both of which help to prevent cellulite.*
Key nutrients: *Saponins, beta-carotene, calcium, vitamins B1, B2, and C.*
How to drink: *Drink a cup daily. Add 1–2 tsp dried gotu kola leaf to ¾ cup of boiling water and steep for 10–15 minutes.*

MORE SUPERFOODS

Berries
The dark pigment in berries, such as blueberries, blackberries, raspberries, and blackcurrants, indicates high levels of antioxidants, which help the body to eliminate toxins and enhance the production of collagen to help renew skin tissue and keep it supple and smooth.
Key nutrients: *Vitamins B2, B6, C, and E, potassium, folate, manganese, copper.*
How to eat: *A handful makes part of your five a day. Add raspberries, strawberries, blueberries, or blackberries to cereal or oatmeal each morning, or snack on a handful.*

Papaya
This is one of the best sources of vitamin C, which is essential for strong connective tissue to keep skin firm and toned. Some studies have shown a digestive enzyme, papain, in the fruit helps to break up proteins and prevent the tissue damage under the skin that can lead to cellulite.
Key nutrients: *Vitamin C, B vitamins, potassium, copper, magnesium.*
How to eat: *Eat a papaya once a week.*

Nuts
Full of collagen-building protein, nuts help the body to digest and expel food to avoid a build-up of the toxins that can contribute to cellulite.
Key nutrients: *Vitamins B and E, calcium, iron, zinc, potassium, magnesium.*
How to eat: *Enjoy a handful of nuts daily.*

Oily fish
Oily fish such as salmon, mackerel, and trout, stimulate collagen production and are anti-inflammatory, helping to reduce cellulite.
Key nutrients: *Omega-3.*
How to eat: *Add 2–3 tsp of nuts and seeds at meals daily or eat oily fish 2–3 times a week.*

For supplements, see page 249.

Water retention

Also known as oedema, this occurs when fluid builds up in the body's tissues, causing swelling in the hands, feet, ankles, and legs. Inactivity, pregnancy, some medical conditions, a poor diet, and a lack of fluids can be causes. Potassium-rich foods relieve symptoms by increasing urine output and by decreasing sodium levels, and proteins support cell structure to prevent fluid leaking out into surrounding tissues.

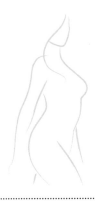

Superfood recipe suggestions...**Fruity quinoa breakfast** p169   **Blueberry and chia pancakes** p171
Avocado on toast with mixed-herb pesto p180   **Hot nuts!** p194   **Japanese ocean soup** p201   **Ratatouille** p207

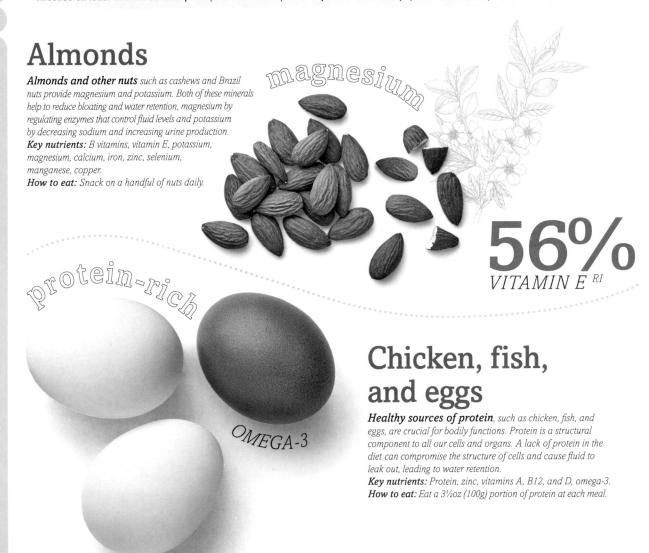

Almonds

Almonds and other nuts such as cashews and Brazil nuts provide magnesium and potassium. Both of these minerals help to reduce bloating and water retention, magnesium by regulating enzymes that control fluid levels and potassium by decreasing sodium and increasing urine production.
Key nutrients: B vitamins, vitamin E, potassium, magnesium, calcium, iron, zinc, selenium, manganese, copper.
How to eat: Snack on a handful of nuts daily.

magnesium

56%
VITAMIN E ^RI

protein-rich

OMEGA-3

Chicken, fish, and eggs

Healthy sources of protein, such as chicken, fish, and eggs, are crucial for bodily functions. Protein is a structural component to all our cells and organs. A lack of protein in the diet can compromise the structure of cells and cause fluid to leak out, leading to water retention.
Key nutrients: Protein, zinc, vitamins A, B12, and D, omega-3.
How to eat: Eat a 3½oz (100g) portion of protein at each meal.

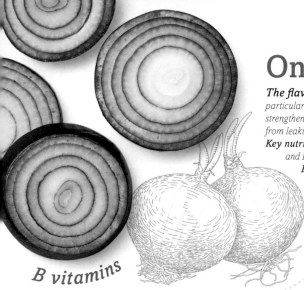

Onions

The flavonoid quercetin, whose levels are particularly high in red onions, is thought to strengthen capillary walls, preventing fluids from leaking out into the surrounding tissues.
Key nutrients: Folate, vitamins B1, B2, C, and E, fiber, potassium, magnesium, copper.
How to eat: Add an onion to salads and use as a flavor base in meals daily.

B vitamins

QUICK FIX

Flush out excess fluids with this salad. Finely slice a red onion. Toss with 2 bunches of watercress, a drizzle of olive oil, a pinch of Himalayan pink salt, parsley, and a squeeze of lemon.

POTASSIUM

Watercress

This nutrient-dense salad leaf is a rich source of potassium, which acts as a natural diuretic, drawing out excess fluids. It is also low in calories, so a great dietary addition.
Key nutrients: Vitamins A, C, E, and B vitamins, magnesium, phosphorus, potassium, manganese.
How to eat: Eat a handful daily in a salad or snack.

vitamins A, B, C, E

Lemon

The diuretic effect of lemons is largely due to its vitamin C content. Antibacterial and cleansing, lemon helps to flush out excess fluids and toxins from the body to restore a healthy fluid balance.
Key nutrient: Vitamin C.
How to eat: Start each day with a hot water and lemon drink.

72%
VITAMIN C RI

MORE SUPERFOODS

Celery
This versatile vegetable has natural diuretic properties that help to reduce excess fluid. It is also an incredibly low-calorie food choice.
Key nutrients: Vitamin C, potassium, magnesium.
How to eat: Eat daily either chopped up on a salad, as a snack with hummus, or add to meals or smoothies.

Avocado
This is an excellent natural diuretic to help combat water retention. It provides a boost to potassium levels, helping to ensure the body has the right balance of sodium and potassium needed to regulate fluid levels.
Key nutrients: Potassium, omega-9, vitamin E, B vitamins, and folic acid.
How to eat: Eat 1 medium avocado 2–4 times a week.

Dandelion
This has a long history in natural medicine as a healthy natural diuretic, helping to flush out excess fluids.
Key nutrients: Potassium, calcium, iron, manganese, magnesium, vitamins C and A.
How to drink: Add the leaves to salads or drink daily as a tea: add 1–2 tsp of dried leaves to 1 cup of boiling water.

Pineapple
Made up of 85 percent water and rich in vitamin C and manganese, pineapple hydrates and detoxifies, helping flush out toxins. An enzyme, bromelain, in pineapple is anti-inflammatory, helping to calm bloating.
Key nutrients: Vitamins B1, B2, B6, and C, manganese, copper, potassium.
How to eat: Enjoy 1 large slice of pineapple after meals or add to smoothies.

For supplements, see page 249

Meal planner Fluid rebalancing

Our bodies are made up of around 60 percent water. If we are dehydrated, toxins can build up, leading to water retention and cellulite. This fluid-rebalancing meal planner, drawing on recipes from the book with additional meal ideas, is designed to provide hydrating, detoxifying foods and the essential nutrients required to help the body regulate its fluid levels.

Your fluid-rebalancing week This nutritionally balanced, one-week meal planner will start you on your fluid-rebalancing diet. To get the best results, continue for four weeks, using the additional ideas, opposite, for variety. Start each day with a hot water and lemon drink to aid digestion.

Monday

Breakfast
Grapefruit and pear juice (p.243) with whole-wheat toast and nut butter

Snacks
Coconut smoothie (p.235)

Lunch
Salmon pâté (p.193) on rye bread with a watercress salad

Dinner
Roasted broccoli and cauliflower with couscous (p.206)

Tuesday

Breakfast
Green smoothie (p.244)

Snacks
Rye bread with hummus

Lunch
Gazpacho with watermelon (p.188)

Dinner
Roasted sea bass with tomato salsa (p.212)

Wednesday

Breakfast
Natural live yogurt with mixed berries

Snacks
Nuts and apricots

Lunch
Winter salad (p.185, variation)

Dinner
Japanese ocean soup (p.201)

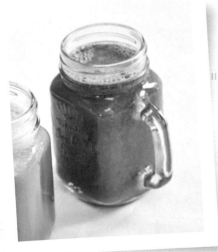

Grapefruit and pear juice (p.243)

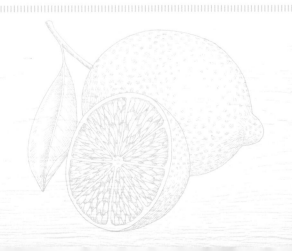

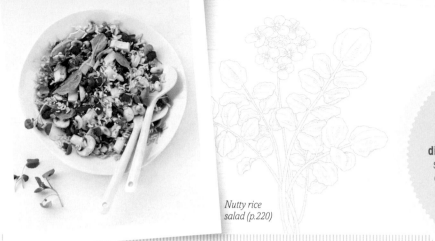

Nutty rice salad (p.220)

NATURAL DIURETICS

Dandelion acts as a **gentle diuretic**, unlike caffeinated drinks such as coffee, which although diuretic, are also addictive and overstimulating. A daily cup of dandelion tea helps to reduce water retention.

Thursday

Breakfast
Poached egg on rye bread

Snacks
Red berry smoothie (p.235)

Lunch
Pasta salad with avocado, mixed beans, cucumber, lemon, olive oil, and basil

Dinner
Lemon and herb-roasted chicken (p.210)

Friday

Breakfast
Cashew butter on rye bread

Snacks
Two oat cakes with nut butter and celery sticks

Lunch
Summer asparagus salad (p.189)

Dinner
Nutty rice salad (p.220)

Saturday

Breakfast
Poached egg on spelt or whole-wheat toast

Snacks
Handful of nuts and raisins

Lunch
Apple, pear, celery, and hazelnut salad with a tablespoon of hummus

Dinner
Salmon with samphire (p.215)

Sweet treat
Coconut yogurt with baobab and goldenberries (p.226)

Sunday

Breakfast
Cucumber and kale juice (p.243) with whole-wheat toast and nut butter

Snacks
Two corn cakes with hummus and celery sticks

Lunch
Cherry tomatoes with olives and basil leaves

Dinner
Japanese ocean soup (p.201)

Coconut yogurt with baobab and goldenberries (p.226)

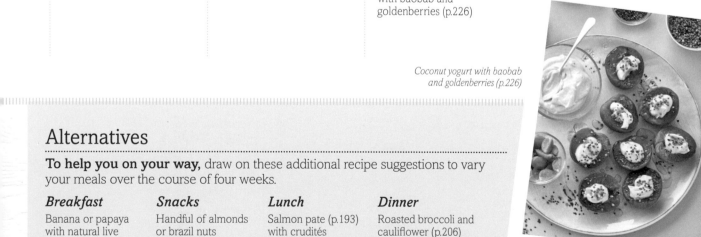

Alternatives

To help you on your way, draw on these additional recipe suggestions to vary your meals over the course of four weeks.

Breakfast
Banana or papaya with natural live yogurt

Snacks
Handful of almonds or brazil nuts

Celery sticks

Lunch
Salmon pate (p.193) with crudités

Gazpacho with watermelon (p.188)

Dinner
Roasted broccoli and cauliflower (p.206)

Pasta with dairy-free pesto (p.187, variation)

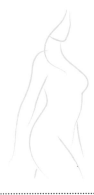

Saggy skin

As we age, a loss of skin tone and extra weight can cause skin to sag, typified by "chicken wings," areas of underarm skin that wobble when shaken! Obesity, lack of fitness, and a drop in testosterone with age worsen upper arm definition. Healthy proteins and unrefined carbohydrates build muscle tone, while vitamin C–rich foods support skin-firming collagen and elastin, and omega-3 boosts testosterone levels to restore muscle.

Superfood recipe suggestions... Overnight oats with superberry compote p168   Fruity quinoa breakfast p169
Gazpacho with watermelon p188   Baked stuffed squash p203   Salmon with samphire p215   Berry nice skin! p238

Oats

These provide a wide range of nutrients including minerals such as silica, which boosts the production of collagen and elastin for firmer, more toned, and supple skin. Silica is also a crucial component of hyaluronic acid, a substance that bathes collagen and elastin in moisture, keeping them flexible so the skin remains supple and firm.
Key nutrients: Silica, copper, biotin, fiber, vitamin B1, magnesium, chromium, zinc.
How to eat: Eat up to ¼ cup daily. Use to make oatmeal or add to your morning smoothie.

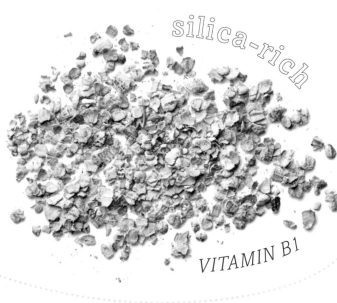

silica-rich

VITAMIN B1

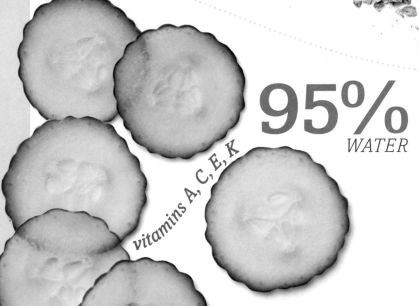

vitamins A, C, E, K

95%
WATER

Cucumber

As well as its high water content, which rehydrates skin, cucumber contains silica, which boosts collagen and keeps skin firm; sulfur, which strengthens the skin; and vitamin K, which supports the elasticity of blood vessels, supporting circulation to the skin.
Key nutrients: Vitamins A, C, E, and K, silica, sulfur.
How to eat: Eat ¼ cucumber daily as a snack or in a salad.

Berries

All types of berries are high in vitamin C, which the body uses to boost the production of collagen, whose production decreases naturally with age. Also, an antioxidant called anthocyanin in berries has skin-protecting properties, helping to keep skin cells healthy and skin toned.
Key nutrients: Vitamins C and E, omega-3, potassium, magnesium.
How to eat: Aim to eat ¼ cup or 2 handfuls of berries each day.

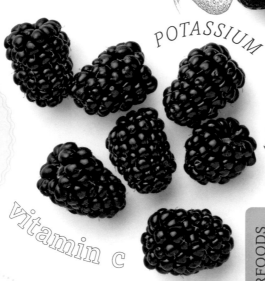

POTASSIUM

vitamin c

QUICK FIX

For a **skin-firming** start to the day, add a berry compote to your daily oatmeal. Gently heat fresh or frozen berries with a sprinkle of water until warm, then add to cooked oatmeal.

39%
FOLATE RI

Quinoa

Made up of almost 22 percent protein, quinoa has all the essential amino acids needed for muscle repair and renewal, plus a variety of skin-firming vitamins and minerals, including silica, to build collagen and promote skin elasticity.
Key nutrients: Manganese, phosphorus, copper, magnesium, silica, folate, zinc, protein, vitamins B1, B2, B6, and E.
How to eat: Have a ¼-cup serving a couple of times a week.

MORE SUPERFOODS

Salmon
This is a fantastic source of the essential fat omega-3. Omega-3 has anti-inflammatory properties that help to keep skin soft and supple and, in turn, well conditioned.
Key nutrients: Vitamins B12 and D, omega-3.
How to eat: Aim to eat oily fish 2–3 times a week.

Turmeric
This contains a powerfully anti-inflammatory antioxidant called curcumin, which also increases levels of an enzyme, glutathione S-transferase, an important antioxidant that helps to eliminate toxins to keep skin clear, firm, and toned.
Key nutrients: Iron, manganese, vitamin B6, curcumin, potassium.
How to eat: Flavor meals with ½ tsp of ground turmeric or add to a smoothie.

Matcha tea
Matcha is rich in catechin polyphenols—compounds with a high antioxidant activity that offer protection against the aging process and an anti-inflammatory effect that improves skin elasticity and resilience.
Key nutrients: Vitamin A, polyphenols, epigallocatechin gallate (EGCG).
How to eat: Have a matcha tea daily.

10 ways to... Avoid overeating

Many of us eat more food than our body really needs. Taking time to prepare, cook, and eat delicious, nutrient-rich meals and snacks is enjoyable and has many benefits for your health, beauty, and well-being. Eat enough of the right foods and eliminate unhealthy eating habits and you will reap the beauty rewards with a toned body and well-nourished, glowing skin and hair.

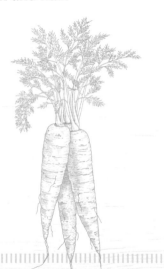

1 Time your eating

Maintain your blood sugar levels throughout the day by eating approximately every two to three hours. Eat nutrient-dense main meals and healthy snacks. Both snacks and main meals should include protein and carbohydrates—this combination slows the release of sugar from carbohydrates into your bloodstream, preventing hunger pangs and providing a steady supply of energy for your body.

2 Don't diet

Low-calorie diets can often cause more harm than good, causing you inevitably to overeat to make up for deprivation. Your body isn't designed to work on minimal energy supplies, and can go into survival mode if it's deprived of basic nutrients—this can mean holding on to weight, slowing your metabolism, and increasing your cravings for unhealthy food.

6 Concentrate on your food

Instead of sitting on the sofa or looking at your phone while eating, make the effort to cook a wholesome, nutritious meal from scratch. Eat sitting at the table, and concentrate on your food. This may feel a little forced at first, but it will soon begin to feel natural. Taking the time to focus on and savor food decreases the likelihood that you will overeat.

7 Use a small plate

Most of us eat much more than we really need to function. Eating from a smaller plate is a simple way to decrease your portion sizes. Research shows that people eat more when presented with larger portions—this can contribute to overeating and weight gain. Try to cook only as much as you need, eat a healthy portion, and don't go back for seconds.

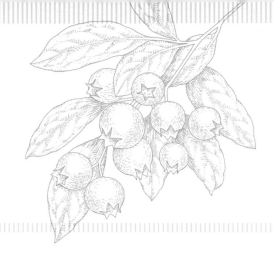

3 Check for **thirst**

If you start craving a snack, try drinking a glass of water instead. The hormones that trigger food cravings and thirst are the same, so we often confuse hunger and thirst. Drinking more fluids will keep the skin hydrated and healthy.

4 Don't eat **on the run**

Eating while on the move signals to your body that time is scarce and that you are under pressure. This causes your body to produce stress hormones, which makes your digestive system sluggish as the energy needed for your digestive system is diverted elsewhere. Instead, take your time to eat meals sitting down. Digestion starts in your mouth, so savor your food and chew every mouthful thoroughly before swallowing.

5 Watch what you **drink**

Drinking caffeinated drinks, alcohol, and fizzy drinks can cause spikes in blood sugar levels, as well as damaging your skin and dental health. Alcohol is also an antinutrient that depletes your body of vitamins and minerals. Fruit juice can also cause a sugar hit, so drink it only occasionally, and in small quantities— no more than 5fl oz (150ml) at a time.

8 Read **the label**

Studies show that most of us are confused by the nutritional labels on premade meals. Often, we assume that the nutritional information on the label is for the whole contents of the package, rather than a half- or quarter-portion. This means that we eat far more food than we need to. Always check the label for the portion or serving size, or—even better— cook your meal from scratch yourself to maximize your intake of beauty-boosting nutrients.

9 Understand **portions**

Portion size is the amount of food that you should eat in each sitting. Portions of meat or fish should be about the size of the palm of your hand. Portions of grains or pasta should fit in one cupped hand. A portion of cheese should be the size of a matchbox. Medium-sized fruit, such as apples, pears, and oranges, should be eaten one per serving, and smaller fruit, such as kiwis and plums, two per serving. A portion of vegetables is the equivalent of 3 tablespoons. Butter or oil should be used only a teaspoon per serving.

10 Don't **eat out often**

People who eat out regularly are more likely to have an increased calorie intake, which can lead to weight gain and obesity. Studies show that this is true of both eating out at restaurants and eating out at fast-food establishments. If you eat at home, you're more likely to use healthy ingredients, fewer unhealthy fats, and you have more control over your portion size, which will help to keep your body toned and reduce problems such as cellulite that can accompany weight gain.

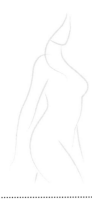

Stretch marks

These reddish, wavy stripes can appear on the abdomen, buttocks, breasts, and thighs when rapid weight gain, for example in pregnancy, overstretches skin. Zinc- and vitamin C–rich foods boost skin-firming collagen, promoting skin elasticity, which can help to prevent stretch marks, while vitamins A and E and omega-3 have an anti-inflammatory action that keeps skin cells healthy and skin supple, helping to reduce the appearance of stretch marks.

Superfood recipe suggestions... **Berry, seed, and nut granola** p166 **Blueberry and chia pancakes** p171
Fall flavors soup p178 **Huevos rancheros** p184 **Salmon pâté** p193 **Black lentil and coconut curry** p204

Tomatoes

Tomatoes are high in vitamin C, *crucial for collagen formation to keep skin firm and supple. The carotenoid lycopene found in tomatoes helps to neutralize the harmful effects of UV rays, reducing sun damage, which can emphasize stretch marks.*
Key nutrients: *Vitamins A, B3, C, E, and K, folate, lycopene, potassium, manganese, phosphorus.*
How to eat: *Eat 3oz (85g) tomatoes daily.*

QUICK FIX

Boost your vitamin C by including tomatoes in your diet regularly. Add them to salads or drizzle with olive oil, sprinkle with oregano, and roast them. Tomatoes release more lycopene the longer they're cooked.

10%
IRON RI

Lentils

The skin is 75 percent collagen, *which helps to keep it smooth and flexible. Lentils are a top source of healthy protein, essential for collagen production.*
Key nutrients: *Iron, protein, vitamins B1, B5, and B6, zinc, potassium.*
How to eat: *Aim to eat a ½-cup portion of lentils at least once a week.*

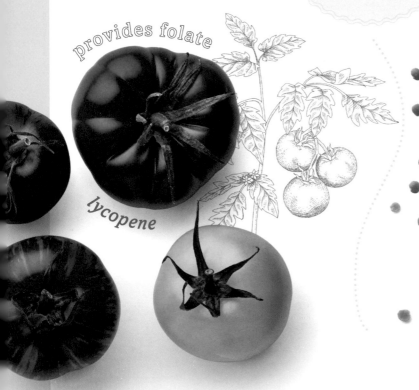

provides folate

lycopene

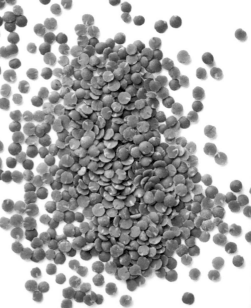

Oily fish

Oily fish, such as mackerel and salmon, *are a top source of the essential fatty acid omega-3, which can only be obtained through the diet. Omega-3 helps to promote cell growth and skin repair, keeping skin moisturized and reducing inflammation.*
Key nutrients: *Omega-3, vitamins B12 and D, selenium.*
How to eat: *Aim to eat oily fish 2–3 times a week.*

74%
SELENIUM RI

vitamin B12

vitamin D

GOOD SOURCE OF OMEGA-3

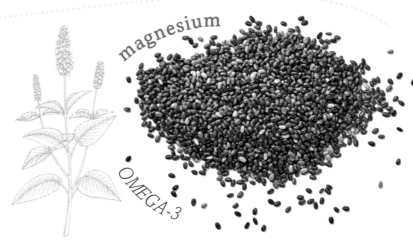

magnesium

OMEGA-3

Chia seeds

These are high in vitamin E, *which acts as an anti-inflammatory antioxidant that helps to keep skin soft and increase its elasticity. Chia seeds also contain eight times more omega-3 than salmon, so are fantastic anti-inflammatories.*
Key nutrients: *Vitamin E, magnesium, omega-3, protein.*
How to eat: *Add 1 tbsp of chia seeds to oatmeal or a smoothie daily.*

MORE SUPERFOODS

Eggs
These are an excellent source of protein, which is essential for building collagen and elastin to improve the quality of skin, helping to make it more supple and stretchy and prevent stretch marks from developing in the first place.
Key nutrients: *Vitamin A, carotenes, lutein, zinc.*
How to eat: *Eat 1 boiled or poached egg up to 4 times a week.*

Avocados
These are an excellent source of healthy fats. Incorporating healthy fats into your diet boosts skin elasticity and helps the body to absorb antioxidants from other nutrient-dense foods. Avocados are also packed full of nutrients themselves, including skin-protecting vitamin E and a range of B vitamins.
Key nutrients: *Potassium, omega-9, vitamin E, B vitamins, folic acid.*
How to eat: *Eat an avocado daily.*

Cucumbers
Around 95 percent water, these hydrate the body and skin and promote elasticity and collagen formation to help to prevent stretch marks. Staying well hydrated also helps to flush out toxins, which in turn keeps skin conditioned.
Key nutrients: *Vitamins C, B5, B6, biotin, magnesium, potassium, phosphorus.*
How to eat: *Eat ¼ cucumber, or more, daily in your diet, as a snack, or in salads.*

Berries
High in antioxidants, berries protect the body from free radical damage caused by the sun, which can exaggerate the appearance of stretch marks. High in vitamin C, berries also support collagen formation for supple, flexible skin.
Key nutrients: *Vitamin C, potassium.*
How to eat: *Eat a handful daily, added to smoothies or oatmeal or eaten as a snack.*

For supplements, see page 249.

Meal planner Skin firming

Our skin is made up of connective tissues, fibers, and other components that can stretch or contract, often as a result of aging, weight loss, or poor nutrition. This skin-firming meal plan, based on the recipes in this book with additional meal ideas, includes foods to promote elastin and collagen production, giving skin elasticity, firmness, and helping to prevent sagging.

Your skin-firming week
This nutritionally balanced one-week meal plan sets you off on your skin-firming diet. Continue for four weeks for the best skin results, using the alternatives, opposite, for variety. Start each day with a hot water and lemon drink to aid digestion.

Monday

Breakfast
Spiced apple oatmeal (p.170)

Snacks
Vitamin C boost (p.245)

Lunch
Mixed salad with cherry tomatoes and avocado

Dinner
Thai chicken and noodle soup (p.214)

Tuesday

Breakfast
Cacao and chia chocolate "pudding" (p.174)

Snacks
Coconut smoothie (p.235) and protein power beauty bites (p.195)

Lunch
Salmon pâté (p.193) with rye bread

Dinner
Sweet potato and mackerel mash (p.219, variation) with watercress and arugula salad

Wednesday

Breakfast
Fruity quinoa breakfast (p.169)

Snacks
Pineapple smoothie (p.239)

Lunch
Scrambled tofu (p.181) with cucumber slices

Dinner
Lamb tagine (p.208)

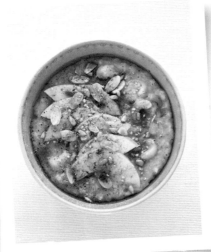

Spiced apple oatmeal (p.170)

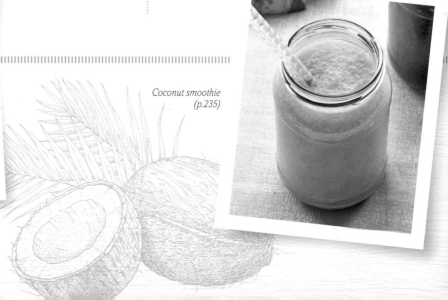

Coconut smoothie (p.235)

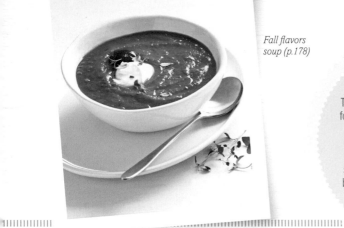

Fall flavors soup (p.178)

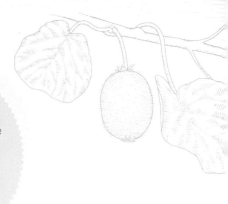

SILICA

This important mineral, found in foods such as oats, supports the manufacture of **elastin and collagen**, helping to keep skin toned, supple, and firm. Other sources of silica include green beans, asparagus, strawberries, and cucumber.

Thursday

Breakfast

Berry nice skin! (p.238)

Snacks

Apple slices spread with almond butter

Lunch

Fall flavors soup (p.178)

Dinner

Barley vegetable risotto (p.200)

Friday

Breakfast

Rye bread with almond butter

Snacks

Natural live yogurt with berries

Lunch

Spring veggie salad (p.183)

Dinner

Thai chicken and noodle soup (p.214)

Saturday

Breakfast

Mixed berry and kiwi fruit salad with natural live yogurt and ground flaxseeds

Snacks

Handful of brazil nuts and apricots

Lunch

Huevos rancheros (p.184)

Dinner

Lemon and herb-roasted chicken (p.210)

Sunday

Breakfast

Superfood spread (p.172) with rye bread

Snacks

Protein power beauty bites (p.195)

Lunch

Summer asparagus salad (p.189)

Dinner

Roasted sea bass with tomato salsa (p.212)

Sweet treats

Salted goldenberry chocolate cups (p.225)

Alternatives

To help you on your way, draw on these additional recipe suggestions to vary your meals over the course of four weeks.

Breakfast

Poached egg on rye toast

Rye toast with nut butters

Snacks

Red berry smoothie (p.235)

Lunch

Winter veggie slaw (p.185)

Gazpacho with watermelon (p.188)

Dinner

Miso-glazed tofu with quinoa (p.218)

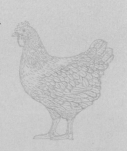

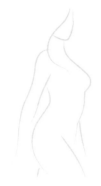

Dry body skin

A good balance of natural oils and moisture is crucial for smooth skin. A host of factors strip skin of moisture, including diuretics such as alcohol and caffeine and heat-processed oils. Foods high in omega-3 reduce the inflammation and redness common in dry skin; vitamin C–rich foods aid collagen production, keeping skin supple; and vitamin A and sulfur-high foods support connective tissues, keeping skin smooth and nourished.

Superfood recipe suggestions...**Spiced apple oatmeal** p170 **Cacao and chia chocolate "pudding"** p174 **Huevos rancheros** p184 **Chile guacamole** p190 **Potato mash with veggie mix** p219 **Nutty rice salad** p220

Oily fish

Oily fish, such as sardines, *provide the essential fatty acid omega-3, whose anti-inflammatory action soothes the redness that often accompanies dry skin. Other oily fish include salmon and mackerel.*
Key nutrients: *Omega-3, vitamin D, selenium.*
How to eat: *Try to eat oily fish 2–3 times a week.*

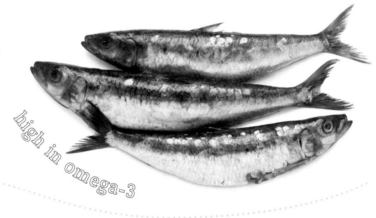

high in omega-3

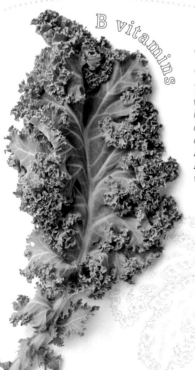

B vitamins

Kale

This cruciferous vegetable is high in vitamin C, *which promotes collagen synthesis and protects the skin's barrier to lock in moisture and help alleviate dry skin conditions. Other cruciferous vegetables such as broccoli, cabbage, and cauliflower are also high in vitamin C.*
Key nutrients: *Vitamins B and C, potassium, calcium.*
How to eat: *Include a 3½oz (100g) serving of a cruciferous vegetable in your diet at least 2–3 times a week.*

110%
VITAMIN C *RI*

QUICK FIX

Moisturize skin with a delicious kale and cilantro salad. Add other vegetables of your choice and serve with quinoa, a drizzle of olive oil, a squeeze of lemon, and seasoning.

Sweet potato

This nutrient-dense alternative to white potatoes is high in vitamin A, vital for strengthening and protecting skin tissue.
Key nutrients: Vitamins A, B5, B6, and C, manganese, copper.
How to eat: Have a 3oz (85g) serving of steamed or boiled sweet potatoes 2–3 times a week.

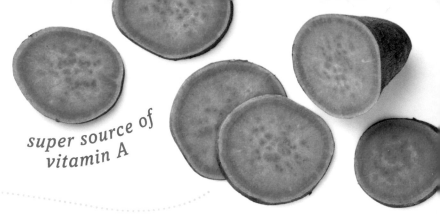

super source of vitamin A

Marigold herbal tea

Caffeine-free herbal infusions boost hydration levels. Marigold, from the calendula family, has skin-moistening and healing properties.
Key nutrients: Lutein, zeaxanthin, lycopene.
How to eat: Drink a daily infusion, made by pouring 1 cup of boiling water over 1–2 tsp of the flowers. Cover and steep for 10–15 minutes, then strain and drink.

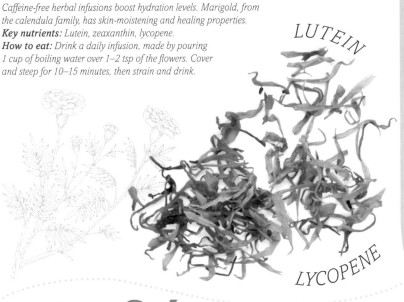

LUTEIN

LYCOPENE

34%
VITAMIN C RI

Cilantro

A healthy intake of vitamin C is linked to decreased levels of dry skin as the vitamin boosts collagen production, vital for healthy, supple skin. Fresh herbs such as cilantro, chives, thyme, basil, and parsley contain useful levels of vitamin C.
Key nutrients: Vitamins A, B1, C, and E, zinc.
How to eat: Add fresh herbs to meals to supplement other vitamin C–rich foods, such as bell peppers and broccoli.

MORE SUPERFOODS

Avocados
These are full of the healthy fats and oils that provide vital moisture and keep skin supple and nourished.
Key nutrients: Omega-9, B vitamins, magnesium, iron, potassium, vitamin E.
How to eat: Eat 1 a day for nourished skin.

Nuts and seeds
These are a great source of zinc, needed for the normal functioning of the oil-producing sebaceous glands in the skin and to help repair damage, keeping skin soft and supple.
Key nutrients: B vitamins (including folate), vitamin E, calcium, iron, zinc, potassium, magnesium, selenium, manganese, copper.
How to eat: Eat around 3 tbsp of nuts and/or seeds a day, as a snack or sprinkled on cereal, oatmeal, and salads.

Coconut oil
Coconut oil has an anti-inflammatory effect that helps to smooth dry skin on the body. It's also a good source of fatty acids, which means it has inherent moisturizing properties that help to repair and nourish dry skin.
Key nutrients: Essential fatty acids, vitamins E and K, iron.
How to eat: Add 1 tsp of coconut oil to a smoothie or use daily in cooking.

Eggs
As well as being a source of healthy protein, vital for strong, conditioned skin, egg whites provide sulfur, which boosts the development of connective tissues, helping skin to hold its structure and stay well nourished.
Key nutrients: Vitamins A, B2, B12, and D, selenium, iodine, sulfur.
How to eat: Eat a boiled or poached egg 2–3 times a week.

For supplements see page 249.

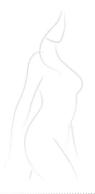

Skin bumps

A number of skin conditions can cause bumpy skin, including keratosis pilaris, a common condition where bumps appear on the arms, which is exacerbated by a lack of vitamin A, and cold weather. Hydrating foods and foods high in omega-3 oils nourish and condition skin, keeping it smooth. Vitamin A supports tissue repair, and zinc aids the synthesis of vitamin A, while vitamin C boosts collagen production and conditions skin.

Superfood recipe suggestions...Berry, seed, and nut granola p166   Winter veggie slaw p185
Summer asparagus Psalad p189   Black lentil and coconut curry p204   Green smoothie p244

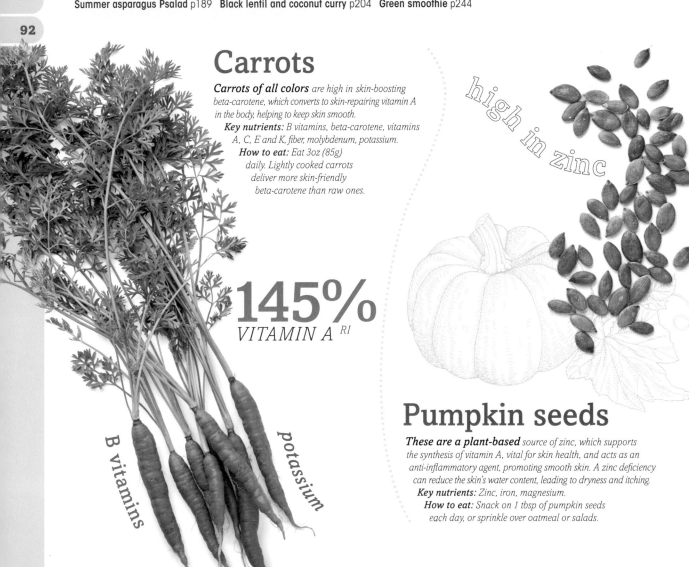

Carrots

Carrots of all colors are high in skin-boosting beta-carotene, which converts to skin-repairing vitamin A in the body, helping to keep skin smooth.

Key nutrients: B vitamins, beta-carotene, vitamins A, C, E and K, fiber, molybdenum, potassium.

How to eat: Eat 3oz (85g) daily. Lightly cooked carrots deliver more skin-friendly beta-carotene than raw ones.

145%
VITAMIN A RI

B vitamins

potassium

high in zinc

Pumpkin seeds

These are a plant-based source of zinc, which supports the synthesis of vitamin A, vital for skin health, and acts as an anti-inflammatory agent, promoting smooth skin. A zinc deficiency can reduce the skin's water content, leading to dryness and itching.

Key nutrients: Zinc, iron, magnesium.

How to eat: Snack on 1 tbsp of pumpkin seeds each day, or sprinkle over oatmeal or salads.

Oranges

These are a top source of vitamin C, crucial for building the structural protein collagen, which "holds" skin together, promoting smooth skin. A lack of vitamin C can cause follicles to become damaged, making skin appear rough and bumpy.
Key nutrients: Vitamin B1 and C, folate, potassium.
How to eat: Eat 3–4 oranges a week.

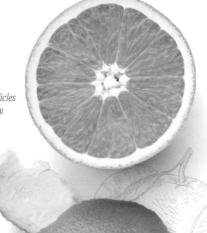

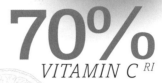

70%
VITAMIN C ^{RI}

QUICK FIX

Boost **skin-smoothing** vitamin C with this quenching juice. Peel 4 carrots and peel and remove the pith from 2 oranges. Process in a blender, then add 1 tbsp chia seeds, and serve immediately.

SUPPLIES FOLATE

POTASSIUM

Burdock root tea

Burdock root has diuretic and anti-inflammatory actions that can improve the body's immune system and flush out toxins that can contribute to uneven skin tone.
Key nutrients: Vitamins C and E, potassium.
How to eat: Have 2–4ml of burdock root tincture a day, added to drinks or taken directly.

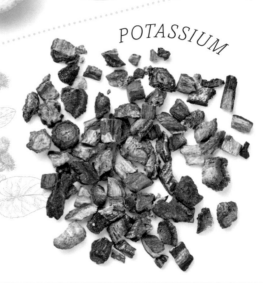

MORE SUPERFOODS

Sweet potatoes
These are full of beta-carotene, which converts to vitamin A, essential for skin health.
Key nutrients: Beta-carotene, vitamin C, calcium, folate, potassium.
How to eat: Eat a 3oz (85g) serving of sweet potatoes 2–3 times a week. Boil or bake in their skins to maximize nutrients.

Kale
High in vitamin A for healthy skin-cell growth. Low vitamin A levels affect the cellular makeup of skin, causing a build-up of dead skin cells, affecting oil and sweat glands and causing dry, scaly skin.
Key nutrients: Vitamins A and C, calcium, iron.
How to eat: Eat kale or other cruciferous vegetables such as broccoli 2–3 times a week.

Green leafy vegetables
These provide magnesium, which can help to alleviate the scaly skin condition keratosis pilaris.
Key nutrients: Magnesium, folic acid, vitamin C, potassium.
How to eat: Eat a 3oz (85g) portion daily.

Eggs
Egg protein provides essential amino acids needed to generate skin-strengthening collagen and elastin.
Key nutrients: Vitamin A, carotenes, lutein, zinc.
How to eat: Eat at least 3 poached eggs a week.

Oily fish
Essential fatty acids, found in oily fish, are key to producing sebum. Without enough sebum, the process of "skin shedding" is disrupted and the substance keratin builds up in the skin.
Key nutrients: Omega-3, vitamin D.
How to eat: Eat oily fish 2–3 times a week.

Coconut oil
Ingesting coconut oil, which is antibacterial and anti-inflammatory, is an effective treatment for the bumpy skin complaint keratosis pilaris.
Key nutrients: Omega-3, vitamin D.
How to eat: Add 1 tsp of coconut oil to smoothies or use as a cooking oil.

10 ways to...
Plan a food diary

The best way to discover what may be triggering a health or beauty problem is to keep a record of what you eat each day for a set period of time. A simple and effective way to do this is to plan a food diary. Keeping track of your food intake, exercise, illness, and sleep can help you to spot patterns and links between eating particular foods and your levels of wellness and the condition of your skin, hair, and nails.

1 Make a template

Before you begin to document your eating habits, set up a simple template. You can do this by hand, on a computer, or use an app or template from the internet. The format is up to you—table, list, or note-style—but make sure that there's enough space to document all of your meals, snacks, and drinks, plus health and lifestyle information.

2 Be specific

Note down everything that you eat, including as much detail as possible. For example, if you've eaten vegetable curry, note down which vegetables you included, the type of oil you used, and any rice or grains that you served it with. The more ingredients you note down, the better chance you have of pinpointing food sensitivities and eliminating foods that may be exacerbating your skin.

6 Record any symptoms

Make a note of how you feel after eating your food. This could include positive symptoms, such as feeling full, sated, or energized. Watch out for fatigue, stomach discomfort (such as bloating), heartburn, itchy skin, nausea, or insomnia. If you notice that you're regularly having negative symptoms after eating a certain food, you may have a food sensitivity, meaning that your body struggles to digest this particular food.

7 Keep track of digestion

Record your bowel movements, including any changes. Daily, regular, normal bowel movements are important for your digestive health and for the health of your whole body. Constipation can cause excess toxins in your system, which can manifest themselves in skin problems. If you have had periods of either loose or constipated bowels, you may need to seek advice from a healthcare professional.

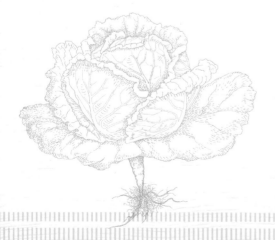

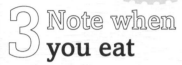

3 Note when **you eat**

Make a note of your eating times, including main meals and any snacks. This will help you to monitor if you are eating too frequently or not frequently enough. Aim to eat three meals per day, and one or two snacks to keep skin nourished throughout the day. Too long between meals can lead to a dip in energy and a craving for a sugary snack.

4 Record your **drinks**

Record everything that you drink, as well as foods. Make a note of how much water you're drinking each day, and check how it compares with the recommended fluid intakes (see p.42). If you're drinking alcohol, record what you drink and how much. This will help you track if you are drinking more than the recommended amount.

5 Keep track for **a month**

Keep your food diary for at least four to six weeks. This will allow for hormonal variations and imbalances throughout the month, which can impact on your skin. The longer you collect information, the better chance you have of spotting links between your habits and symptoms.

8 Record **your cycle**

Alongside your food and drink notes, keep track of your menstrual cycle. Your body, and particularly your skin, can be influenced by fluctuations in hormones throughout your monthly cycle. A poor diet—especially one high in sugars and starches—can throw off the balance between estrogen and testosterone, exacerbating skin problems. Being aware of your cycle can help you to avoid trigger foods at certain times.

9 Monitor **lifestyle**

Lifestyle factors such as sleep, stress, and exercise play a significant role in how much—and what types of—foods our bodies want to consume. Research shows that sleep deprivation triggers a chemical reaction that increases hunger levels and cravings for salty and sweet snacks. Sleep deprivation also has a negative impact on your skin, causing a decrease in blood flow to the skin surrounding your face.

10 Be **honest**

A food diary is your personal record, so try to be as honest as possible. Make a note of everything that you eat, including any extra snacks or less-than-healthy foods. Knowing when you're tempted to reach for a chocolate bar or a package of chips can help you spot connections between these and other eating habits—perhaps you're not including enough protein or slow-release carbohydrates in your main meals, so are craving a quick energy hit.

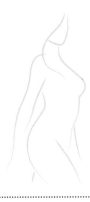

Eczema

Also referred to as dermatitis, this produces red, scaly, dry, flaky skin that itches and weeps. An imbalance of good and bad gut bacteria can be a factor, and dairy and gluten can exacerbate eczema. Foods with lubricating fatty acids help to replenish moisture, while sulfur- and chlorophyll-rich foods help reduce redness, and skin-calming vitamin B and anti-inflammatory antioxidant-rich foods soothe sore skin.

Superfood recipe suggestions...**Fruity quinoa breakfast** p169 **Superfood spread** p172 **Fall flavors soup** p178
Avocado on toast with mixed-herb pesto p180 **Spring veggie salad** p183 **Greek vegetable mezze** p198

Brightly colored vegetables and fruits

Yellow, orange, and red pigments *indicate antioxidants called carotenoids, which are fat-soluble and key to reducing inflammation in the skin. Fiber-rich root vegetables, such as squash and sweet potatoes, are also good prebiotics, helping to populate the gut with "good" bacteria.*
   Key nutrients: *Carotenoids, fiber, prebiotic.*
   How to eat: *Eat a 2oz (60g) portion of a bright fruit or vegetable each day.*

FIBER-RICH

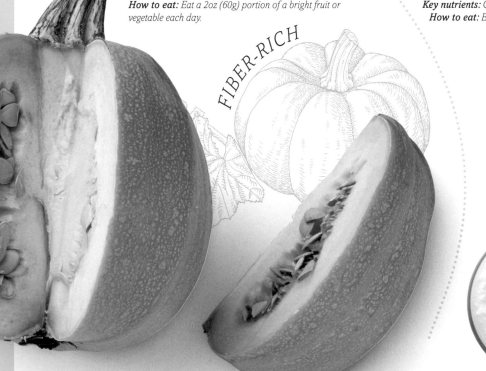

Fermented and cultured foods

Cultured dairy foods, *such as natural live yogurt and kefir yogurt (below, bottom) and kefir milk (below, top), help to heal the gut by destroying harmful bacteria that exacerbate eczema. Fermented foods such as miso, sauerkraut, and kimchi contain probiotics that introduce healthy gut bacteria.*
   Key nutrients: *Calcium, vitamin B2, potassium, protein.*
   How to eat: *Eat 5½oz (150g) yogurt daily.*

CALCIUM

potassium

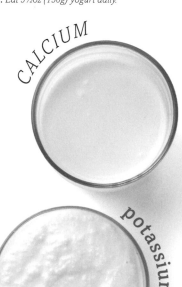

Turmeric

This contains curcumin, *a powerful anti-inflammatory antioxidant that helps to calm skin and relieve the itching that accompanies eczema.*
Key nutrients: *Curcumin, beta-carotene, iron, manganese, vitamin B6.*
How to eat: *Add ½ tsp to smoothies, juices, soups, and while cooking meals.*

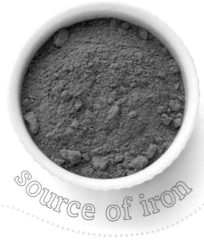

source of iron

QUICK FIX

Enjoy a **skin-soothing** smoothie. Add 2 tbsp flaxseeds to 3 tbsp kefir yogurt and ¾ cup water. Add 1 cup of summer berries and blend until smooth and creamy.

Flaxseeds

Flaxseeds *are a great source of omega-3, a powerful anti-inflammatory that helps soothe dry, itchy skin. Other seeds such as chia, pumpkin, and sunflower seeds are also high in omega-3.*
Key nutrients: *Omega-3, manganese, vitamin B1.*
How to eat: *Add 2–3 tsp daily to a drink or meal.*

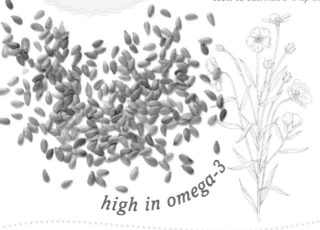

high in omega-3

Berries

All types of berries *are low in sugar, yet full of potent skin antioxidants, such as anthocyanins, quercetin, and resveratrol, that protect the skin and blood vessels. Think goldenberries, goji berries, mulberries, and summer berries.*
Key nutrients: *Quercetin, resveratrol, anthoyanins, vitamins C and E, omega-3, potassium, magnesium.*
How to eat: *Have a handful daily as a healthy snack.*

ANTIOXIDANTS

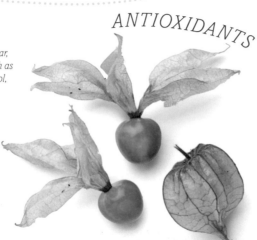

Nuts
Plentiful in omega-3 fatty acids, these balance sebum and promote skin repair, helping to prevent scarring from eczema.
Key nutrients: *Zinc, protein, vitamin E, fatty acids, fiber, magnesium.*
How to eat: *Snack on a handful each day.*

Leafy greens
These have a range of skin-protecting vitamins, omega-3, chlorophyll and sulfur, which nourish the blood and help reduce redness.
Key nutrients: *Fiber, vitamin C, beta-carotene, quercetin, omega-3.*
How to eat: *Eat as a side vegetable or in salads.*

Avocados
With omega-3, -6, and -9, and vitamins, these regenerate skin, reducing redness from eczema.
Key nutrients: *Lutein, beta-carotene, omega-3, -6, and -9, copper, vitamins B5, B6, C, E, and K, folate, potassium.*
How to eat: *1 medium avocado 2–4 times a week.*

Garlic
Raw, this contains a fiber, inulin, a prebiotic that promotes good bacteria. They also have skin-calming sulfur, and natural antibiotic properties that speed skin healing.
Key nutrients: *Sulfur, selenium, vitamin B6.*
How to eat: *Add 1–2 cloves daily to meals.*

Buckwheat
This contains the skin-strengthening antioxidant rutin and anti-inflammatory quercetin.
Key nutrients: *Rutin, quercetin, fiber, magnesium, protein.*
How to eat: *Eat up to ⅓ cup daily.*

Bee pollen
Nutritionally dense, this is a good source of quercetin, which calms inflamed skin.
Key nutrients: *B complex vitamins, amino acids, fatty acids, protein.*
How to eat: *Add 1 tsp daily to food. Do not give to young children, or take if you have an allergy to honey or bee stings, or if you're pregnant or breastfeeding.*

Spirulina
This has anti-inflammatory GLA (gamma linolenic acid), which soothes dry skin.
Key nutrients: *Protein, antioxidants, fatty acids, GLA, B vitamins, calcium.*
How to eat: *Start with ¼ teaspoon daily in a meal or drink and build up to 1 teaspoon.*

For supplements, see page 249.

Bruises

When tissues underlying the skin are injured, tiny blood vessels can rupture and blood leaks out, resulting in a blue-black mark. A tendency to bruise can indicate a nutritional deficiency, notably vitamin C, which aids collagen production. Smoking and anemia also increase bruising. Foods with vitamins C and E and bioflavonoids boost blood vessel health, and zinc- and vitamin K–rich foods strengthen blood vessels to aid clotting.

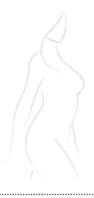

Superfood recipe suggestions...**Berry, seed, and nut granola** p166   **Spiced apple oatmeal** p170   **Huevos rancheros** p184
Greek vegetable mezze p198   **Japanese ocean soup** p201   **Pineapple smoothie** p239

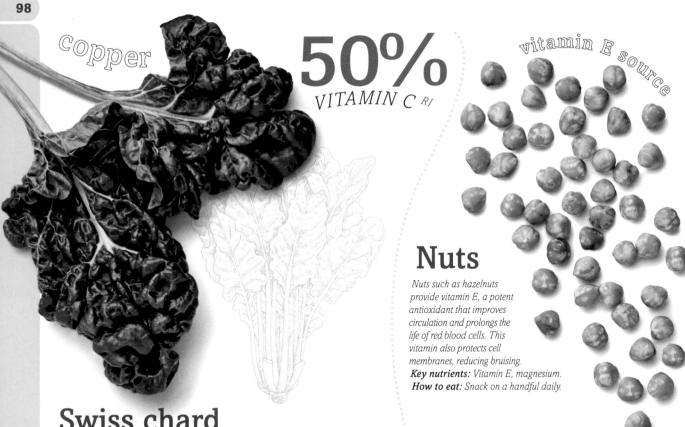

copper

50%
VITAMIN C RI

vitamin E source

Nuts

Nuts such as hazelnuts provide vitamin E, a potent antioxidant that improves circulation and prolongs the life of red blood cells. This vitamin also protects cell membranes, reducing bruising.
***Key nutrients:** Vitamin E, magnesium.*
***How to eat:** Snack on a handful daily.*

Swiss chard

This is a prime source of healing vitamin K. *A deficiency in vitamin K can result in slow blood clotting and cause skin to bruise more easily.*
Key nutrients: *Vitamins A, C, E, and K, magnesium, copper, manganese, potassium, iron.*
How to eat: *Eat a daily 3oz (85g) portion, steamed, or boiled for 3 minutes.*

40%
MAGNESIUM RI

Sunflower seeds

A good source of iron, these help prevent iron-deficiency anemia, which makes skin more prone to bruising.
Key nutrients: *Iron, manganese, selenium, phosphorus, magnesium, vitamins B3 and B6, folate.*
How to eat: *Sprinkle 1 tbsp on salads or over cereal or oatmeal daily.*

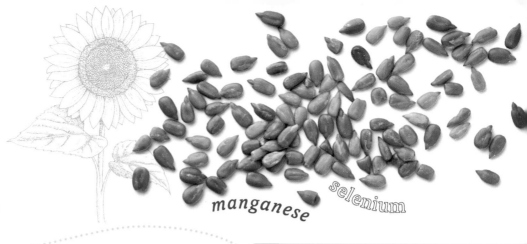

manganese   selenium

Sesame seeds

These supply the body with zinc, which helps to strengthen the skin and blood vessels to prevent bruising.
Key nutrients: *Zinc, calcium, magnesium, iron, phosphorus, vitamin B1, selenium.*
How to eat: *Sprinkle 1 tbsp over salads or breakfast each day.*

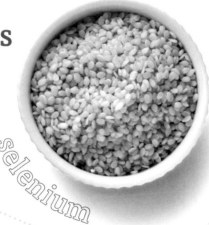

selenium

QUICK FIX

Add **healing alfalfa seeds** to a spinach salad, or mash up with an avocado for a nutrient-dense snack that has impressive **skin-healing** properties.

Alfalfa sprouts

Alfalfa supplies beneficial minerals and vitamin K, which promotes healing.
Key nutrients: *Vitamin K, B vitamins, magnesium.*
How to eat: *Add to meals up to 3 times a week. Rinse well before eating.*

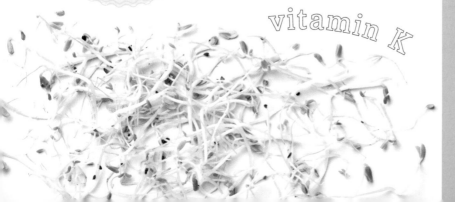

vitamin K

MORE SUPERFOODS

Spinach
This leafy green is high in folate, necessary for healthy skin renewal. A regular intake of folate encourages and promotes accelerated skin healing after bruising.
Key nutrients: *Folate, vitamins A, B2, B6, C, E, and K, magnesium, iron, calcium, potassium.*
How to eat: *Try to eat a generous handful of fresh spinach each day in a salad, or add ½ handful of spinach to meals.*

Pineapple
This tropical fruit is especially high in vitamin C, helping to heal wounds and repair damaged tissues. Vitamin C isn't stored in the body, so it needs to be eaten regularly to replenish sources.
Key nutrients: *Vitamin C, manganese.*
How to eat: *Aim to eat 2–3 slices of pineapple daily as a snack or add to a smoothie or salad.*

Eggs
These supply the body with vitamin B12, which supports platelet production to promote healthy blood clotting, giving the vitamin skin-healing properties that can help to hasten the healing of bruises.
Key nutrients: *Protein, vitamins B2, B12 and D, phosphorus.*
How to eat: *Eat 1 large egg each day, either poached or boiled.*

Avocados
Versatile avocado contains a range of skin-healing and blood vessel–boosting vitamins, including vitamins C and K.
Key nutrients: *Lutein, beta-carotene, omega-3, vitamins A, B6, C, E, and K, folate, copper, potassium.*
How to eat: *Eat 1 large egg each day, poached or boiled.*

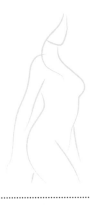

Sun damage

Excessive exposure to UVA and UVB rays can damage all the layers of the skin, increasing the risk of skin cancer. Prevention is key to sun damage. Antioxidant-rich foods help to protect skin from the sun's rays by neutralizing the damage to cells, while hydrating foods quench affected skin. Foods with omega-3 help to calm inflammation caused by sun damage, and healthy proteins are essential to help repair tissue damage.

Superfood recipe suggestions...**Overnight oats with superberry compote** p168 **Winter veggie slaw** p185
Greek vegetable mezze p198 **Roasted broccoli and cauliflower with couscous** p206 **Potato mash with veggie mix** p219

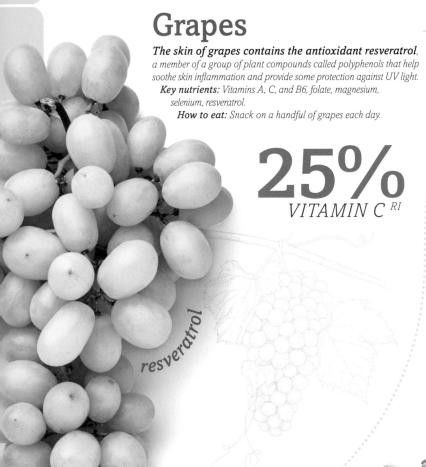

Grapes

The skin of grapes contains the antioxidant resveratrol, *a member of a group of plant compounds called polyphenols that help soothe skin inflammation and provide some protection against UV light.*
Key nutrients: *Vitamins A, C, and B6, folate, magnesium, selenium, resveratrol.*
How to eat: *Snack on a handful of grapes each day.*

resveratrol

25%
VITAMIN C ^RI

QUICK FIX

There are plenty of ways to enjoy **skin-soothing** oats. Vary oatmeal by adding favorite fruits, nuts, or seeds, add oats to smoothies, or make delicious homemade oat-milk.

Oats

Rolled oats contain a natural plant chemical *called tocotrienol, a member of the vitamin E family, that helps to soothe skin. Tocotrienols neutralize free radical damage to the body and are thought to help offer the skin some protection against harmful UV rays.*
Key nutrients: *Vitamins B1 and E, magnesium, zinc, protein.*
How to eat: *Eat oats for breakfast 2–3 times a week.*

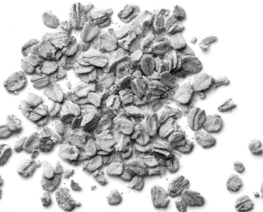

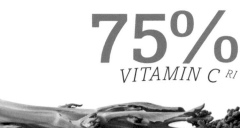

75%
VITAMIN C RI

source of folate

Pomegranate

This colorful fruit *contains powerful antioxidant polyphenols, including catechins and anthocyanins, which strengthen the skin's upper layers, increasing its protection.*
Key nutrients: *Vitamins B6 and C, magnesium, zinc, polyphenols.*
How to eat: *Sprinkle a handful of the seeds on a salad or add to your breakfast in the morning.*

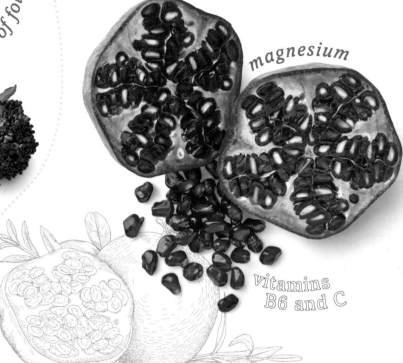

magnesium

vitamins B6 and C

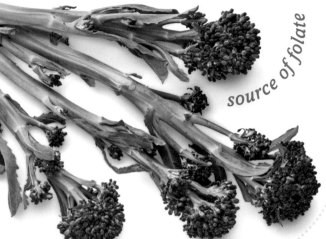

Broccoli

Rich in the antioxidant sulforaphane, *this helps to protect skin by inhibiting the growth of unhealthy cells caused by UV damage. Other cruciferous vegetables include kale, cauliflower, and Brussels sprouts.*
Key nutrients: *Vitamins A, B1, B5, B6, C, and E, chromium, folate, manganese, phosphorus, choline, potassium.*
How to eat: *Eat cruciferous vegetables at least 2–3 times a week. Steam broccoli or eat raw.*

MORE SUPERFOODS

Tomatoes
Bright red tomatoes contain lycopene, a carotenoid that helps protect the skin against sunburn.
Key nutrients: *Vitamins A, B3, B6, C, and K, biotin, lycopene, potassium, manganese, folate.*
How to eat: *Eat 7 cherry tomatoes or 1 medium tomato a day.*

Pumpkin seeds
These have protein and zinc, an antioxidant and anti-inflammatory that protects against UV rays.
Key nutrients: *Zinc, iron, phosphorus, magnesium, manganese, copper.*
How to eat: *Sprinkle 1 tbsp of pumpkin seeds daily on cereal or add to salads.*

Carrots
A good source of antioxidant carotenoids, which reduce the negative effects of UV. The pigment carotenes is used by plants as a sunscreen and can activate melanin.
Key nutrients: *Carotenoids, B vitamins, vitamins C and E, potassium.*
How to eat: *Have a daily 3oz (85g) serving.*

Avocado
These are packed with healthy monounsaturated fats, which help hydrate skin.
Key nutrients: *Potassium, omega-9, vitamin E, B vitamins, folic acid.*
How to eat: *Eat 1 a day for vibrant skin.*

Brussels sprouts
These are a great source of vitamins A and C, which promote collagen and folate, all of which helps to protect the skin against UV rays.
Key nutrients: *Vitamins A, B1, B6, and C, folate, omega-3.*
How to eat: *In season, make Brussel sprouts a regular vegetable during the week.*

Spirulina
This has a skin-protecting carotenoid astaxanthin.
Key nutrients: *Protein, antioxidants, essential fatty acids, B vitamins, calcium.*
How to eat: *Start with ¼ tsp daily in a meal or drink and build up to 1 tsp.*

Meal planner Skin smoothing

Our skin is made up of trillions of cells, which require the right nutrients to promote healthy, smooth, contoured skin. This skin-smoothing meal planner, which uses recipes in the book with additional meal ideas, has been designed to include the nutrients needed to keep skin supple and firm, and to renew cells speedily, protecting skin from UV damage.

Your skin-smoothing week This nutritionally balanced meal plan will set you off on your skin-smoothing diet. For best results, continue for four weeks, using the alternatives, opposite, for variety. Start each day with a hot water and lemon drink to aid digestion.

Monday

Breakfast
Green smoothie (p.244)

Snacks
Handful each of sunflower seeds and grapes

Lunch
Avocado on toast with mixed-herb pesto (p.180) and vitamin C boost (p.245)

Dinner
Salmon with samphire (p.215)

Tuesday

Breakfast
Cacao and chia chocolate "pudding" (p.174)

Snacks
Sweet garden pea dip (p.190) with carrot sticks

Lunch
Cannellini beans, bok choy, and arugula salad with cherry tomatoes and olives

Dinner
Potato and veggie bake (p.211)

Wednesday

Breakfast
Fruity quinoa breakfast (p.169)

Snacks
Pineapple smoothie (p.239)

Lunch
Zucchini noodles with basil pesto (p.186) and cherry tomatoes

Dinner
Summer salad with pomegranate and pistachio (p.202)

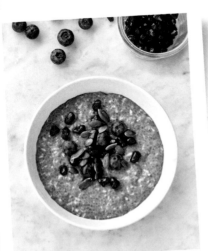

Cacao and chia chocolate "pudding" (p.174)

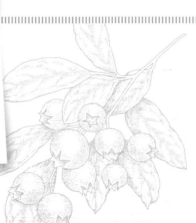

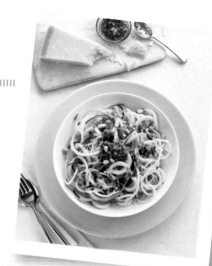

Zucchini noodles with basil pesto (p.186)

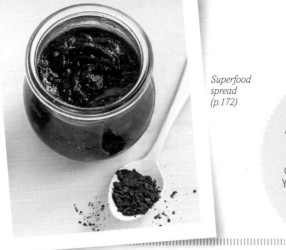

Superfood spread (p.172)

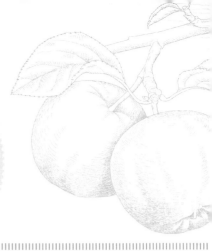

POLYPHENOLS

Antioxidant polyphenols help to **strengthen the skin's upper layers**, which can help protect against UV damage from the sun. You can find polyphenols such as catechins and anthocyanins in pomegranates and green tea.

Thursday

Breakfast

Berry nice skin! (p.238)

Snacks

Hummus and oat cakes with a sprinkle of alfalfa sprouts

Lunch

Crunchy apple, radish, and carrot salad

Dinner

Ratatouille (p.207) with quinoa

Friday

Breakfast

Rye bread with almond butter and orange segments

Snacks

Superfood spread (p.172) on a slice of toasted rye bread and handful of grapes

Lunch

Huevos rancheros (p.184)

Dinner

Sweet potato and mackerel mash (p.219, variation) with broccoli

Saturday

Breakfast

Mixed berry and kiwi fruit salad with natural live yogurt and ground flaxseeds

Snacks

Handful of Hot nuts! (p.194) and Cacao comfort (p.237)

Lunch

Spinach salad with avocado

Dinner

Lamb tagine (p.208) with broccoli

Sunday

Breakfast

Poached egg on rye bread with orange segments

Snacks

Two slices of pineapple with coconut yogurt

Lunch

Potato mash with veggie mix (p.219)

Dinner

Black lentil and coconut curry (p.204)

Sweet treat

Cashew and goji berry cheesecake (p.230)

Alternatives

To help you on your way, draw on these additional recipe suggestions to vary your meals over the course of four weeks.

Breakfast

Oatmeal with mixed seeds and dates

Hemp seed butter (p.172) on rye bread toast

Snacks

Poached egg on rye bread toast

Lunch

Two-egg omelet with a rainbow salad

Chile guacamole (p.190) with rye bread

Dinner

Lemon and herb-roasted chicken (p.210)

Polenta and grilled vegetables (p.216)

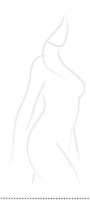

Scars

Following an injury, burn, acne, or surgery, you are likely to notice a scar where collagen builds up over damaged tissue. Scars fade over time, and the right foods can speed this process. Healthy proteins provide essential amino acids to rebuild tissues, while foods with zinc reduce inflammation, and vitamin E helps to fade out stubborn acne scars. A hydrating, antioxidant-rich diet keeps skin well-nourished, helping accelerate healing.

Superfood recipe suggestions...**Fruity quinoa breakfast** p169   **Fall flavors soup** p178   **Fava bean soup** p182
Huevos rancheros p184   **Hot nuts!** p194   **Japanese ocean soup** p201

Peas

Sweet garden peas are high in vitamin A, which promotes the production of connective tissue such as collagen and nourishes skin cells, helping skin to heal.
Key nutrients: Vitamins A, B1, folate, fiber, iron.
How to eat: Eat up to 3oz (85g) daily, as a side vegetable or added to salads.

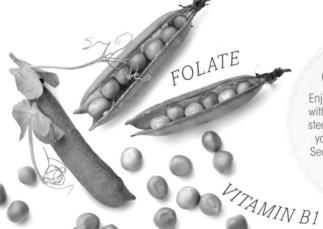

FOLATE

VITAMIN B1

QUICK FIX

Enjoy a **skin-nourishing** salad with sweet garden peas, lightly steamed broccoli, and a mix of your favorite summer herbs. Season and drizzle with some extra-virgin olive oil.

potassium

Broccoli

Broccoli and other cruciferous vegetables contain vitamin C, essential for the healing process because it promotes the production of collagen protein, which heals cuts by forming a grid of tissue that allows new skin to grow.
Key nutrients: Vitamins A, B1, B5, B6, C, and E, chromium, folate, manganese, phosphorus, choline, potassium.
How to eat: Eat cruciferous vegetables 2–3 times a week. Ideally steam broccoli for 3–4 minutes.

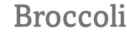

75% VITAMIN C ᴿᴵ

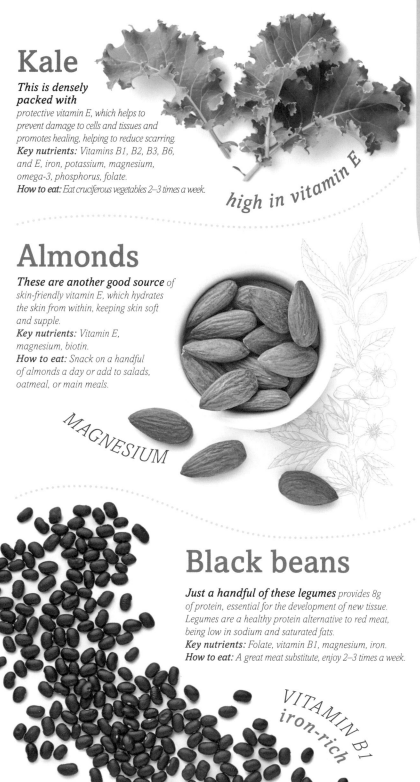

Kale

This is densely packed with protective vitamin E, which helps to prevent damage to cells and tissues and promotes healing, helping to reduce scarring.
Key nutrients: Vitamins B1, B2, B3, B6, and E, iron, potassium, magnesium, omega-3, phosphorus, folate.
How to eat: Eat cruciferous vegetables 2–3 times a week.

high in vitamin E

Almonds

These are another good source of skin-friendly vitamin E, which hydrates the skin from within, keeping skin soft and supple.
Key nutrients: Vitamin E, magnesium, biotin.
How to eat: Snack on a handful of almonds a day or add to salads, oatmeal, or main meals.

MAGNESIUM

Black beans

Just a handful of these legumes provides 8g of protein, essential for the development of new tissue. Legumes are a healthy protein alternative to red meat, being low in sodium and saturated fats.
Key nutrients: Folate, vitamin B1, magnesium, iron.
How to eat: A great meat substitute, enjoy 2–3 times a week.

VITAMIN B1 iron-rich

Oily fish
The oils from oily fish such as salmon, mackerel, sardines, and trout contain a large amount of omega-3 fatty acids, which interact with omega-6 fatty acids to reduce the body's inflammatory response. Oily fish have a good ratio of omega-3 and omega-6 fats, which helps to optimize their skin-nurturing benefits.
Key nutrients: Omega-3 and -6, vitamin D.
How to eat: Aim to eat a 5½oz (150g) portion of oily fish 2–3 times a week.

Seeds
Like oily fish, seeds such as chia and flaxseeds have a plentiful supply of omega-3 fatty acids. Just 1 tsp of freshly ground flaxseeds yields nearly 1.8g of omega-3 fatty acids.
Key nutrients: Omega-3, vitamin B1, magnesium, phosphorus, selenium.
How to eat: Try snacking on 1 tbsp of flaxseeds each day, or sprinkle over oatmeal or salads.

Sweet potato
Eating vitamin A–rich foods such as sweet potatoes activates genes that help specialized skin cells known as keratinocytes, which move toward the skin's surface to promote wound healing. This in turn accelerates the healing process of scars.
Key nutrients: Vitamins A and C, calcium, folate, potassium.
How to eat: Have a 3oz (85g) serving of sweet potatoes 2–3 times a week. Steam, bake, or boil sweet potatoes, ideally with their skin on to maximize nutrients.

Spinach
This provides vitamin C, essential for the healthy production of collagen, which helps to build new skin tissue to heal skin.
Key nutrients: Vitamins A and C, B vitamins, potassium, iron.
How to eat: Enjoy spinach raw in salads, add to smoothies, and add wilted spinach to meals.

Oranges
Citrus fruits such as oranges and grapefruit provide collagen-building vitamin C to promote skin healing.
Key nutrients: Vitamins B1 and C, folate, potassium.
How to eat: Eat an orange after a meal, add to juices and smoothies, and flavor meals with the juice.

For supplements, see page 249.

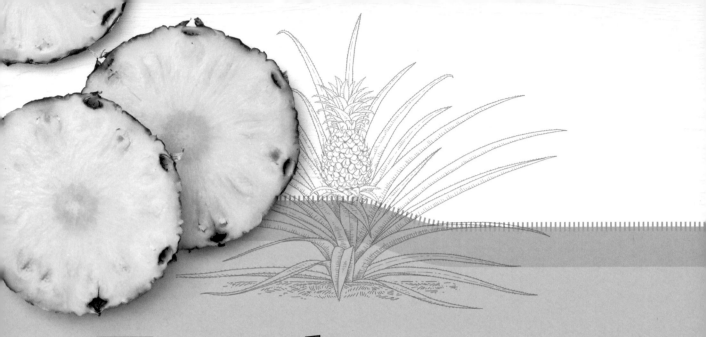

Foods
for the hair

A lustrous head of hair is a great indicator of a healthy diet and lifestyle. Discover the very best nutrients for strengthening and conditioning hair, and follow a nutritionally balanced meal plan designed to optimize hair health, improving its texture and leaving you with glossy, voluminous locks.

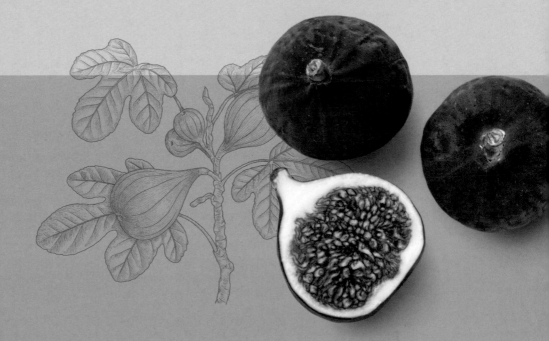

Eat for beauty: hair

Lustrous hair that looks and feels wonderful requires a whole spectrum of healthy beauty nutrients to keep it **well conditioned**, healthy, and **strong**. Discover the key nutrients you need to feed and nourish your hair, ensuring that it looks wonderful and is in great condition.

Nutrients for your hair

Before you explore the foods for specific hair concerns in this chapter, find out why certain key nutrients are essential for healthy, beautiful-looking hair.

Iron As with our skin, healthy hair is dependent on a diet that is rich in a range of beneficial nutrients, and deficiencies in our diet can impact the condition of our hair and scalp. The roots of our hair are fed by an extensive network of tiny blood vessels in the scalp, which carry oxygen and nutrients to the scalp cells. If our diets are lacking in iron, carried around the body in red blood cells, the scalp may not receive adequate nutrients and oxygen and hair can appear dull and become brittle. It's vital therefore to include good sources of iron in your daily diet from leafy greens, nuts, seeds, fish, oats, whole grains, and legumes.

Antioxidants These protective plant compounds help to strengthen the tiny capillaries near the surface of our skin. This in turn promotes healthy circulation to the scalp, nourishing the hair shaft and keeping hair looking glossy and feeling strong. Antioxidants are found most abundantly in brightly colored fresh fruit and vegetables, such as berries and intensely pigmented beets, peppers, squash, and tomatoes.

Vitamins B and C B vitamins have an important role to play in hair because they help to promote strong hair growth, while antioxidant vitamin C is essential for forming collagen, the structural protein that holds the hair together. Hair follicles, blood vessels, and the scalp all need collagen to stay healthy, and even a moderate lack of vitamin C can have a detrimental effect on our hair, leaving it dry,

brittle, and lackluster. Good sources of B vitamins include almonds and eggs, while vitamin C is found in a range of fruit and vegetables, such as citrus fruits, kiwi, berries, broccoli, kale, and sweet potatoes.

Essential fatty acids These important fats help to balance sebum production in the body, which in turn keeps the scalp healthy and hair looking glossy and well conditioned. As our bodies can't make omega-3 and omega-6, we need to eat foods that are plentiful in these essential fats, such as chia, flaxseeds, hemp, pumpkin, and sunflower seeds, avocado, nuts, microalgae such as seaweed, and oily fish. The right balance of omega-3 and omega-6 is also important. While both support a healthy cell structure, too much omega-6 from unhealthier sources such as meat and cereal grains, can have an

The health of your hair reflects the foods you eat. A diet rich in essential beauty nutrients will ensure beautiful, glossy, well-conditioned hair.

inflammatory effect, which can increase sebum production and leave hair feeling greasy.

High-quality protein Protein is the building block of hair, and is essential for healthy growth and

29%

of our daily zinc needs is met by ½ cup pumpkin seeds.

strength. Insufficient protein can slow hair growth and lead to brittle hair strands. Sources of healthy proteins include hemp seeds, legumes, miso, fish, and lean meat.

Sulfur This important beauty mineral helps to build strong, healthy hair. Sulfur is essential for holding keratin, the main hair protein, in shape, strengthening hair and aiding the absorption of other important proteins. You can up your intake of sulfur by eating vegetables from the brassica family, such as cauliflower, cabbage, broccoli, and Brussels sprouts, and by including onions and garlic regularly in your diet.

Zinc This key mineral helps to balance the production of sebum from the sebaceous glands at the base of the hair follicle, which in turn encourages hair growth, promotes a healthy, flake-free scalp, and ensures hair is well conditioned. For a good supply of zinc eat plenty of unrefined grains, nuts such as cashews, pumpkin and sesame seeds, lentils, and, more occasionally, lamb.

Silica A vital mineral for hair health, this is essential for the production of the protein collagen. We have silica in abundance when we're young, but the mineral reduces with age, so we need to ensure we get reliable sources from our food. Silica helps the body absorb other vital minerals and vitamins, taking nutrients to the peripheries of the body and ensuring the hair follicles are supplied with all the nourishment needed for hair growth. This in turn prevents hair thinning and restores vitality to hair. Top sources of silica include whole-grain cereals, apples, cherries, almonds, oranges, fish, oats, and seeds.

Hydration Being well hydrated is essential for a moisturized scalp and frizz-free hair. As well as drinking up to 2 liters daily, eat hydrating foods and try mineral-rich vegetable juices.

What affects our hair?

Lifestyle factors, hormonal swings, periods of stress and illness, and harsh hair products can all affect the health of your hair and scalp. Finding the root cause of a hair problem will help you make some dietary adjustments that can restore luster to hair.

Diet and lifestyle A lack of nutrients and poor lifestyle choices tend to show in our hair. Excessive amounts of sugar can hamper the absorption of healthy proteins needed for hair growth. Eliminate sugar, or replace white, low-mineral sugars with mineral-rich alternatives such as maple syrup (in moderation). Avoid, too, hydrogenated fats in fast and processed foods, which clog pores on the scalp, making the scalp greasy and leading to hair loss. Replace these fats with essential fatty acids and olive oil. Too much red meat, dairy, and salt can also mean hair isn't getting the best nutrients. Swap processed table salt for Himalayan pink salt, and reduce your meat and dairy intake. Alcohol lowers the body's zinc levels, a vital mineral for hair growth, and dehydrates hair, making it brittle, while carbonated diet drinks contain aspartame, which affects the absorption of nutrients and has been linked to hair loss. Stimulants, such as excess caffeine, smoking, and alcohol, also impact hair health, drying hair and leaving it looking dull.

Stress, illness, and hormones Anxiety and stress contribute to graying hair and hair loss. Stress depletes the body of key nutrients as it uses them to create the stress hormones adrenaline and cortisol. Eat foods with calming nutrients such as B vitamins, vitamin C, zinc,

Eat for your age

As we grow older, hair inevitably changes. Life events, such as pregnancy and illness, can change hair texture and volume, and from our 40s onward, hair starts to thin and to lose its natural color. Eating a nourishing and balanced diet will support your hair though each stage of life, helping hair to remain healthy and vital. A multivitamin and mineral supplement supports hair health in each decade.

In your 20s

In our 20s, collagen production is high, which keeps hair strong and gives it structure, and hair can appear thick, glossy, and healthy. Sometimes, though, we may still be battling oily hair from adolescence in this decade, which can be a problem for finer hair especially. A hectic lifestyle or yo-yo dieting can mean key nutrients for healthy hair are lacking. **Eat:** A diet high in antioxidant-rich, brightly colored fruit and vegetables to provide essential nutrients. Healthy proteins support healthy collagen production, so include protein from eggs, fish, legumes, nuts and seeds, and lean meats.

In your 30s

In this decade, hormones may change subtly, which can have an effect on hair. Growth hormone starts to fall in your 30s, which can make hair weaker. If pregnant, higher estrogen levels keep hair in an extended growth phase so it looks thick and glossy, but when estrogen returns to normal after childbirth there may be a period of greater hair loss as the hair that wasn't shed in pregnancy is lost. **Eat:** Continue to eat a diet with a good range of antioxidants from fresh fruit and vegetables and healthy proteins from fish, lean meats, legumes, and nuts and seeds to support hair regrowth.

110%

of the vitamin C we need each day is supplied by a 3½oz (100g) serving of kale.

magnesium, and chromium. Illness can also cause hair loss, with hair follicles going into a resting phase and growth temporarily ceasing, and chemotherapy medications can cause hair to fall out. Healthy

proteins and antioxidant-rich foods support regrowth. Hormonal imbalances are one of the biggest causes of hair loss and thinning. Foods derived from soy can help to rebalance hormones.

Hair products and treatments
Harsh hair products and daily washing can strip the scalp of precious natural oils, which in turn causes the scalp to produce more sebum to compensate. Synthetic silicones in hair products can clog pores, overcoloring can alter the texture of hair, making it brittle, and frequent blow-drying or use of heated curling irons dehydrates hair and causes split ends. Juices and smoothies are a good way to get a lot of hair-loving nutrients in one dose, and raw foods contain live enzymes and beneficial nutrients that help to nourish hair.

In your 40s

Hair is often thinner and has a different texture in our 40s. We lose approximately 100 hairs every day, and as regrowth slows, this can impact our hair volume. Collagen production decreases, which further weakens hair, and hair may start to lose color and turn increasingly gray. Gray hair tends to have a coarser texture and can look dull and frizzy.
Eat: Copper-rich foods, such as almonds, pineapples, and blackberries, can help to maintain natural color. Eat healthy proteins, and vitamin C–rich foods such as kiwi, broccoli, and kale.

In your 50s

As oil glands shrink over time, hair becomes drier and more brittle, and as pigment is reduced, the color of hair becomes progressively more gray. For some, thyroid problems can lead to changes in hair texture and growth, thinning hair and slowing regrowth. Collagen continues to decline now, which can weaken the hair shaft and make hair more brittle.
Eat: Foods such as flaxseeds and oily fish provide both healthy omega-3 fats and protein, to moisturize and strengthen hair. Include bright fruit and vegetables for vitamins, and almonds eggs for vitamin B.

60s plus

Hair continues to thin—each strand becomes smaller in diameter—and become finer as we reach our 60s. The rate of regrowth slows and hair follicles start to rest, which means there can be less scalp coverage. Hair increasingly loses elasticity, which can make it harder to manage and style. Gray hair may be extensive now and can gradually become whiter.
Eat: Foods with the B vitamin biotin help to strengthen hair and encourage growth; include eggs, salmon, and nuts. Eat iron-rich foods such as lentils, and plenty of fresh fruits and vegetables.

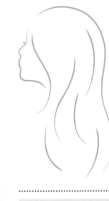

Hair loss and thinning

Baldness or hair loss is called alopecia and can be a distressing condition. Alopecia areata, when the hair falls out in patches, is usually temporary. Hair loss can be down to hormonal changes, a medical condition, stress, and nutritional deficiencies. Eat foods with antioxidant flavonoids to strengthen hair follicles, iron-rich foods to boost red blood cells, and protein- and silica-rich foods to promote hair growth and healthy hair.

Superfood recipe suggestions...Berry, seed, and nut granola p166   Avocado on toast with mixed-herb pesto p180
Huevos rancheros p184   Summer asparagus salad p189   Japanese ocean soup p201   Pineapple smoothie p239

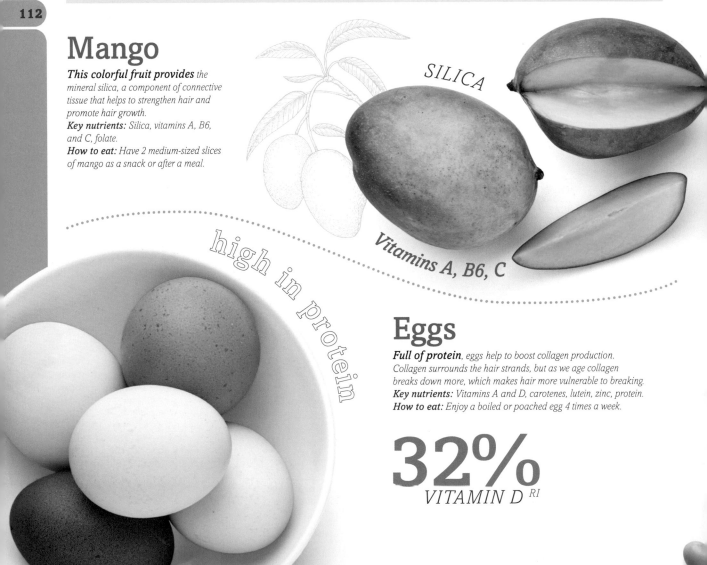

Mango

This colorful fruit provides *the mineral silica, a component of connective tissue that helps to strengthen hair and promote hair growth.*
Key nutrients: *Silica, vitamins A, B6, and C, folate.*
How to eat: *Have 2 medium-sized slices of mango as a snack or after a meal.*

SILICA

Vitamins A, B6, C

high in protein

Eggs

Full of protein, *eggs help to boost collagen production. Collagen surrounds the hair strands, but as we age collagen breaks down more, which makes hair more vulnerable to breaking.*
Key nutrients: *Vitamins A and D, carotenes, lutein, zinc, protein.*
How to eat: *Enjoy a boiled or poached egg 4 times a week.*

32%
VITAMIN D RI

Figs

Figs are a great source of iron, essential for healthy hair growth and shiny locks. Other good sources include dried fruit and berries.
Key nutrients: Iron, potassium, magnesium, vitamins A and E.
How to eat: Eat 2 figs a day.

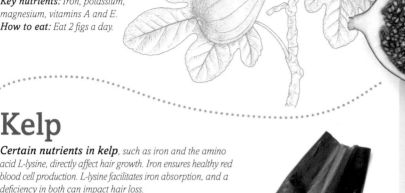

POTASSIUM

Kelp

Certain nutrients in kelp, such as iron and the amino acid L-lysine, directly affect hair growth. Iron ensures healthy red blood cell production. L-lysine facilitates iron absorption, and a deficiency in both can impact hair loss.
Key nutrients: Iron, L-lysine, vitamins B2 and B5, zinc, folate, magnesium.
How to eat: Have 10g daily to reach your nutrient quota or try a kelp supplement.

30%
MAGNESIUM ^{RI}

provides iron

Soybeans

Foods derived from soy, such as soybeans and tempeh, are thought to inhibit the formation of a hormone called dihydrotestosterone, an imbalance of which is thought to contribute to hair loss.
Key nutrients: Iron, omega-3, vitamin B2, magnesium.
How to eat: Aim for at least one 2½oz (75g) portion a week.

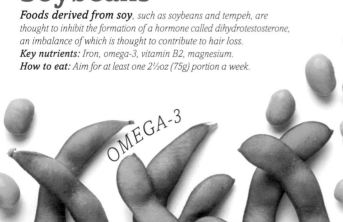

OMEGA-3

MORE SUPERFOODS

Flaxseeds
High in omega-3, these help nourish hair and prevent it from drying out and becoming weak and easily broken .
Key nutrients: Omega-3, vitamin B1, magnesium, phosphorus, selenium.
How to eat: Eat up to 1 tbsp a day, either as a snack or sprinkled over meals.

Pumpkin seeds
These protein-rich seeds provide zinc, which supports cellular reproduction and enhances immunity, in turn promoting hair growth.
Key nutrients: Zinc, iron, phosphorus, magnesium, manganese, copper.
How to eat: Eat up to 1 tbsp a day. Combine with flaxseeds for a nutritious mix.

Berries
Naturally high in collagen-boosting vitamin C, berries aid iron absorption. Vitamin C boosts scalp circulation, and its antioxidant action protects follicles from free-radical damage.
Key nutrients: Vitamin C, potassium.
How to eat: Have a handful each day.

Avocado
Creamy avocados supply vitamin E, which increases oxygen uptake, improving circulation to the scalp to promote healthy hair growth.
Key nutrients: Vitamin E, potassium, omega-9, B-vitamins, folic acid.
How to eat: Eat 1 medium avocado 2–4 times a week.

Leafy greens
Greens, such as Swiss chard, watercress, spinach, and cabbage, promote keratin, a hair protein that strengthens the follicles.
Key nutrients: Vitamins A, C, and K, B vitamins, potassium, folate.
How to eat: Eat a 3½oz (100g) portion of leafy greens daily in a salad or a meal.

For supplements, see page 249.

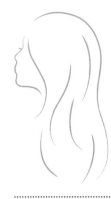

Fragile hair

Hair can become dry, frizzy, and break easily. Strong hair depends on the strength of the hair shaft and a healthy scalp and follicles. Overuse of hair products, sun, illness, and poor diet can all weaken hair. Eating the right foods can restore lustrous hair: the B vitamin biotin boosts scalp health, healthy proteins provide keratin to strengthen hair strands, and beta-carotene converts to cell-building vitamin A in the body.

Superfood recipe suggestions...**Spiced apple oatmeal** p170 **Beet and chickpea soup** p192 **Japanese ocean soup** p201 **Salmon with samphire** p215 **Pineapple smoothie** p239

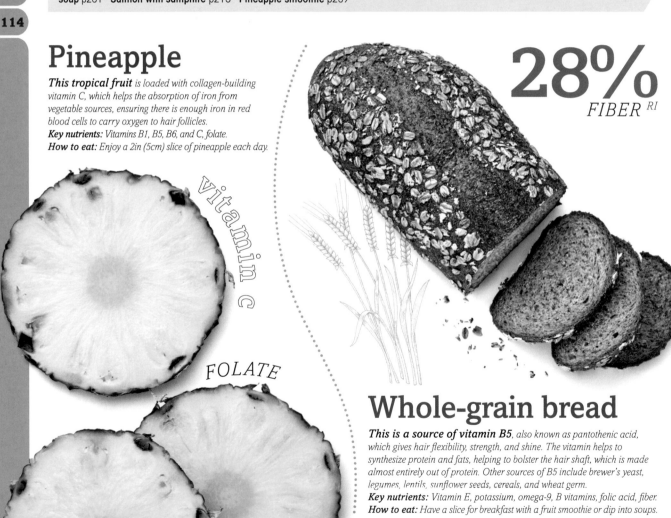

Pineapple

This tropical fruit is loaded with collagen-building vitamin C, which helps the absorption of iron from vegetable sources, ensuring there is enough iron in red blood cells to carry oxygen to hair follicles.
Key nutrients: Vitamins B1, B5, B6, and C, folate.
How to eat: Enjoy a 2in (5cm) slice of pineapple each day.

vitamin c

FOLATE

28%
FIBER RI

Whole-grain bread

This is a source of vitamin B5, also known as pantothenic acid, which gives hair flexibility, strength, and shine. The vitamin helps to synthesize protein and fats, helping to bolster the hair shaft, which is made almost entirely out of protein. Other sources of B5 include brewer's yeast, legumes, lentils, sunflower seeds, cereals, and wheat germ.
Key nutrients: Vitamin E, potassium, omega-9, B vitamins, folic acid, fiber.
How to eat: Have a slice for breakfast with a fruit smoothie or dip into soups.

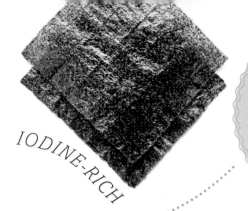

Seaweed

Seaweeds such as dulse, *bladder wrack, kelp, and nori are high in iodine. A deficiency in iodine can contribute to the condition hypothyroidism, associated with dry, brittle hair.*
Key nutrients: *Iodine, iron, zinc, folate, magnesium, vitamins B2 and B5.*
How to eat: *Add 1 tbsp dried seaweed daily to food, or soak seaweed sheets to use in meals.*

IODINE-RICH

QUICK FIX

Try this **hair-boosting** sushi. Add a splash of tamari to cooked sushi rice, then layer on nori sheets with some smoked salmon. Roll the sheets and cut into bite-sized sushi treats.

Almonds

These sweet nuts contain *vitamin E, an antioxidant that helps to stabilize and strengthen cell membranes in hair follicles to promote healthy hair.*
Key nutrients: *Vitamin E, magnesium, biotin.*
How to eat: *Snack on a handful of almonds daily.*

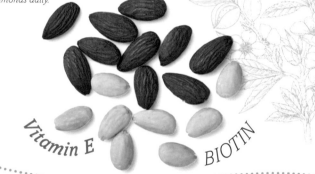

Vitamin E   *BIOTIN*

Wild salmon

This fish supplies vitamin B12, *which supports the formation of red blood cells. At the base of each hair follicle, blood vessels connect to each strand. Red blood cells carry oxygen to the living portion of the hair strands. Without adequate oxygen, hair can't sustain healthy growth.*
Key nutrients: *Vitamin B12 and D, selenium, omega-3.*
How to eat: *Aim to eat 2–3 portions of oily fish a week.*

74%
SELENIUM RI

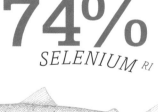

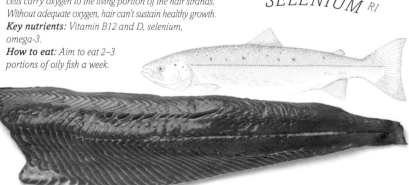

MORE SUPERFOODS

Chickpeas

These provide vitamin B6. This vitamin is involved in the creation of oxygen-carrying red blood cells. A lack of B6 can compromise the hair cells, resulting in hair being shed, slow growth, or weak hair that is prone to breaking.
Key nutrients: *Vitamin B6, folate, iron, zinc.*
How to eat: *Aim for a ½-cup portion of chickpeas 4 times a week.*

Broccoli

This cruciferous vegetable is high in the B vitamin folate, essential for cell regeneration and repair. A folate deficiency can cause the hair to become fragile and brittle.
Key nutrients: *Vitamins A, B1, B5, B6, C, and E, chromium, folate, choline, manganese, phosphorus, potassium.*
How to eat: *Include cruciferous vegetables in your weekly menu at least 2–3 times.*

Eggs

Protein-rich eggs help to build and strengthen cells. A lack of protein in the diet, or low-quality protein, can produce weak and brittle hair.
Key nutrients: *Vitamin A, carotenes, protein, lutein, zinc.*
How to eat: *Have a poached egg for breakfast, or try a boiled egg as a snack at least 3 times a week.*

Edamame

These soft soybeans are a good source of iron, necessary for the oxygenation of body tissues, which in turn helps to strengthen the hair shaft. Eat vitamin C–rich foods alongside vegetable sources of iron, as this improves the body's ability to absorb iron from plant sources.
Key nutrients: *Iron, folate, magnesium.*
How to eat: *Eat a 2½oz (75g) portion at least 2 times a week, as a healthy snack or added to salads.*

10 ways to...
Eat seasonally

Eating with the seasons is a habit most of us have forgotten. We are so used to being able to buy any food at any time of year that it can be easy to lose touch with seasonality. However, foods that have been grown in another country are often processed to make them last longer and contain lower nutrient levels than local fare. Eat fresh, local, seasonal produce in order to maximize nutrients and beauty benefits.

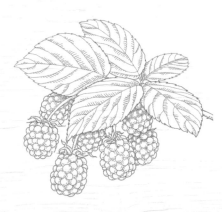

1 Choose carefully

When buying food in a grocery store or market, pick fruit that smells ripe, juicy, and sweet, with a firm, plump texture. Vegetables should be firm and crisp—this shows that they've ripened naturally in the sun, making them perfect to eat and full of skin-boosting antioxidants.

2 Grow your own

Get a farm share. Food straight from the earth is unbeatable for freshness and taste, and encourages you to make the most of seasonal bounty and its higher nutritional value. If you find yourself overwhelmed with too much of one food, freeze or preserve it just after harvesting to conserve nutrients.

6 Grow at home

If a farm share is too ambitious or time-consuming for you, create a smaller vegetable plot in your garden or, if you don't have much outdoor space, grow vegetables in containers. A hanging basket of strawberries or tomatoes, a pot filled with green beans, or a sack of potatoes takes up very little space or time, and can provide you with nutrient-rich, seasonal foods for your table.

7 Try foraging

A fun way to get more seasonal foods into your diet is to go foraging in your local area. Foraging can make you more aware of which foods are naturally ready when—try hunting for blackberries in early fall or elderberries in summer. Always be certain that what you are picking is safe to eat, that it is growing away from railroad lines and roads, and that It is on public property.

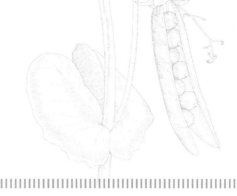

DID YOU KNOW?

A recent study found that fewer than one in ten adults knows when foods are in season. Get to know which fruits and vegetables are ripe at which times of year to maximize their beauty benefits.

3 Pick in Spring

In springtime, enjoy sweet, new vegetables, herbs, leaves, and roots, such as:

• asparagus • cauliflower • new potatoes • purple-sprouting broccoli • broccoli • radishes • Savoy cabbage • sorrel • spinach • spring greens • kale • fava beans • carrots • scallions • watercress • rhubarb • nettles • dandelion greens

4 Eat organic

Where possible, always eat organic. Nonorganic produce is likely to have been sprayed with pesticides, leaving toxic byproducts that often can't be removed by washing, scrubbing, or peeling. Research suggests that organic foods contain higher levels of nutrients and antioxidants than their nonorganic counterparts—so choose organic produce to promote glowing, healthy-looking skin and hair.

5 Pick in Summer

In summer, enjoy an abundance of fruits and vegetables, including:

• fava beans • broccoli • carrots • zucchini • cucumbers • fennel • peas • garlic • green beans • lettuce • new potatoes • radishes • arugula • green beans • onions • eggplant • beets • sorrel • tomatoes • watercress • blueberries • currants • plums • raspberries • strawberries

8 Pick in Fall

Enjoy the harvest foods during the fall months, including:

• beets • carrots • celeriac • fennel • mushrooms • kale • leeks • squash • potatoes • pumpkin • arugula • sorrel • corn • tomatoes • watercress • lettuce • apples • blackberries • elderberries • pears • plums

9 Shop locally

Head to a farmers' market, or shop at your local farm stand to benefit from freshly picked, ripe fruit and vegetables. These foods will be packed with nutrients and antioxidants, making them taste incredible and giving your body the tools it needs to keep your skin looking beautiful and your body toned and conditioned.

10 Pick in Winter

During the colder months, look out for slow-cooking vegetables, greens, and hard fruits, such as:

• beets • Brussels sprouts • cabbage • cauliflower • celeriac • chicory • fennel • Jerusalem artichokes • kale • chard • leeks • parsnips • potatoes • red cabbage • rutabaga • turnips • apples • pears

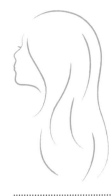

Dry hair and scalp

Scalp psoriasis and seborrheic dermatitis are common conditions that affect the scalp, causing dry, flaky skin and redness. A dry scalp in turn lacks oil to moisturize the hair. Nutritional shortfalls, including a lack of healthy fats, can contribute to dry, stringy hair. Eat healthy proteins to strengthen hair and a range of colorful fruits and veggies for antioxidants and vitamins A and C, which boost sebum production to condition hair.

Superfood recipe suggestions...Berry, seed, and nut granola p166   Avocado on toast with mixed-herb pesto p180
Huevos rancheros p184   Black lentil and coconut curry p204   Lemon and herb-roasted chicken p210   Green smoothie p244

Spinach

This contains vitamins B, C, and E, as well as potassium, calcium, iron, and magnesium, all of which help to nourish hair. The iron content in particular supports red blood cells, enabling them to carry oxygen to the hair follicles.
Key nutrients: *Vitamins B1, B2, B6, C, and E, folate, potassium, calcium, iron, magnesium.*
How to eat: *Have a generous handful of fresh spinach, or a small handful of cooked spinach each day.*

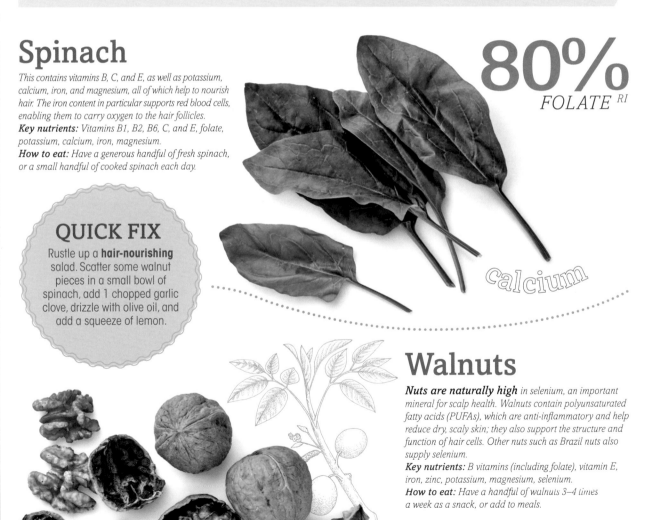

80%
FOLATE RI

calcium

QUICK FIX
Rustle up a **hair-nourishing** salad. Scatter some walnut pieces in a small bowl of spinach, add 1 chopped garlic clove, drizzle with olive oil, and add a squeeze of lemon.

Walnuts

Nuts are naturally high *in selenium, an important mineral for scalp health. Walnuts contain polyunsaturated fatty acids (PUFAs), which are anti-inflammatory and help reduce dry, scaly skin; they also support the structure and function of hair cells. Other nuts such as Brazil nuts also supply selenium.*
Key nutrients: *B vitamins (including folate), vitamin E, iron, zinc, potassium, magnesium, selenium.*
How to eat: *Have a handful of walnuts 3–4 times a week as a snack, or add to meals.*

Parsley

This provides vitamin A, needed by the body to make sebum, the oily substance secreted by the sebaceous glands that is a natural scalp conditioner.

Key nutrients: Carotenoids, B vitamins, vitamins A, C, and E, potassium.

How to eat: Add a handful of chopped parsley leaves and stems to salads and meals.

POTASSIUM

vitamin A

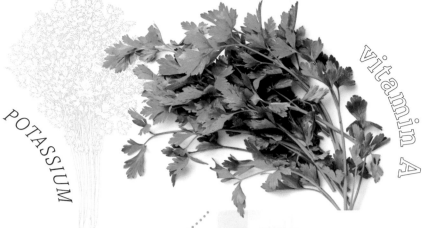

Sardines

Oily fish such as sardines, trout, and salmon provide omega-3, protein, vitamin B12, and iron, all essential nutrients for a healthy scalp and hair.

Key nutrients: Omega-3, vitamin B12 and D, iron.

How to eat: Try to eat a 5½oz (150g) portion of oily fish 2–3 times a week.

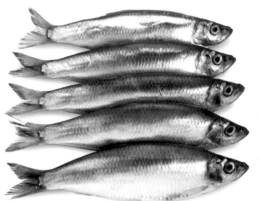

high in omega-3

16%
IRON RI

Flaxseeds

These are a great source of plant-based omega-3 fats, essential to support a healthy scalp and hair.

Key nutrients: Omega-3, vitamin B1, magnesium, phosphorus, selenium.

How to eat: Sprinkle 1 tbsp on oatmeal or in a smoothie daily.

omega-3
SELENIUM

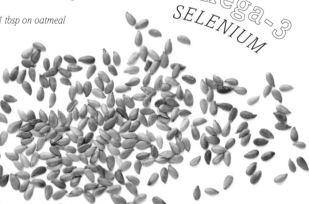

MORE SUPERFOODS

Chicken

Chicken is a great source of healthy protein, essential for hair health. Ensuring you have enough protein in your diet is crucial for strong, vibrant, nourished hair.

Key nutrients: Protein, selenium, vitamins B6 and B12, phosphorus.

How to eat: Eat 5½oz (150g) portion of chicken up to 3 times a week.

Sweet potatoes

These are packed full of beta-carotene, which is converted by the body into vitamin A, a lack of which can result in dry and brittle hair that consequently breaks easily. For a nourished scalp, incorporate plenty of beta-carotene into your diet from a range of brightly colored fruit and vegetables.

Key nutrients: Vitamin C, calcium, folate, potassium, beta-carotene.

How to eat: Add a 3oz (85g) serving of sweet potatoes, ideally steamed or boiled, to meals at least 2–3 times a week. Leave the skins on to maximize nutrients.

Eggs

As well as being high in protein, eggs also contain the B vitamin biotin, which is essential for scalp health and well-conditioned hair.

Key nutrients: Biotin, vitamins A, B2, B12, and D, choline, selenium, phosphorus, zinc.

How to eat: Eat a poached or boiled egg 3–4 times a week.

Avocado

As well as providing a range of hair-conditioning vitamins, avocados are full of healthy fats to keep the hair shaft nourished and hair conditioned.

Key nutrients: Vitamin E, potassium, omega-9, B vitamins, folic acid.

How to eat: Have 1 medium avocado 3–4 times a week.

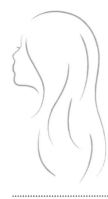

Greasy hair

Greasy hair is directly related to the overproduction of sebum, the waxy substance designed to keep hair supple, soft, and waterproof. Hormonal changes in puberty can cause greasy hair and dietary factors can lead to overactive sebaceous glands. Eat nourishing healthy fats and up your intake of anti-inflammatory foods and foods with vitamins B2 and B6 and zinc, all of which help to balance the production of sebum.

Superfood recipe suggestions...**Overnight oats with superberry compote** p168 **Fruity quinoa breakfast** p169
Scrambled tofu p181 **Bell pepper and tomato dip** p190 **Barley vegetable risotto** p200 **Salmon with samphire** p215

Chamomile tea

Calming chamomile is well known for promoting relaxation and sleep and relieving the symptoms of stress, which in turn can help to control greasy hair because stress is linked to an overproduction of sebum. Caffeine-free and high in antioxidants, chamomile has anti-inflammatory properties that help to calm sebum production.
Key nutrients: Vitamin A, calcium, magnesium, zinc.
How to drink: Drink daily as a wind-down beverage.

VITAMIN A

QUICK FIX

Make a **hair-conditioning** salad by adding nutrient-dense black-eyed peas to a mixed or green salad. Dress with olive oil, a squeeze of lemon, and a pinch of Himalayan pink salt.

Black-eyed peas

Packed full of protein, zinc, and B vitamins, black-eyed peas contain many of the nutrients needed to regulate sebum production and keep the hair shaft healthy.
Key nutrients:, Zinc, folate, B vitamins, vitamin C, iron, protein.
How to eat: Add 3 heaping tbsp to salads or meals 2–3 times a week.

vitamin C and iron

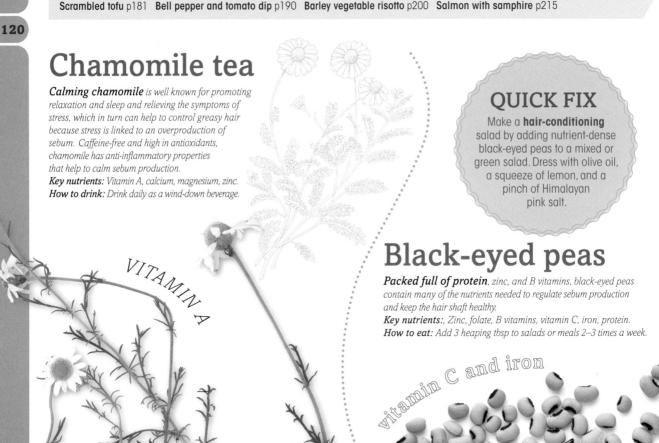

Barley

Barley has a low glycemic index (GI) rating. *Foods with a high GI rating are broken down quickly by the body, which leads to a spike in glucose levels and an overproduction of insulin, and excess insulin leads to a chain of reactions that increases sebum production. In contrast, low-GI foods take longer to digest, resulting in a steady rise in blood glucose and insulin levels.*
Key nutrients: *Vitamin B1, magnesium, selenium.*
How to eat: *Aim for a ½-cup portion of barley a week. Add a handful to a salad or a soup.*

109%
MAGNESIUM RI

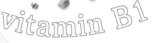

vitamin B1

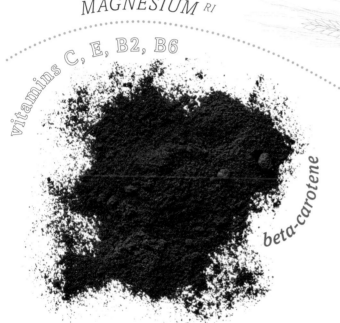

vitamins C, E, B2, B6

beta-carotene

Paprika

This spice is packed with the antioxidant beta-carotene, *which converts to vitamin A in the body, as well as vitamins E and C, all of which help to condition and balance hair. Paprika is also one of the most concentrated sources of B vitamins, particularly sebum-regulating vitamins B2 and B6.*
Key nutrients: *Vitamins C, E, B2, and B6, beta-carotene.*
How to eat: *Add 1 tbsp to cooking to flavor meals or to a smoothie.*

MORE SUPERFOODS

Oats
These are the best plant-based source of the mineral zinc, healthy levels of which help to control the production of sebum.
Key nutrients: *Copper, biotin, vitamin B1, magnesium, chromium, zinc.*
How to eat: *Make a ⅓-cup portion of oats a part of your daily diet.*

Almonds
Concentrated in sebum-regulating vitamin B2, a handful of whole almonds provides more than 40 percent of your daily needs of this vitamin. They also contain vitamin B6, aiding the uptake of zinc, and essential fatty acids.

Key nutrients: *Vitamins B2 and B6, omega-6.*
How to eat: *Eat a small handful of nuts daily as a snack or added to meals.*

Salmon
These provide omega-3, protein, vitamin B12, and iron, all vital for hair. Foods high in healthy fats help to balance the oil-producing sebaceous glands to ensure there isn't an overproduction of sebum. Iron boosts the production of red blood cells, helping to ensure that nutrients reach the hair. Try also mackerel, sardines, and trout.
Key nutrients: *Omega-3, vitamin D.*
How to eat: *Have a 5½oz (150g) portion of oily fish 2–3 times a week.*

Sunflower seeds
These nutritious seeds are an excellent source of vitamins B2 and B6, and are also high in zinc, providing all the key nutrients needed for balanced, healthy hair. Pumpkin and sesame seeds also provide B vitamins to promote hair health and condition the scalp.
Key nutrients: *Vitamins B6, B2, and E, zinc, omega-6, magnesium.*
How to eat: *Add 1 tbsp to oatmeal each morning or sprinkle over salads. Grinding the seeds helps to release the essential fats.*

For supplements, see page 249.

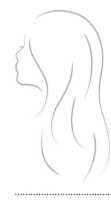

Dull, lifeless hair

Lackluster hair appears frizzy, lifeless, and without sheen. Natural oils in the outer layer of the hair reflect light, adding shine. If this layer breaks down and there's a lack of moisture, hair appears dull. Thyroid problems and a diet low in nutrients can affect hair health. Hydrating foods, antioxidant-rich fresh produce, and foods with omega-3 and -6 nourish the hair shaft, improving texture and adding shine to hair.

Superfood recipe suggestions...Berry, seed, and nut granola p166   Huevos rancheros p184   Summer asparagus salad p189
Baked stuffed squash p203   Roasted sea bass with tomato salsa p212   Nutty rice salad p220

Oily fish

Omega-3 fatty acids, protein, vitamin B12, and iron, are all found in fish sources and help to liven dull hair. About 3 percent of the hair shaft is made up of omega-3, and these are also found in cell membranes on the scalp and in the natural oils that keep the scalp and hair hydrated.
Key nutrients: Omega-3, vitamins B12 and D, iron.
How to eat: Aim to eat a 5½oz (150g) portion of oily fish 2–3 times a week.

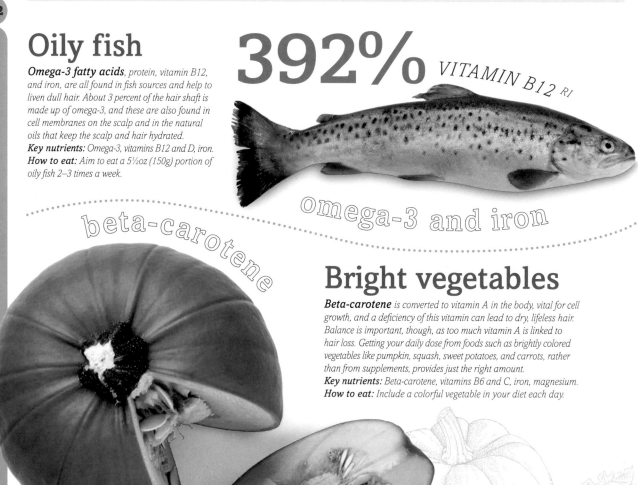

392% VITAMIN B12 RI

omega-3 and iron

beta-carotene

Bright vegetables

Beta-carotene is converted to vitamin A in the body, vital for cell growth, and a deficiency of this vitamin can lead to dry, lifeless hair. Balance is important, though, as too much vitamin A is linked to hair loss. Getting your daily dose from foods such as brightly colored vegetables like pumpkin, squash, sweet potatoes, and carrots, rather than from supplements, provides just the right amount.
Key nutrients: Beta-carotene, vitamins B6 and C, iron, magnesium.
How to eat: Include a colorful vegetable in your diet each day.

Leafy greens

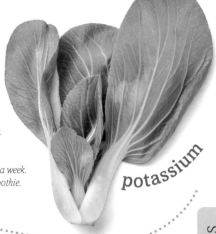

Dark green leafy vegetables, such as bok choy, spinach, broccoli, kale, and Swiss chard, provide a boost for hair, with nutrients such as iron, beta-carotene, folate, and vitamin C, keeping hair follicles healthy and hair looking vibrant.

Key nutrients: Beta-carotene, vitamins C and B, potassium, calcium, folate, iron.

How to eat: Eat a 3oz (85g) portion at least 2–3 times a week. Either steam for 3–4 minutes or add raw to a green smoothie.

potassium

QUICK FIX

For a **hydrating** salad or side dish, lightly steam your choice of leafy green vegetable, then add a squeeze of lemon, 1 finely chopped garlic clove, and a pinch of Himalayan pink salt.

Avocado

The important B vitamin biotin, found in avocados, is necessary for healthy hair growth. While a deficiency of biotin is rare, eating biotin-rich foods supplements the vitamin manufactured in the body to improve hair strength and prevent breakage so hair looks thicker and healthier.

Key nutrients: Omega-9, B vitamins, magnesium, iron, potassium, vitamin E.

How to eat: Eat 1 medium avocado 3–4 times a week.

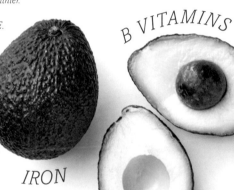

B VITAMINS

IRON

Salad foods

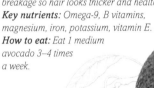

Around 20 percent of our daily water intake comes from solid foods, and hydrating salad vegetables such as celery and cucumber are a key source of fluids, supporting hydration in the body.

Key nutrients: Vitamin C, B vitamins, potassium, calcium.

How to eat: Eat 3½oz (100g) or more of fresh raw salad vegetables daily.

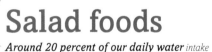

7%
POTASSIUM RI

MORE SUPERFOODS

Asparagus

This provides silica, a mineral that is essential for strong, healthy, shiny hair.

Key nutrients: Vitamins A, B2, B3, B5, B6, C, and K, folate, copper, selenium, manganese, phosphorus, potassium, choline, zinc, iron, protein.

How to eat: Add 3–4 asparagus spears to salads, either raw or lightly steamed, or eat as a side vegetable.

Walnuts

These truly delicious nuts contain copper, a mineral that helps keep natural hair color rich and vibrant. Nuts also contain high amounts of selenium, which is fantastic for hair vitality and lustrous locks.

Key nutrients: Copper, selenium, alpha-linoleic acid, zinc.

How to eat: Snack on a small handful of walnuts daily.

Eggs

Full of protein, eggs also have four key hair minerals: zinc, selenium, sulfur, and iron. Hair is nearly all protein, so protein-rich foods provide the building blocks for hair, keeping the hair cells healthy and hair strands strong and conditioned.

Key nutrients: Protein, vitamins B2, B12 and D, phosphorus, zinc, selenium, sulfur, iron.

How to eat: Eat a daily egg, poached or boiled, for breakfast or as a snack.

Flaxseeds

These provide alpha-linoleic acid, a hair-boosting essential fatty acid, and zinc, which conditions and helps reduce hair loss.

Key nutrients: Magnesium, phosphorus, selenium, vitamin B6, iron, potassium, copper, zinc, fatty acids.

How to eat: Sprinkle 1 tsp of flaxseeds onto your morning oatmeal or add to a smoothie blend.

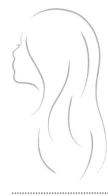

Dandruff

This common scalp condition occurs when dead skin is shed, producing white flakes. Stress, illness, hormonal imbalance, and an overconsumption of sugar and refined carbohydrates can all be triggers. Eating raw foods and fermented products helps to cleanse blood, and foods high in vitamin B, selenium, and essential fats can be lacking with dandruff. Zinc-rich foods are also vital as zinc promotes the healthy functioning of hair follicles.

Superfood recipe suggestions...Huevos rancheros p184   Bell pepper and tomato dip p190   Greek vegetable mezze p198
Japanese ocean soup p201   Ratatouille p207   Roasted sea bass with tomato salsa p212   Nutty rice salad p220

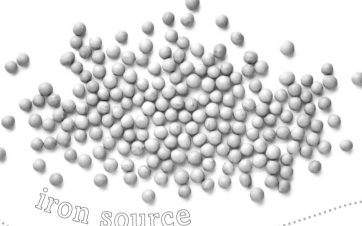

iron source

Soybeans

These are a top source of biotin, *an essential nutrient necessary for cell growth and the metabolism of fats and amino acids, which promotes a healthy scalp to help remedy dandruff. Biotin also enhances the immune system response and the functioning of the nervous system.*
Key nutrients: *Biotin, iron, omega-3, vitamins B2 and K, magnesium, potassium.*
How to eat: *Add ½ cup of cooked soybeans to a salad or while cooking twice a week.*

Bell pepper

These supply vitamin B6 *(pyridoxine), thought to help reduce dandruff. An inefficient metabolism of carbohydrates and fatty acids could be one of the underlying causes of dandruff, and B-complex vitamins help to support metabolic processes in the body.*
Key nutrients: *Vitamins A, B6, and C, copper.*
How to eat: *Snack on a handful of raw bell pepper sticks daily or add to salads.*

85%
VITAMIN A [R1]

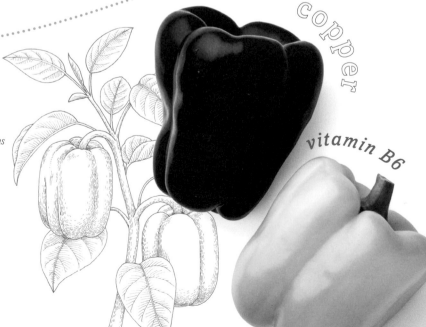

copper

vitamin B6

Brazil nuts

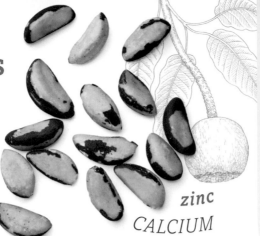

These contain selenium, an important antioxidant that helps to condition the scalp.
Key nutrients: Selenium, copper, magnesium, manganese, potassium, calcium, iron, phosphorus, zinc.
How to eat: Snack on a handful of Brazil nuts daily.

zinc
CALCIUM

QUICK FIX

Boost scalp health with this stir-fry. Heat 1 tbsp oil in a wok. Add 2oz (60g) tempeh, 1 garlic clove, and ginger; cook for 2–3 minutes. Add slices of 1 red bell pepper and tamari sauce; cook for 2 more minutes.

Tempeh

Tempeh contains vitamin B2, which promotes the growth of new cells and is needed for healthy skin and hair.
Key nutrients: Phosphorus, vitamin B2, magnesium.
How to eat: A serving of 5½oz (150g) can be eaten daily, or aim for at least 1 portion a week.

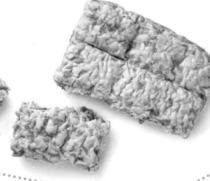

VITAMIN B2

25% MANGANESE RI

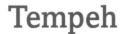

Kidney beans

These succulent beans are a fantastic source of zinc, involved in tissue growth and repair, and in helping the oil glands around the hair work properly.
Key nutrients: Manganese, phosphorus, protein, zinc, vitamin B1, iron, potassium, magnesium.
How to eat: Add a handful of cooked kidney beans to a salad or use as a protein base for a meal.

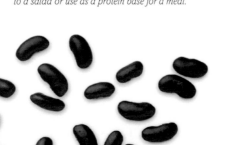

Flaxseeds

These contain omega-3, which can help to relieve the itching that can exacerbate dandruff, and also have anti-inflammatory properties to help balance sebum.
Key nutrients: Omega-3, vitamin B1, magnesium, phosphorus, selenium.
How to eat: Sprinkle 1 tbsp on oatmeal or in a smoothie daily. Grinding the seeds releases more of their essential oils.

Oily fish

Oily fish such as salmon, mackerel, and sardines are full of omega-3, a deficiency of which can cause dandruff.
Key nutrients: Omega-3, iron.
How to eat: Try to eat a 5½oz (150g) portion of oily fish 2–3 times a week.

Eggs

These are a good source of vitamin A, which is essential for skin and hair health. Vitamin A also plays an important role in the circulatory and immune systems and supports the maintenance and function of skin cells, which can improve scalp health; all of these can help to condition the scalp and in turn alleviate dandruff.
Key nutrients: Vitamins A, B2, B12, and D, choline, selenium, phosphorus.
How to eat: Eat a poached or boiled egg as a snack daily.

Seaweed

Seaweed such as kelp and nori supplies much-needed minerals and iodine, which helps hair to grow healthfully and heals the scalp. Kelp contains the highest natural concentration of calcium of any food, which supports a healthy scalp and hair.
Key nutrients: Vitamins A, B1, B2, C, D, and E, iodine, zinc, magnesium, iron, potassium, copper, calcium.
How to eat: Sprinkle 1 tsp dried daily on salads, add to cooking or eat as a snack.

Kiwi fruit

This fruit is high in vitamin C, so it supports the immune system. Vitamin C helps prevent conditions that can be triggered by weakened immunity, such as dandruff. Vitamin C is also an antioxidant that helps to prevent tissue damage to the scalp and aids healing.
Key nutrients: Vitamins C and E, potassium, folate, manganese.
How to eat: Try to eat at least 1 kiwi daily. Eat after meals or add to salads, smoothies, or juices.

For supplements, see page 249.

Meal planner
Hair conditioning

The cells that make up each hair strand need key nutrients to keep the hair shaft healthy. This meal plan uses recipes from the book and meal ideas to provide nutrients that help to condition hair and optimize hair health.

Your hair-conditioning week This nutritionally balanced one-week meal planner will start you on your hair-conditioning diet. Continue for four weeks for optimum results, using the alternative meal ideas, opposite, for variety. Start each day with a hot water and lemon drink to aid digestion.

Monday

Breakfast
Berry, seed, and nut granola (p.166)

Snacks
Pineapple smoothie (p.239)

Lunch
Green salad with avocado

Dinner
Sweet potato and mackerel mash (p.219, variation)

Tuesday

Breakfast
Green smoothie (p.244)

Snacks
Handful of Hot nuts! (p.194)

Lunch
Japanese ocean soup (p.201)

Dinner
Barley vegetable risotto (p.200)

Wednesday

Breakfast
Cacao and chia chocolate "pudding" (p.174)

Snacks
Coconut smoothie (p.235) and handful of sunflower seeds

Lunch
Crunchy apple, carrot, and radish salad

Dinner
Roasted sea bass with tomato salsa (p.212)

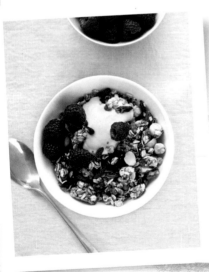

Berry, seed, and nut granola (p.166)

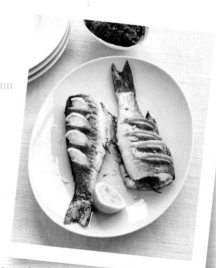

Roasted sea bass with tomato salsa (p.212)

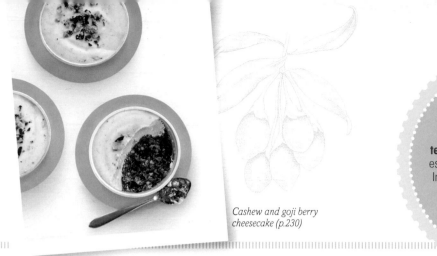

Cashew and goji berry
cheesecake (p.230)

Thursday

Breakfast
Poached egg on rye bread with a kiwi

Snacks
Chile guacamole (p.190) on two oat cakes and a fig

Lunch
Mashed avocado on rye bread with a green salad

Dinner
Thai chicken and noodle soup (p.214)

Friday

Breakfast
Cashew butter on rye bread with kiwi

Snacks
Red bell pepper sticks with hummus

Lunch
Dairy-free pesto (p.186, variation) with gluten-free pasta and a green salad with slices of tempeh

Dinner
Potato and veggie bake (p.211)

Saturday

Breakfast
Fruity quinoa breakfast (p.169)

Snacks
Apple slices spread with nut butter

Lunch
Huevos rancheros (p.184)

Dinner
Salmon with samphire (p.215)

Sweet treat
Cashew and goji berry cheesecake (p.230)

Sunday

Breakfast
Blueberry and chia pancakes (p.171)

Snacks
Two figs and a handful of almonds

Lunch
Mixed salad with avocado

Dinner
Lamb tagine (p.212)

Alternatives

To help you on your way, draw on these additional recipe suggestions to vary your meals over the course of four weeks.

Breakfast
Nutty overnight oats (p.168, variation)

Oatmeal with mixed seeds and sliced apricot

Snacks
Mixed fruit salad with natural live yogurt and a handful of almonds

Lunch
Beet and chickpea soup (p.192)

Baked potato, tomato salsa (p.212), and goat cheese

Dinner
Salmon with coconut rice (p.215, variation)

Poached chicken with rice noodles and mango

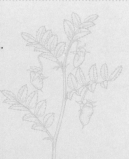

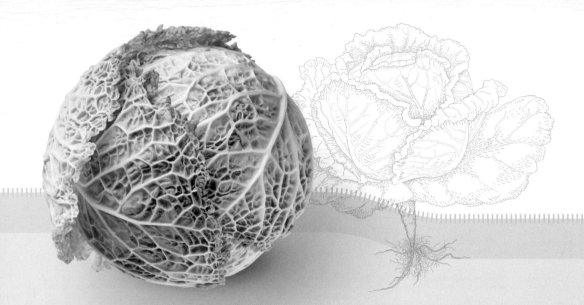

Foods for the
hands and feet

Our hands, feet, and nails are often the first areas to show signs of wear and tear, so they demand a bit of extra care to keep them in good condition. Find out how the foods you eat can form part of your daily hand- and foot-care regime, and follow a nutritionally tailored meal plan for strong, beautifully glossy nails.

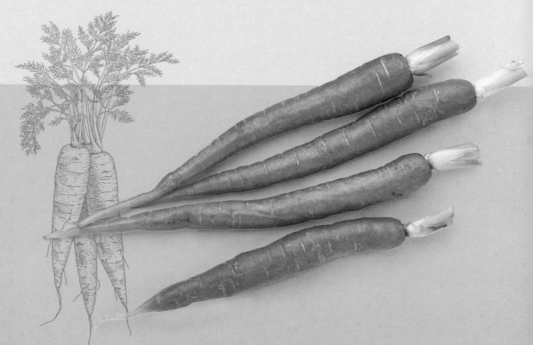

Eat for beauty: hands and feet

For strong, **glossy** nails, and **beautifully conditioned**, smooth skin on our hands and feet, we need to eat a diet that is high in **skin-nourishing**, protective nutrients. Discover the top nutrients to nourish your hands, feet, and nails to keep these looking wonderful.

Nutrients for your hands and feet

Before you explore the foods for the specific beauty concerns in this chapter, discover the key nutrients that help to keep hands and feet in great condition.

Zinc A small, steady supply of this essential mineral is needed by the body to support the growth of cells. Zinc is especially important for areas where cells grow and divide rapidly, such as in our fingernails and toenails, where this mineral facilitates chemical reactions in cells, in turn promoting the healthy growth of new nail tissue. A zinc deficiency will often show up first in our nails, causing nails to become dry and brittle, and charactersitic white specks may appear. Occasionally, foot odor is also due to a zinc deficiency. You can increase and maintain your zinc levels by eating unrefined grains, nuts such as cashews, pumpkin and sesame seeds, eggs, and, occasionally, lamb.

Essential fatty acids We often notice dry skin first on exposed areas such as our hands and feet. While some of us have a natural tendency to dry skin, the problem is often exacerbated by a lack of essential fatty acids in the diet, or by a diet that is high in unhealthy saturated fats, which dehydrate skin. The essential fatty acids omega-3 and omega-6 provide moisture for the skin's oil-producing glands, supporting the skin cell membranes and reducing water loss through the outer layer of the skin. Our bodies can't synthesize omega-3 and omega-6 fatty acids, so we need to obtain these via our diet. On the whole, we need more omega-3 than omega-6, since too much omega-6 can have an inflammatory effect.

A top source of omega-3 fatty acids is oily fish, and eating fish such as salmon or mackerel just 2–3 times a week can make a noticeable difference to the condition of the skin on the hands and feet over time. Other good sources of omega-3 include flax and hemp seeds, nuts, avocados, and dark green leafy vegetables. Omega-6 is also found in nuts and seeds, and in grapseed oil, as well as in meat and cereal grains.

Betacarotene, vitamin E, and biotin The delicate skin on the hands is constantly exposed to the elements and vulnerable to damage from harmful UV rays. Foods rich in the antioxidants betacarotene, which converts to vitamin A in the body, and vitamin E help to protect skin against UV sun damage and speed skin repair. Vitamin E also promotes healthy red blood cells, helping oxygen

Your hands, feet, and nails bear the brunt of daily wear and tear. Treating them to nourishing nutrients each day helps them to look beautiful and cared for.

and nutrients to reach the nails to strengthen them and give them a sheen. Include leafy greens, nuts seeds, and avocados in your diet for vitamin E, and vegetables such as squash, sweet potato, kale, and carrots to ensure you are getting

20%

of our daily water intake comes from solid foods.

enough betacarotene. The water-soluble B vitamin biotin is essential for the breakdown and distribution of fatty acids, which is important for healthy skin, hair, and nails.

Protein Nails are made of structural proteins called keratin, so it's essential to include plenty of high-quality proteins in your diet each day, since an adequate supply of dietary protein is needed to provide the building blocks for strong nails. The skin also needs protein for collagen production, which helps ensure skin elasticity and strength, making it especially beneficial to the fragile skin on the tops of the hands. Sources of healthy proteins include beans and legumes, fish, lean meat, and eggs.

Sulfur, silica, and allicin These minerals play an important role in nail health. Sulfur, found in foods such as garlic and red onions, boosts circulation, in turn promoting nail growth. Silica, found in alfalfa beans, oats, asparagus, barley, broccoli, seaweed, and strawberries, is a component of collagen, essential for strong

tissues, and helps to carry other vital nutrients to the peripheral parts of the body such as the nails. Garlic contains a substance called allicin, which has anti-microbial and antifungal properties, making it a useful complementary treatment for fungal infections such as athlete's foot.

Hydration Being sufficiently hydrated is essential for all the body's tissues and cells. If our nails lack hydration they can become weak and brittle and start to split and peel. As well as drinking up to 2 liters of water daily, include hydrating foods in your diet each day. Around 20 percent of our daily water intake comes from solid foods, especially fruits and vegetables, and these also provide us with essential nutrients. Eat hydrating foods such as celery, cucumber, and watermelon, and enjoy raw salads and fresh fruits.

What affects our hands and feet?

Our hands and feet are subject to a great deal of wear and tear, and require a bit of extra care. Being aware of the various factors that can affect our hands and feet and how diet can help to counter their effects can help you to keep them in the best possible condition.

Diet and lifestyle Processed foods, sugar, caffeine, alcohol, poor-quality cooking oils, and too much red meat can leave the body lacking in nutrients, with a negative impact on skin and nails. Nails are made up of protein, so you can support them by eating good-quality proteins with every meal. Ensure, too, that you eat a range of fruit and vegetables for minerals such as magnesium, zinc, copper, and silica to help keep nails strong.

Poor diet and lifestyle choices affect circulation, too, which can result in pale and cold hands and feet. Alcohol and smoking have a negative impact on circulation. Try to stop smoking altogether, and cut out alcohol or reduce its consumption to below the advised limit of 5 drinks a week. If poor circulation is a problem, eat foods that boost circulation. Vitamin E–rich foods protect blood vessel cells, optimizing blood flow, and omega-3 foods have anti-inflammatory properties that aid circulation. Foods with vitamin C, such as citrus fruits, help to generate new cells and protect blood vessels from damage.

Sun damage We often neglect our hands when protecting our skin from the sun, even though these are very exposed. As a result the skin on our hands can age faster than the rest of the body. Eat to protect your hands by including

Eat for your age

As we get older, our hands and feet bear the brunt of daily wear and tear. From our 30s onward, skin starts to thin and lose its elasticity, and the skin on both the hands and feet can become dry and more fragile. Eating a healthy, well-balanced diet is essential to protect your feet at all ages to support the fragile skin on your hands, and keep nails robust. A multivitamin and mineral supplement will also benefit the hands, feet, and nails.

In your 20s

Healthy collagen production in our 20s means that hands, feet, and nails usually look well conditioned and healthy. However, wear and tear and the effects of sunlight gradually start to show later on in this decade.
Eat: Plenty of antioxidant-rich fruit and vegetables, especially foods with skin-strengthening vitamins C and E, such as tomatoes, citrus fruits, green leafy vegetables, and carrots. Oily fish, eggs, and nuts and seeds are important to provide essential omega-3 fats, and garlic and onions provide important minerals to keep nails healthy.

In your 30s

In our 30s, skin cell production decreases by around 10 percent, which means the skin becomes less efficient at repairing itself. The tops of the hands in particular, where the skin is thin, can be the first place to show noticeable signs of aging, and as skin starts to lose plumpness with the loss of collagen and elastin, veins and knuckles can look more prominent.
Eat: Healthy proteins from eggs, fish, legumes, nuts and seeds, lean meats; betacarotene-rich yellow and orange foods such as peppers, carrots, and squash provide sun protection.

86%

of our daily omega-3 needs are included in a 5½oz (150g) portion of salmon.

omega-3 fats in your diet and vitamins C and E, and betacarotene. Green tea contains a polyphenol antioxidant, catechin, that increases the skin's resistance to UV rays, helping to reduce and repair DNA damage from UV rays and prevent premature skin aging.

Exposure to chemicals Our hands are frequently exposed to substances that can irritate the skin, leaving them red, chapped, and dry. Try to identify the source of an irritation and avoid it or protect your hands. Omega-3 has an anti-inflammatory effect that can protect the skin against irritants.

Infections Fungal infections of the nails or between the toes, where skin is moist, are common. A poor diet feeds the infection-causing bacteria. If you're prone to infections, avoid processed foods, alcohol, wheat, gluten, and sugar, and eat raw or steamed vegetables, fermented foods, such as miso, and sea vegetables, such as kelp.

In your 40s

During our 40s, hormonal changes can affect the skin. A drop in estrogen can mean skin loses moisture and firmness, which means skin on hands may appear less firm and skin on the feet can harden and become dry. The cumulative effects of sun on the hands can mean that age spots, or liver spots, appear.
Eat: Increase your intake of antioxidant-rich fruit and vegetables such as red peppers, tomatoes, squash, berries, kiwi, and oranges, and eat foods that provide zinc, such as nuts and seeds, lentils, and whole grains.

In your 50s

Age spots may become increasingly noticeable now. The skin on the back of the hands is much thinner than on the face and neck, so it's more susceptible to the aging process in general. A drop in sebum production can affect the skin on the feet, too, and skin can become drier, harden, and sometimes start to crack around the heels. Nails may be weaker now as collagen production also continues to decline.
Eat: Plenty of detoxifying foods to support the liver and help prevent age spots, such as citrus fruits, brightly colored vegetables, and whole grains.

60s plus

Our reservoir of silica, which helps to support the structure of our skin and nails, declines steadily as we age. Changes in metabolism can mean that nails thicken on the hands and feet now and problems such as corns, calluses, and fungal infections can become more common. Nails may also start to peel more as lower sebum levels removes conditioning moisture.
Eat Healthy oils, such as coconut oil, flaxseed, olive, and hemp seed oils, and foods with zinc, vitamin C, and biotin, such as egg yolks, kale, sweet potatoes, and nuts and seeds.

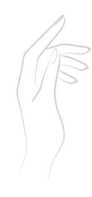

Weak nails

These tend to be thin, and peel and break easily, which can result in painful splits. Aging and some medical conditions can weaken nails, and nutritional deficiencies can compromise nail health. Fresh foods high in vitamins and nutrients such as sulfur and silica strengthen nails, good-quality proteins boost collagen for robust, healthy nails, and iron- and zinc-rich foods provide the nutrients nails need to grow well.

Superfood recipe suggestions...Fall flavors soup p178   Avocado on toast with mixed-herb pesto p180   Huevos rancheros p184   Gazpacho with watermelon p188   Salmon with samphire p215 Homemade oat milk p241

Eggs

These are one of the few dietary sources of vitamin D, and their protein content is crucial for strong fingernails. Unlike meat, the protein in eggs is highly digestible and easily taken up by the body. Eggs also contain the B vitamin biotin, which helps to increase fingernail thickness.
Key nutrients: Vitamin D, iron, biotin.
How to eat: Aim to eat a poached or boiled egg daily.

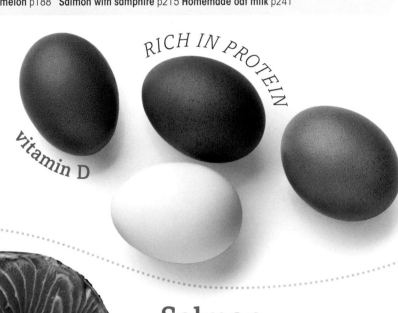

RICH IN PROTEIN

vitamin D

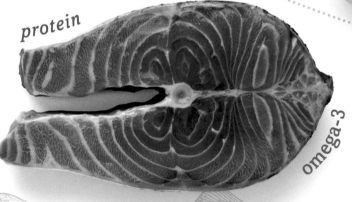

protein

omega-3

Salmon

This is a good source of biotin and protein, as well as omega-3, which promote healthy, moisturized nails. Omega-3s' anti-inflammatory properties support nails; inflammation impairs the development of the nail plate, leading to weak nails.
Key nutrients: Omega-3, biotin, vitamins B12 and D, protein.
How to eat: Have a 5½oz (150g) portion of oily fish such as salmon 2–3 times a week.

392%
VITAMIN B12 RI

Carrots

Carrot provide beta-carotene, which converts to vitamin A in the body, needed for the body to utilize protein and essential for strong, healthy nails. Carrots are also high in calcium and phosphorus, which both help to strengthen nails.
Key nutrients: *Beta-carotene, B vitamins, vitamins C, E, and K, fiber, molybdenum, potassium, calcium, phosphorus.*
How to eat: *Aim to eat a 3oz (85g) serving daily.*

calcium

Alfalfa sprouts

Alfalfa is a great source of silica, which helps to strengthen nails.
Key nutrients: *Silica, vitamin K, B vitamins.*
How to eat: *Add a handful to salads, meals, or heat very briefly in stir-fry. Eat daily if you wish, or aim to eat this three times a week.*

QUICK FIX

Strengthen nails with a nutrient-boosting juice or smoothie. Drink fresh carrot juice daily or add to a smoothie blend. For a flavor kick, add a little freshly grated ginger.

HIGH IN SILICA

38%
VITAMIN B1 RI

Oats

These contain micronutrients such as copper, zinc, manganese, silica, and B vitamins, all of which promote healthy nails.
Key nutrients: *Copper, biotin, vitamin B1, magnesium, chromium, zinc.*
How to eat: *Have a ⅓-cup portion daily in oatmeal or add to a smoothie.*

biotin

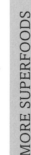

MORE SUPERFOODS

Sunflower seeds
These crunchy seeds contain essential vitamins and zinc, which provide nails with the nutrients they need for healthy growth.
Key nutrients: *Vitamins B1, B3, B6, and E, zinc, manganese, selenium, phosphorus, magnesium, folate.*
How to eat: *Have up to 1 tbsp a day, as a snack, sprinkled over your breakfast or added to salads. Soaking the seeds in 3 tbsp of water overnight will release beneficial oils, making these more readily available.*

Tomatoes
High amounts of biotin and lycopene in tomatoes help nails to grow, thicken, and shine. They are also full of vitamins A and C, both beneficial for healthy, strong nails that grow well.
Key nutrients: *Biotin, lycopene, vitamins A and C.*
How to eat: *Have 1 medium tomato or 7 cherry tomatoes daily, added to a meal or eaten as a snack.*

10 ways to...
Preserve nutrients

We often learn to cook from our parents and use the same cooking methods throughout our lives, but these techniques may not be the most effective at preserving nutrients and maximizing the beauty benefits of our food. The way we prepare and cook food has a significant impact on nutritional content. High temperatures, long cooking times, and cooking with large quantities of water can all cause a loss of nutrients.

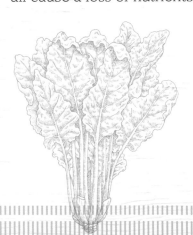

1 Steam vegetables

Steaming is one of the best methods to preserve nutrients and flavor. Use a steamer, or try this method that uses minimal added water to steam vegetables in their own juices:

Preheat a heavy-bottomed pan over medium-high heat and add the prepared vegetables, along with 2 tablespoons of water. Bring the water to the evaporating point, then reduce the heat and cover the pan. Cook until the vegetables are just cooked, still firm, and brightly colored.

2 Limit boiling

Boiling, poaching, or simmering vegetables causes them to lose nutrients into the water. Significant quantities of nutrients are lost after only two minutes in boiling water, and vitamin C is destroyed at high temperatures. If you boil veg, use the least amount of water possible, cook only for as long as necessary, and reuse the water in sauces, stocks, or gravies, so you don't waste nutrients.

6 Eat raw foods

Rich in enzymes and unadulterated vitamins and minerals, raw foods are a beauty-boosting addition to your diet. Eating foods raw removes the risk of introducing carcinogens during cooking, and reduces the chance of consuming oxidized foods that can cause visible signs of aging. Try adding thinly sliced raw fennel or beets to a salad, basing your breakfast smoothie on kale or apple, or dipping sticks of red bell pepper and celery in hummus for a quick snack.

7 Soak and sprout

Soaking and sprouting foods before eating activates their nutrients and beneficial enzymes, and increases levels of some vitamins. Try sprouting your own seeds, beans, and legumes at home, and soaking grains in cold water for two to three hours before cooking.

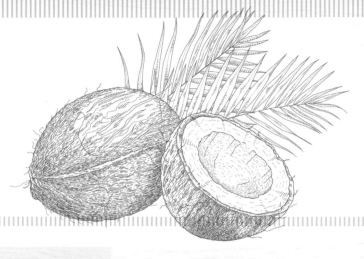

DID YOU KNOW?

Your body absorbs more of certain nutrients, including carotenoids, when they are served with a little healthy oil or fat. Carotenoids in carrots, squashes, bell peppers, and tomatoes improve skin color and tone.

3 Sauté with care

Sautéing, or fying, foods can seal in beneficial skin nutrients, flavors, and juices. Make sure you use the right cooking oil or fat for the job—coconut oil and ghee are both stable at high temperatures and produce fewer aldehydes (toxins linked with cancer). Avoid overheating while cooking, as this can oxidize oil, making it acidic, and reduce the nutrient content of the food.

4 Cook at low temperatures

Roasting, baking, and slow cooking can be particularly appealing during the colder months. Make sure that you cook at lower temperatures over a long period of time to conserve skin-healthy vitamins. Avoid burning or charring baked and roasted foods, as this can create harmful carcinogens and dietary toxins that can be aging for skin.

5 Make soups

Soups, broths, and casseroles are all healthy ways to prepare foods. Even though water is usually used, water-soluble nutrients are then consumed with the meal, making it a healthier choice than boiling. These types of dishes retain nutrients and may make foods easier to digest.

8 Cook from scratch

Cooking your meals yourself—rather than buying premade meals or takeout food—ensures that you know exactly what is in the foods you are eating. This includes how much sugar and salt is added, and which oils and cooking methods are used, all of which helps to conserve nutrients and promotes radiant skin and healthy hair and nails.

9 Prepare fruits and veggies

Avoid buying prepared packs of fruit and vegetables—instead, prepare these yourself, just before cooking, to avoid nutrient loss. As most of the nutrients in vegetables are found just beneath the skin, scrub them clean using a vegetable brush, rather than peeling them. This will also help eliminate surface chemicals in nonorganic foods.

10 Freeze fresh

If you find yourself with a plethora of fruits or vegetables, freezing is a good option—it will keep you from wasting food and locks in nutrients. Choose good-quality, freshly harvested foods, and freeze them as soon as possible after buying or picking. Vegetables and fruits should be frozen for a maximum of six months. Where possible, cook from frozen, as thawing causes some nutrients to degrade, including antioxidant, collagen-boosting vitamin C.

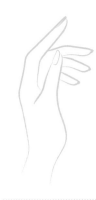

Age spots

Our hands are often first to show signs of aging, when age spots, or areas of darker pigmentation, appear. A lack of good nutrients, stress, and exposure to sun can trigger free radical damage that ages skin. Antioxidant vitamins C and E help to protect the skin from damaging UV rays, cleansing foods and foods that support liver health help to flush out toxins, while collagen-boosting foods help to keep skin firm and toned.

Superfood recipe suggestions...Overnight oats with superberry compote p168   **Fall flavors soup** p178   **Zucchini noodles with basil pesto** p186   **Summer salad with pomegranate and pistachio** p202   **Red berry smoothie** p235   **Matcha beauty shot** p236

Matcha

Made from powdered *green tea leaves, matcha has 10 times the antioxidant value of green tea. Catechins, the active antioxidant found in green tea, are thought to increase the skin's resistance to UV radiation from the sun's rays, helping to prevent and repair DNA damage.*
Key nutrients: *L-theanine, catechins, epigallocatechin gallate (EGCG), vitamins A and K.*
How to drink: *Add 1 scant tsp daily to drinks.*

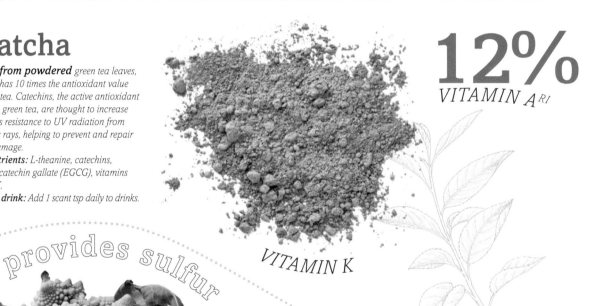

12%
VITAMIN A RI

VITAMIN K

provides sulfur

Brassicas

Cabbage, kale, Brussels sprouts, *broccoli, cauliflower, and other brassicas contain sulfur, which increases an antioxidant in the body, intracellular glutathione, which reduces skin pigmentation.*
Key nutrients: *Fiber, vitamin C, beta-carotene, quercetin, omega-3, sulfur.*
How to eat: *Try alternating members of the brassica family, incorporating them into one of your meals each day.*

Berries

Blackberries, cranberries, goji berries, mulberries, raspberries, and strawberries are a great source of ellagic acid, a natural phytochemical that helps to prevent an excessive production of melanin, in turn evening out and brightening skin tone.
Key nutrients: Flavonoids, vitamins A, C, and E, ellegic acid, omega-3, potassium, magnesium.
How to eat: Add a small handful of berries to muesli or oatmeal daily.

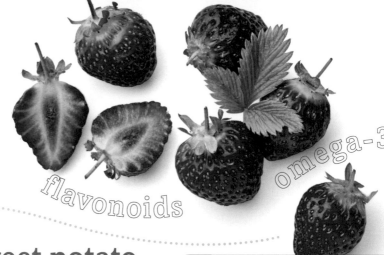

flavonoids

omega-3

QUICK FIX

Boost **skin-protecting** antioxidants. Steam a chopped sweet potato with its skin on. Mix with some lightly steamed kale, then drizzle with olive oil and add a squeeze of lemon.

Sweet potato

These contain antioxidant carotenoids such as beta-carotene, lutein, and lycopene. Beta-carotene protects and helps repair damage from UV rays. Carrots, squash, and bell peppers also provide carotenoids.
Key nutrients: Beta-carotenes, lutein, lycopene, vitamins B6, C, and K, biotin, fiber, potassium.
How to eat: Eat carotenoid-rich foods daily.

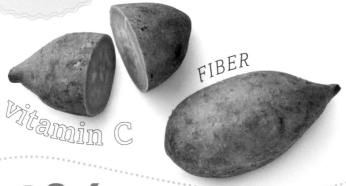

FIBER

vitamin C

56%
VITAMIN C RI

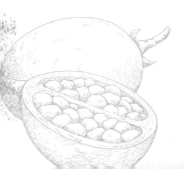

Baobab

Baobab, a powder from the African fruit, stimulates collagen production to keep skin healthy and supple and therefore more resistant to the signs of aging.
Key nutrients: Calcium, vitamins A, B1, B6, and C, potassium, magnesium, zinc, bioflavonoids, fiber.
How to eat: Add 1–2 tsp daily to meals.

MORE SUPERFOODS

Sea buckthorn fruit oil
This oil is a fabulous source of rare omega-7 (palmitoleic acid), a fatty acid that is found naturally in the skin, but which depletes with age and which helps to protect the skin against UV damage. The oil also provides vitamins C and E and beta-carotene, which help to even out and brighten skin tone.
Key nutrients: Omega-7, vitamins C and E, beta-carotene.
How to eat: Add 1 tsp to a juice, smoothie, or yogurt daily.

Miso
This fermented grain or bean paste is a good source of kojic acid, which helps to lighten the skin by inhibiting the action of an enzyme called tyrosinase that hastens the pigmentation of skin, reducing the amount of skin-darkening melanin.
Key nutrients: Kojic acid, vitamin K, zinc, protein, phosphorus, probiotics, fatty acids.
How to eat: Up to 2 tbsp 3–4 times a week.

Leafy greens
These are high in the anti-inflammatory vitamin E. This protective nutrient defends the skin against damaging free radicals.
Key nutrients: Fiber, vitamins C and E, omega-3, beta-carotene, quercetin.
How to eat: Eat a 3oz (85g) portion of leafy greens daily.

Zucchini
These are full of skin-protecting antioxidants, such as beta-carotene and vitamin C.
Key nutrients: Carotenoids, omega-3 and -9, vitamins B6 and C, magnesium, potassium, folate.
How to eat: Have ½ lightly steamed zucchini as a side vegetable, or add raw to salads.

Hard, rough skin

Dry, callused skin is commonly found on the feet and hands, where wear and tear take their toll. A lack of healthy fats can contribute to dry skin. Essential fatty acids and hydrating foods help to restore moisture to the skin, foods that are high in vitamin E speed skin repair, and vitamin A–rich foods help to replenish dry skin. Include, too, foods that facilitate the removal of toxins to help keep skin clear and toned.

Superfood recipe suggestions...**Fruity quinoa breakfast** p169   **Chile guacamole** p190   **Beet and chickpea soup** p192
Protein power beauty bites p195   **Greek vegetable mezze** p198   **Homemade oat milk** p241

Brightly colored fruits and vegetables

Yellow, orange, and red pigments *in foods indicate antioxidants called carotenoids, which convert to vitamin A in the body. These fat-soluble antioxidants are key to reducing skin inflammation, helping to soothe rough skin.*
Key nutrients: *Vitamin A, fiber.*
How to eat: *Have a 3oz (85g) portion of a brightly colored fruit or vegetable each day.*

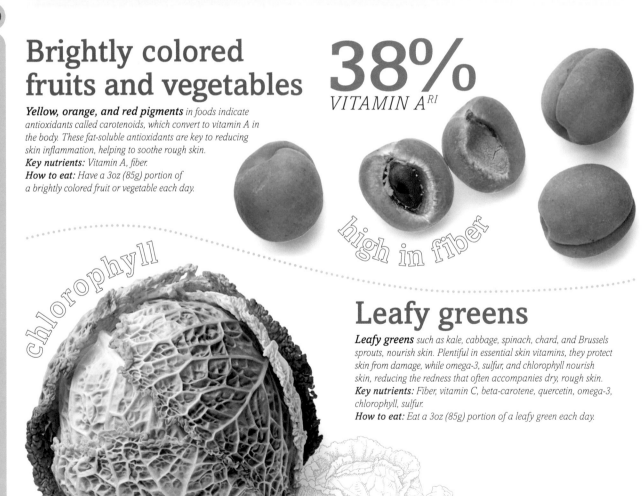

38%
VITAMIN A^{RI}

high in fiber

chlorophyll

Leafy greens

Leafy greens *such as kale, cabbage, spinach, chard, and Brussels sprouts, nourish skin. Plentiful in essential skin vitamins, they protect skin from damage, while omega-3, sulfur, and chlorophyll nourish skin, reducing the redness that often accompanies dry, rough skin.*
Key nutrients: *Fiber, vitamin C, beta-carotene, quercetin, omega-3, chlorophyll, sulfur.*
How to eat: *Eat a 3oz (85g) portion of a leafy green each day.*

Hemp seeds

These contain around 47 percent essential fatty acids, with a perfect ratio of omega fats. Hemp seeds inhibit prostaglandins, which helps to tackle inflammatory dry skin conditions.
Key nutrients: Omega-3, -6, and -9, gamma linolenic acid (GLA), protein, sulfur.
How to eat: Have up to 2 tbsp daily.

provide protein

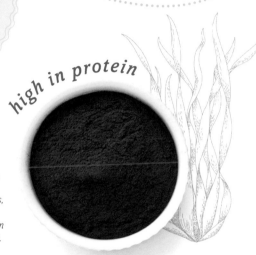

QUICK FIX

Up your "good" fats by adding hemp seeds to meals and desserts. Sprinkle seeds over breakfast muesli and oatmeal, toss a handful in with salads, and add to sweet treats.

Spirulina

high in protein

This algae powder has anti-inflammatory gamma linolenic acid (GLA), which soothes inflamed skin, detoxifying chlorophyll, antioxidants, and protein for skin cell renewal.
Key nutrients: Protein, antioxidants, fatty acids, B vitamins, calcium.
How to eat: Start with ¼ tsp daily in a meal or drink and build up to 1 tsp.

38%
*VITAMIN B1*RI

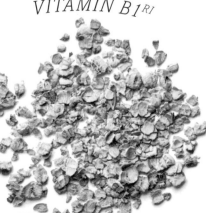

Oats

Rolled jumbo oats are packed with essential fats and minerals, including calcium, zinc, and silica, which the skin requires for repair. They contain B vitamins, beneficial for dry skin, and polysaccharides, which regulate blood sugar levels, while soluble fiber keeps the gut functioning efficiently, ensuring nutrients are circulated in the body to reach the skin.
Key nutrients: Vitamins B1, B5, B6, and E, folic acid, zinc, iron, calcium, magnesium, fiber.
How to eat: ¼–¾ cup daily as oatmeal or add to smoothies.

Chia seeds

These are the richest known vegetarian source of omega-3 fatty acids; flaxseeds are also a good source. Omega-3, which is often lacking in dry skin, helps to normalize fat levels in the skin, keeping skin cells strong and full of moisture. Omega-3 is also anti-inflammatory, helping to calm and smooth irritated skin.
Key nutrients: *Protein, omega-3, calcium, magnesium, iron, zinc, vitamins B, D, and E.*
How to eat: *Add 2–3 tsp daily to juices, smoothies, salad dressings, or oatmeal.*

Pumpkin seeds

These are also full of essential fatty acids, especially omega-3, vital for healthy skin, promoting repair and balancing sebum. They also contain plentiful supplies of antioxidant vitamin E, skin-repairing zinc, and protein. Sunflower seeds have similar nutrients.
Key nutrients: *Fatty acids, fiber, zinc, magnesium, protein, phytosterols.*
How to eat: *Snack on a small handful or sprinkle on oatmeal or salads.*

Avocado

This fruit has the highest healthy fat content, including monounsaturated fats, phytosterols, and omega-3, -6, and -9, all of which help to regenerate the skin and reduce redness and irritation that can result from dry skin. Lutein, a carotenoid contained in avocado, promotes skin hydration and elasticity, reducing the destruction of beneficial skin lipids.
Key nutrients: *Lutein, beta-carotene, omega-3, omega-9, vitamins A, B5, B6, C, D, E, and K, copper, folate, potassium.*
How to eat: *Have 1 medium avocado 2–4 times a week. Add to salads or mash on toast. The nutrients are near the skin, so peel an avocado like a banana to retain the top layer of flesh.*

Coconut oil

This is predominantly made up of healthy saturated fats called medium-chain triglycerides (MCTs). As well as being inherently moisturizing, coconut oil also helps to improve the body's utilization of omega-3 oils. Coconut oil is very stable as it is saturated, staying fresh for long periods even once opened, which is beneficial for the skin as rancid oils contribute to aging.
Key nutrients: *Medium-chain triglycerides.*
How to eat: *Use 2 tbsp daily, for cooking or simply adding to meals.*

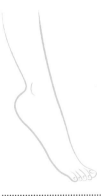

Perspiring feet

Excessive sweating of the feet, or hyperhidrosis, affects 3 percent of the population. An inherited problem with no known cause, it can lead to fungal infections and a bad smell. Eliminating red meat, processed carbohydrates, and yeast reduces body odor. Foods with zinc and leafy green vegetables have nutrients that inhibit odor-releasing compounds in the body, while foods with antifungal properties are also beneficial.

Superfood recipe suggestions...**Spiced apple oatmeal** p170 **Hemp seed butter** p172 **Huevos rancheros** p184 **Winter veggie slaw** p185 **Hot nuts!** p194 **Potato mash with veggie mix** p219 **Pineapple with cacao and coconut sauce** p228 **Sweet green ice cream** p229

Raw apple cider vinegar

Acidic until it's broken down in the digestive system, this condiment is thought to help rebalance the pH ratio in the body, which in turn can help to control body odor that can accompany sweaty feet. The vinegar also acts as a natural prebiotic, promoting a healthy gut, in turn helping to eliminate odor-causing toxins.
Key nutrients: Acetic acid.
How to eat: Dilute 1 tsp in water daily or incorporate into salad dressings.

PREBIOTIC

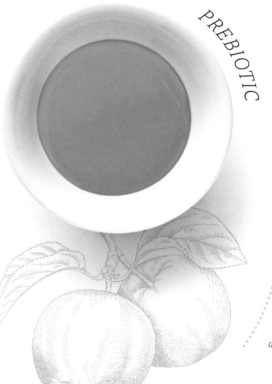

QUICK FIX

Combat foot odor with this salad. Combine 1 tbsp finely chopped sage with 3oz (85g) spinach. Add 1 tbsp sunflower seeds and drizzle with 1 tbsp combined apple cider vinegar and olive oil.

calcium
IRON

Sage

This herb, used traditionally to reduce excessive sweating, has been approved by the German health authorities for the treatment of hyperhidrosis.
Key nutrients: Vitamins A, B6, and C, calcium, iron, magnesium.
How to eat: Drink an infusion made with 1 tbsp of fresh sage or 1 tsp of dried sage 3 times daily and water; allow to cool before drinking. Avoid if pregnant.

Coconut oil

The oil extracted from the kernel *of coconuts contains saturated fats called medium-chain triglycerides (MCTs), which have antifungal properties that can help to promote healthy feet.*
Key nutrients: *MCTs.*
How to eat: *Add up to 2 tbsp to meals daily.*

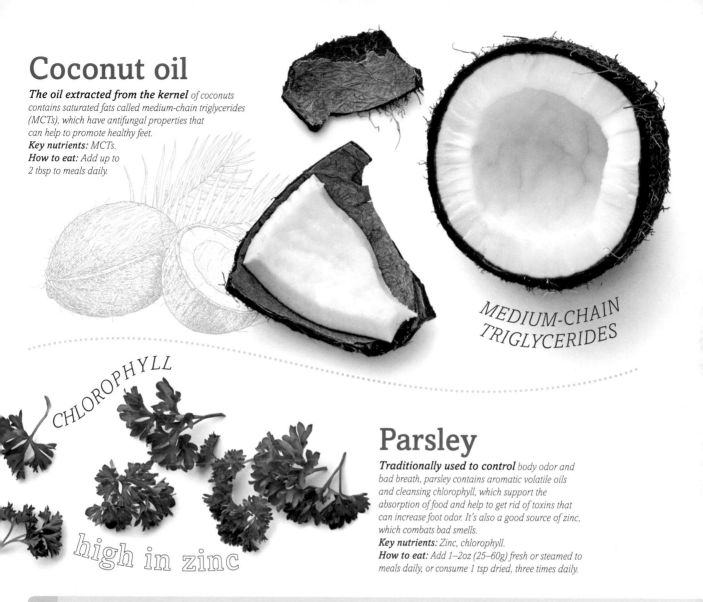

MEDIUM-CHAIN TRIGLYCERIDES

CHLOROPHYLL

high in zinc

Parsley

Traditionally used to control *body odor and bad breath, parsley contains aromatic volatile oils and cleansing chlorophyll, which support the absorption of food and help to get rid of toxins that can increase foot odor. It's also a good source of zinc, which combats bad smells.*
Key nutrients: *Zinc, chlorophyll.*
How to eat: *Add 1–2oz (25–60g) fresh or steamed to meals daily, or consume 1 tsp dried, three times daily.*

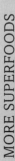

MORE SUPERFOODS

Green tea
Tannins make green tea antimicrobial, which supports digestion and immunity.
Key nutrients: *Antioxidants: catechins, and epigallocatechin gallate (EGCG), L-theanine.*
How to eat: *Drink 1–3 cups daily.*

Leafy greens
Chlorophyll binds to odor-causing compounds in the body, which are then neutralized and removed, controlling foot and body odor.
Key nutrients: *Fiber, chlorophyll, vitamin C, beta-carotene, quercetin, omega-3.*
How to eat: *Include kale, spinach, broccoli, or other leafy greens as one of your five a day.*

Fermented foods
Foods such as yogurt, sauerkraut, and kimchi repopulate the gut with friendly bacteria, which improves gut health and helps remove toxins.
Key nutrients: *Lactobacilli, Bifidobacteria.*
How to eat: *Add 1–2 tbsp to meals.*

Lemons
Lemons are rich in vitamin C, are astringent, helping to cleanse, and have an antimicrobial effect that helps to combat fungal infections.
Key nutrients: *Vitamin C.*
How to eat: *Kickstart the day with a hot water and fresh lemon juice to eliminate toxins from the body.*

Pumpkin seeds
Pumpkin and sunflower seeds are a great source of zinc and magnesium, a lack of which is thought to contribute to excessive sweating and body odor, including smelly feet.
Key nutrients: *Fatty acids, fiber, zinc, magnesium, protein, phytosterols.*
How to eat: *Add a handful to cereal or salads.*

Garlic
This contains an active substance known as allicin, that's produced when fresh garlic is crushed. Allicin is antimicrobial and antifungal.
Key nutrients: *Sulfur, selenium, vitamin B6.*
How to eat: *Have 1–2 cloves daily.*

Meal planner
Nail strengthening

Stress, a poor diet, and lifestyle choices weaken nails. The good news is that nails quickly respond to an improved diet. This meal plan uses recipes from the book and extra ideas to provide the nutrients for strong, glossy nails.

Your nail-strengthening week This nutritionally balanced one-week plan starts your nail-strengthening diet. For best results, continue for four weeks, using the alternatives, opposite, for variety. Start each day with a hot water and lemon drink to aid digestion.

Monday

Breakfast
Fruity chia jam (p.172) with rye bread

Snacks
Pineapple smoothie (p.239)

Lunch
Green salad with red onion and avocado

Dinner
Sweet potato and mackerel mash (p.219, variation)

Tuesday

Breakfast
Berry nice skin! (p.238)

Snacks
Grapefruit and pear drink (p.243) with a piece of rye bread

Lunch
Fava bean soup (p.182)

Dinner
Tomato salsa (p.212) with baked potato

Wednesday

Breakfast
Nutty overnight oats (p.168, variation)

Snacks
Protein power beauty bites (p.195)

Lunch
Crunchy apple, carrot, and radish salad

Dinner
Salmon with samphire (p.215)

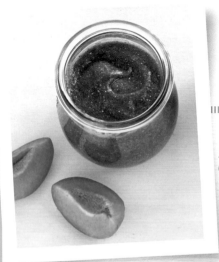

Fruity chia jam (p.172)

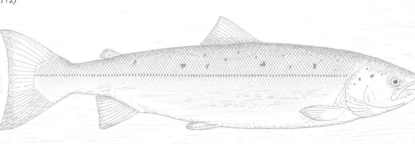

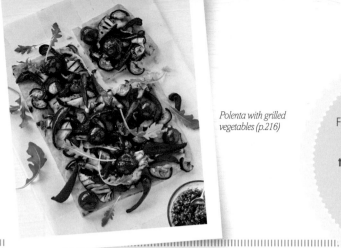

Polenta with grilled vegetables (p.216)

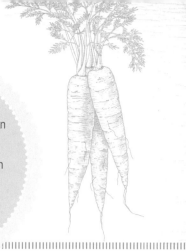

B VITAMIN

Foods that contain the B vitamin **biotin** are beneficial for nails, helping to **strengthen nail tissues**. Good sources of biotin include eggs, nuts such as almonds and walnuts, wild salmon, Swiss chard, and raspberries.

Thursday

Breakfast
Poached egg on rye bread

Snacks
Two slices of fresh pineapple with natural live yogurt

Lunch
Scrambled tofu (p.181)

Dinner
Polenta with grilled vegetables (p.216)

Friday

Breakfast
Cashew butter on rye bread

Snacks
Cherry tomatoes and carrot sticks with hummus

Lunch
Two-egg omelet with arugula and watercress

Dinner
Japanese ocean soup (p.201)

Saturday

Breakfast
Fruity quinoa breakfast (p.169)

Snacks
Natural live yogurt with berries

Lunch
Beet and chickpea soup (p.192)

Dinner
Salmon with coconut rice (p.215, variation)

Sweet treat
Salted goldenberry chocolate cups (p.224)

Sunday

Breakfast
Berry, seed, and nut granola (p.166)

Snacks
Two oat cakes with hummus and carrot sticks

Lunch
Potato mash with veggie mix (p.219)

Dinner
Thai chicken and noodle soup (p.214)

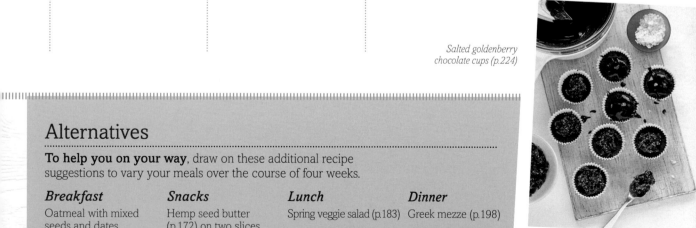

Salted goldenberry chocolate cups (p.224)

Alternatives

To help you on your way, draw on these additional recipe suggestions to vary your meals over the course of four weeks.

Breakfast
Oatmeal with mixed seeds and dates

Mango, pineapple, natural live yogurt, and seeds

Snacks
Hemp seed butter (p.172) on two slices of toasted rye bread

Lunch
Spring veggie salad (p.183)

Winter veggie slaw (p.185)

Dinner
Greek mezze (p.198)

Summer salad with pistachios and pomegranates (p.202)

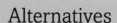

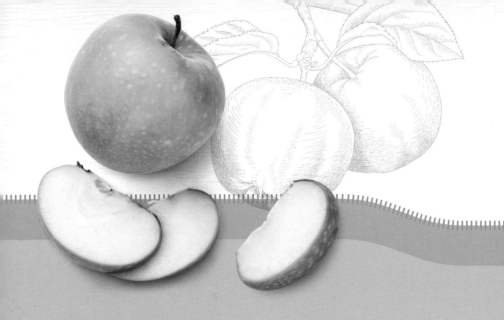

Foods
for the mouth

Your teeth, gums, and oral health are affected by the foods you put in your mouth and the nutrients these foods release once digested. Discover which foods can cleanse your mouth, and follow a specially tailored meal plan designed to provide the optimum nutrients for strong and healthy teeth and gums.

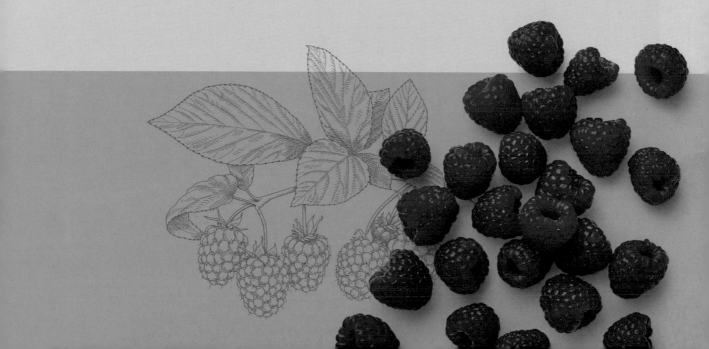

Eat for beauty: mouth

A radiant smile revealing **strong, clean teeth** and healthy-looking gums is supported by the good nutrients we eat daily. Discover which are the **top nutrients** for good oral health and how these help to keep your teeth and gums **refreshed**, strong, and looking like the picture of health.

Foods for the mouth

Before you explore the foods for specific beauty concerns in this chapter, find out why certain nutrients are key to oral health.

Silica This essential mineral has several important benefits for our teeth, gums, and general oral health. Silica supports the growth of the structural protein collagen in our bodies, which helps to keep the teeth and gums strong. It also helps to transport other nutrients to the peripheries of the body, which ensures that the gums and teeth are supplied with all the nutrients they need to stay strong and healthy. Silica is also essential for the absorption of calcium, a vital nutrient for our teeth. Try to include silica in your diet daily from sources such as whole-grain cereals, apples, cherries, almonds, oranges, oats, seeds, and fish.
Sulfur Known as the "beauty"

mineral, sulfur aids the absorption of protein to help build strong, healthy teeth. Good sources of this mineral are found in brassicas, such as broccoli, cauliflower, and Brussels sprouts, as well as in onions and garlic.

Calcium Our teeth and jaws are made up mostly of calcium, so it's crucial that we get sufficient calcium from our diets to help prevent gum disease and tooth decay developing. Good sources of this mineral are found in tofu, sardines, sesame seeds, yogurt, leafy greens, and cheese.

Iron This vital mineral is responsible for healthy red blood cells, which in turn ensure a good supply of nutrients to the gums. The top plant sources of iron include soybeans, lentils and legumes, leafy greens, sesame seeds, and olives. Meat is also

a top source of iron, although meat is acidic, which means it feeds unhealthy bacteria in the mouth, so eat this in moderation only.

Vitamins Vitamin C is essential for the formation of collagen, which holds tissues together, and even a small lack of this vitamin can weaken gums and cause them to bleed. Vitamin C is a water-soluble vitamin, so it isn't stored in the body, which means you need to include it in your diet daily. Excellent sources of vitamin C include berries, kiwi, citrus fruit, kale, and broccoli. Vitamin D helps the body absorb calcium, vital for teeth and gums. Most vitamin D is made in your body from sunlight, and it can be hard to get sufficient quantities from diet alone, so if sunlight is scarce a supplement is advised. Salmon, sardines, milk, eggs, and shiitake

Your teeth are often one of the first features others notice. Providing all the nutrients they need to stay strong will help you smile with confidence.

mushrooms provide some vitamin D. B vitamins, especially B3, B12, and B2, help with the formation of red blood cells, carrying nutrients to the teeth and gums. The best sources are leafy greens, nuts, seeds, whole grains, and legumes.

32%

of our daily vitamin D requirements are supplied by one egg.

Antioxidants A group of antioxidants called anthocyanins helps to prevent harmful bacteria from colonizing the mouth and teeth. Good food sources include blueberries, grapes, red cabbage, black rice, and raspberries. Another group of antioxidants, polyphenols, helps to reduce unhealthy bacteria in the mouth. Polyphenols called catechins are found in green tea and matcha, so drink these regularly to support the teeth and gums.

Co-enzyme Q10 This enzyme enhances blood flow in the body, ensuring that nutrients reach the tissues in the mouth. A deficiency in this enzyme is thought to play a role in the development of periodontal disease. Good food sources include oily fish, sesame seeds, pistachios, broccoli, cauliflower, and strawberries.

Probiotics Foods that contain "good" bacteria help to support a healthy gut flora, which in turn provides a boost to our immune system. Including probiotics in your diet is thought to decrease plaque and gum disease, or gingivitis, as the healthy bacteria in fermented foods suppress the growth of pathogens in the gaps between teeth. Prebiotics can be used alongside probiotics since these help good gut bacteria to thrive. Raise your intake of probiotics by including natural live yogurt and fermented foods such as kefir, saukerkraut, and miso. Prebiotic foods include raw asparagus, garlic, leeks, and onions.

Hydration Staying hydrated is vital for the healthy functioning of every part of your body, including the teeth and gums. Aim to drink up to 2 liters of water daily, and remember that you can increase hydration levels by eating foods with a high water content, such as watermelon, celery, and cucumber.

What affects our mouth?

The mucosal cells in our mouth are renewed frequently, which means that nutrient shortfalls often show up in the mouth first. Problems such as bleeding gums and cracking at the corners of the mouth can be the first indication of a nutritional deficiency in the body, pointing to low levels of nutrients such as vitamins C and B2. Life events such as pregnancy and periods of illness can put added stress on nutrient supplies and impact the health of teeth and gums. Knowing which foods to avoid and which ones help to cleanse the mouth will enable you to support the teeth and gums.

Diet and lifestyle Cavities are caused by regularly eating high-sugar foods and drinking sugary drinks. Sipping sugary drinks means that teeth get repeatedly coated in sugar. Sugar is highly acidic and can leach minerals from the teeth, and energy drinks are especially damaging because they combine a high-sugar content with a very acidic pH. Try to cut out sugars, or avoid refined and highly processed ones, which are low in minerals, and replace with alternatives such as maple syrup (in moderation). Try to replace sugary carbonated drinks with water or a mineral-rich vegetable juice.

Sticky, chewy foods are hard for saliva to wash away and end up sticking to the teeth, providing a breeding ground for bacteria. Alcohol exacerbtes this by reducing the flow of saliva. Try to stop or limit alcohol consumption to below the recommended 5 drinks a week, and avoid foods that stick to teeth, such as raisins.

Carbonated drinks and citrus fruits soften enamel, making it

Eat for your age

Our teeth grow as we do, so nutrients are vital to supply the building materials for them to develop healthfully. Cavities are common in our 20s; as we age, collagen production, needed for strong teeth, slows and we become less efficient at absorbing nutrients. Providing nutrients for healthy teeth for our lifespan is vital. A multivitamin and mineral supplement is helpful, and from our 50s, you can try co-enyzme Q10 and olive leaf supplements.

In your 20s

Collagen production is plentiful during your 20s, which supports the teeth and gums. However, in our 20s we are often less conscious of the need to look after our teeth and gums: our diet may be sugar-rich and lacking key nutrients and we may brush our teeth irregularly, sometimes neglecting to brush teeth before going to bed, which can make teeth prone to cavitites.

Eat: Eat brightly colored veggies and fruit for a range of antioxidants. Oily fish, eggs, and shiitake mushrooms supply vitamin D. Include healthy proteins from eggs, fish, legumes, nuts, seeds, and lean meat.

In your 30s

One of the most common problems during this decade is sensitive teeth, often caused by brushing teeth too hard so that the dentine under the enamel is exposed and gums start to recede. Gum infection (gingivitis) can also cause the gums to pull back. If you're pregnant, you are especially prone to gum disease as gums soften, so it's essential to ensure you have an adequate supply of nutrients to support teeth and gums now.

Eat: Healthy proteins to support collagen, from fish, eggs, legumes, nuts and seeds, and lean meat. Include antioxidant-rich, brightly colored fruits and vegetables.

75%

of the vitamin C we need each day is met by 1 cup of raw broccoli.

more prone to discoloration; coffee, tea, and red wine can also discolor enamel.

A diet that includes plenty of whole foods will provide essential nutrients to support the teeth and

gums. Raw vegetables are loaded with nutrients often destroyed with cooking that help to clean your teeth and prevent discoloration by encouraging saliva to flow and clear away foods.

Pregnancy Hormonal changes during pregnancy can soften and swell gums, making them prone to bleeding and gum disease, so it's important to eat healthy, nutrient-rich whole foods now to support the health of your teeth and gums.

Illness A period of illness can also compromise oral health because nutrients can be used up by other parts of the body that are directly affected. Avoiding sugar and eating an unrefined, varied diet with raw vegetables will give your body a good foundation of nutrients during these times.

In your 40s

Our tooth enamel is porous and discoloration often becomes more apparent during our 40s as the long-term effects of sipping tea, coffee, and red wine take effect. Fillings in your mouth may start to wear down now and become lose or crack, which means that bacteria can set in in the cavities, so frequent checkups are important to avoid problems escalating.
Eat: Raw, crunchy vegetables to encourage saliva flow. Include healthy fats and proteins from fish, lean meat, nuts and seeds, and legumes.

In your 50s

Receding gums may be more of a problem during our 50s as the micocirculation to the gums decreases and plaque build-up increases. Gums may become more swollen and there may be gaps where gums separate from teeth, allowing bacteria to settle. Hormonal changes around this time can also accelerate gum disease. Saliva production starts to decrease, making it harder to wash away bacteria.
Eat: Foods that contain the co-enzyme Q10, which can fight gum disease, found in oily fish, cauliflower, sesame seeds, broccoli, and strawberries.

60s plus

As we get older, taste buds change and foods may become less flavorful, which means we can be tempted to add sugar and salt to increase flavor. Medications can reduce saliva production, which also continues to drop naturally with age. Enamel may wear away more now, leaving teeth increasingly susceptible to discoloration and damage.
Eat: Healthy fats and proteins from sources such as oily fish, lean meat, legumes, nuts and seeds, and eggs. Leafy greens and colorful fruit and vegetables supply essential nutrients.

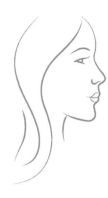

Discolored teeth

Smoking and drinking tea, coffee, red wine, and soft drinks can discolor teeth, and over time stains can set in the cracks and crevices in enamel. Pigments called chromogens that cling to enamel and tannins in drinks such as red wine stain teeth, while acids soften enamel, making it easier to stain. Hydrating fruits and vegetables stimulate saliva to wash bacteria away, and some foods have an abrasive texture that helps to lift staining substances.

Superfood recipe suggestions...**Berry, seed, and nut granola** p166   **Spiced apple oatmeal** p170
Winter veggie slaw p185   **Hot nuts!** p194   **Roasted broccoli and cauliflower with couscous** p206   **Nutty rice salad** p220

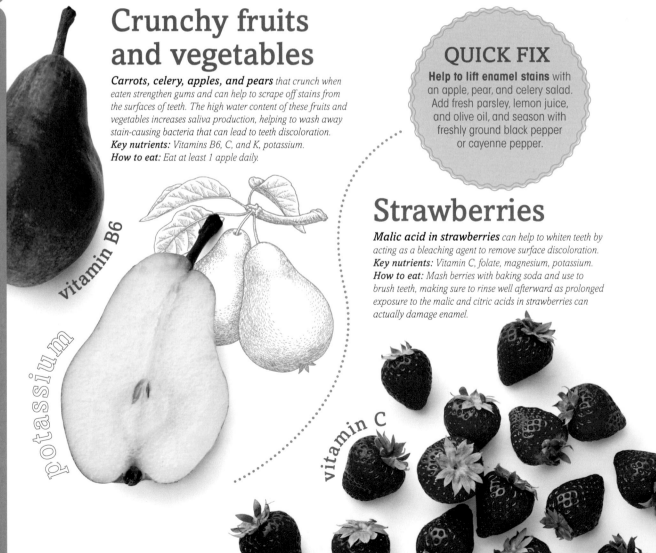

Crunchy fruits and vegetables

Carrots, celery, apples, and pears that crunch when eaten strengthen gums and can help to scrape off stains from the surfaces of teeth. The high water content of these fruits and vegetables increases saliva production, helping to wash away stain-causing bacteria that can lead to teeth discoloration.
Key nutrients: *Vitamins B6, C, and K, potassium.*
How to eat: *Eat at least 1 apple daily.*

vitamin B6

potassium

QUICK FIX

Help to lift enamel stains with an apple, pear, and celery salad. Add fresh parsley, lemon juice, and olive oil, and season with freshly ground black pepper or cayenne pepper.

Strawberries

Malic acid in strawberries can help to whiten teeth by acting as a bleaching agent to remove surface discoloration.
Key nutrients: *Vitamin C, folate, magnesium, potassium.*
How to eat: *Mash berries with baking soda and use to brush teeth, making sure to rinse well afterward as prolonged exposure to the malic and citric acids in strawberries can actually damage enamel.*

vitamin C

Crunchy veggies

Crunchy vegetables, *such as cauliflower and carrots, can help to clean teeth as the chewing action required to break them down gives teeth a natural scrub, helping to remove food lurking in cracks. The vitamin C in cauliflower also promotes collagen to help keep teeth strong.*
Key nutrients: *Vitamin C, folate, magnesium.*
How to eat: *Have a 3oz (85g) portion of a crunchy vegetable 4–5 times a week.*

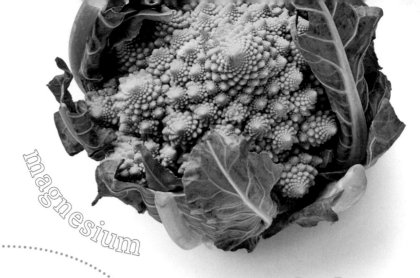

magnesium

Nuts and seeds

The abrasive texture *of nuts and seeds works to remove stains by exfoliation. However, beware of hard nuts that may break teeth if eaten whole. Nuts also provide important minerals for teeth health.*
Key nutrients: *Calcium, phosphorus, magnesium, potassium, zinc.*
How to eat: *Have a handful of chopped nuts daily.*

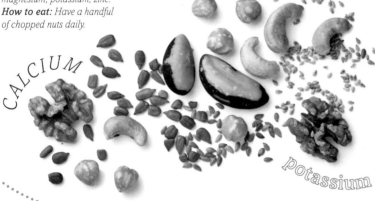

CALCIUM

potassium

38%
VITAMIN C ^RI

MORE SUPERFOODS

Coconut oil
The ancient Indian Ayurvedic practice of "oil pulling"—swishing coconut oil around the mouth after tooth brushing—has recently been revived after studies demonstrated that it could be effective in whitening teeth and reducing gum disease and plaque formation. The lauric acid in the oil has proven antimicrobial and anti-inflammatory effects, and is thought to be responsible for the beneficial effects.
Key nutrients: *Medium-chain triglycerides, lauric acid, caprylic acid.*
How to eat: *Swill 1 tsp around the mouth for several minutes then spit out.*

Mint
Chewing on fresh mint can be a helpful after-dinner cleaner for teeth. As well as being a natural breath freshener, mint has antiseptic properties that can help to clean and refresh the mouth. Chewing on herbs also helps to increase saliva production in the mouth, helping to wash away food and liquids that if left sitting on the teeth can lead to discoloration. Chewing on parsley can also be beneficial.
Key nutrients: *Folate, calcium, vitamin B2, potassium.*
How to eat: *Chew on a couple of mint leaves. Also add to salads and meals. Rinse your mouth with water after chewing.*

Natural live yogurt

vitamin B2

Unsweetened yogurt *has bacteria that helps to reduce levels of plaque and the gum disease gingivitis, and also to lower bad breath–causing hydrogen sulfide levels. Yogurt also helps to increase saliva production to wash away foods and bacteria, and its high calcium levels fortify enamel.*
Key nutrients: *Calcium, protein, vitamin B2.*
How to eat: *Have a ½-cup serving of yogurt daily.*

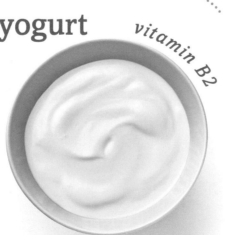

10 ways to... Make smart swaps

It can be easier to spot problems with your diet than to solve them.

A food diary (see pp.94–95) is a great way to highlight foods and eating habits that are detrimental to your health and beauty—once you've identified problem areas, start swapping in healthy options. It's easy to find delicious alternatives so you don't feel deprived. Start making easy swaps to supercharge your diet with all the nutrients you need for a more beautiful you.

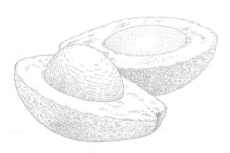

1 Swap sugars

Sugar can aggravate inflamed skin and exacerbate aging, causing the breakdown of the skin proteins collagen and elastin that leads to sagging and fine lines. Choose alternative, minimally processed sweeteners, such as maple syrup, raw honey, molasses, or dates. Stevia is also a good option, as it is much sweeter than sugar, so you need to use only a tiny amount, and it doesn't affect your blood sugar levels.

2 Avoid soft drinks

Soft drinks often contain extremely high levels of added sugar, which can lead to enamel erosion and cavities in your teeth. "Diet" soft drinks are often sweetened with aspartame, an artificial sweetener that can cause skin irritation similar to eczema. Instead, drink water or naturally flavored teas, such as green, matcha, high in anti-aging antioxidants, or herbal teas.

6 Include good fats

Good fats are essential for healthy, glowing skin. Fat also helps your body absorb protective antioxidants and vitamins, strengthens cell membranes, and helps to keep the skin moisturized. Make sure that you include plenty of foods that are rich in healthy omega fats, such as nuts, seeds, oily and cold-water fish, and leafy greens. Choose dairy products from organic, grass-fed animals, as these contain high levels of omega fats.

7 Check gluten

If you're gluten-intolerant, foods containing gluten may cause you to experience digestive issues, inflammation, and skin problems including acne. Choose ancient grains, such as spelt and kamut, in place of pasta, bread, or cereal. These foods contain different forms of gluten from more modern cereals, so they can be easier to digest for those with an intolerance.

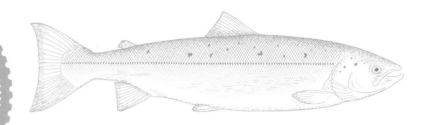

3 Minimize salt

Minimize seep salt consumption. Apart from its effects on blood pressure, too much salt encourages the body to hold onto fluids, causing bloating. Opt for unprocessed, mineral-rich varieties of salt for seasoning. Table salt is rock salt that has been processed and refined, removing beneficial minerals, whereas Himalayan pink salt is toxin-free and packed with minerals to support skin and teeth health.

4 Choose whole grains

Refined carbohydrates, such as white bread, white rice, and pasta, have been stripped of many of their natural nutrients and much of their fiber. These foods provide minimal beauty-boosting nutrients, and will also leave you feeling hungry shortly after eating. Swap these for fiber- and nutrient-rich whole grains, such as brown or black rice, oats, quinoa, or buckwheat.

5 Cook with healthy oils

Hydrogenated and trans fats, including margarine and hydrogenated vegetable oils, promote inflammation and can accelerate skin aging. Avoid cooking with these and opt instead to cook only with unrefined coconut oil. Other cold-pressed plant oils, such as flax, hemp, olive, avocado, coconut, and pumpkin seed can be added to food. These keep your skin nourished and reduce the risk of inflammation and irregular pigmentation.

8 Make your own meals

Premade and takeout foods are usually packed with salt, sugar, and fat, and lacking in nutrients. Cook large batches of food over the weekend, and freeze in individual portions to create your own premade meals. This way, you can control what you're eating and how much, ensuring that your meals are packed with whole grains, fresh fruits and vegetables, lean proteins, and healthy fats.

9 Snack healthily

Keep healthy snacks on hand, so that you're not tempted to reach for a chocolate bar or a package of chips when hunger strikes. Avoid buying unhealthy snacks when you shop, and clear out your cupboards to remove temptation. Choose nutritious light bites or snacks to tide you over until your next meal—vegetable crudités with hummus or oat cakes with nut butter are both good choices.

10 Check dairy

Commercially produced milks often contain hormones that can cause your skin to become oily, so if you are experiencing skin issues it can be a good idea to limit or cut out dairy products. Try using nut, seed, or oat milks in place of animal milks. Coconut yogurt is also a good, dairy-free option. Many people are unknowingly allergic or intolerant to proteins in animal milks—try keeping a food diary to check your food sensitivities (see pp.94–95).

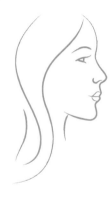

Weakened teeth

Tooth decay occurs when acids erode the enamel on teeth. Sugary, acidic, soft, and fruity drinks, a high-carbohydrate diet, acid reflux, and genetics can all lead to tooth erosion. A balanced diet supplies the essential nutrients required to promote healthy teeth. Many basic nutrients, including vitamins A, C, and D, and minerals such as calcium and phosphorus, are vital for oral health and maintaining strong teeth.

Superfood recipe suggestions...**Overnight oats with superberry compote** p168 **Fall flavors soup** p178 **Winter veggie slaw** p185 **Salmon pâté** p193 **Potato mash with veggie mix** p219 **Matcha latte** p236 **Vitamin C boost** p245

Camu camu

The fruit and leaves of Peruvian camu camu have traditionally been used to treat gum and teeth problems. It is high in vitamin C, essential for healthy gums and for reducing the incidence of bleeding gums and gingivitis, in turn promoting healthy teeth.
Key nutrients: *Iron, vitamins B1 and B2, phosphorus, potassium, beta-carotene, calcium, amino acids.*
How to eat: *Add 1 tsp of powder to smoothies or juices.*

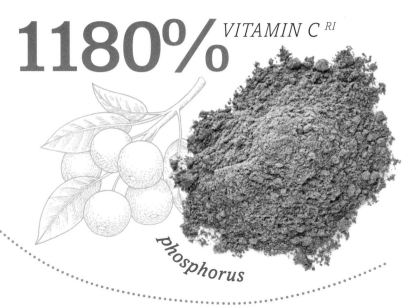

1180% *VITAMIN C* RI

phosphorus

vitamin C

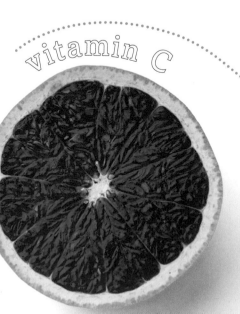

Citrus fruits

Although acidic, *citrus fruit increases saliva flow. While the acidity can be damaging to enamel, the fruits contain a lot of water, so help to wash away bacteria.*
Key nutrients: *Vitamins A, B1, B5, and C, folate, potassium, copper, calcium.*
How to eat: *Try to eat at least 2 servings of citrus fruit weekly.*

QUICK FIX

Make a **vitamin C– and calcium-boosting** fruit salad. Mix raspberries, strawberries, blackberries, and blueberries with natural live yogurt, then top with a good squeeze of lemon juice.

Oily fish

Foods high in omega-3 fatty acids
such as salmon, mackerel, trout, and other oily fish, reduce inflammation and may protect against gum disease.
Key nutrients: *Vitamin B12, omega-3.*
How to eat: *Eat a 5½oz (150g) portion of oily fish 2–3 times a week.*

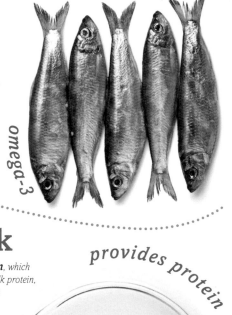

omega-3

Organic milk

Milk encourages saliva production, *which neutralizes mouth acids, while casein, a milk protein, coats enamel to protect it from acids. Calcium and phosphorus also strengthen the teeth.*
Key nutrients: *Calcium, potassium, protein, iodine, phosphorus, vitamins B2 and B12.*
How to drink: *Have a glass of milk daily.*

provides protein

25%
CALCIUM *RI*

16%
VITAMIN C *RI*

Berries

All types of berries *are high in vitamin C, essential for collagen production. Collagen helps to strengthen gums and teeth. An important connective tissue, it also helps to prevent root decay, gum inflammation, and tooth sensitivity. Vitamin C also inhibits the formation of plaque and tartar.*
Key nutrients: *Flavonoids, vitamins C and E, omega-3, potassium, magnesium.*
How to eat: *Eat 2 handfuls of berries every day.*

potassium
FLAVONOIDS

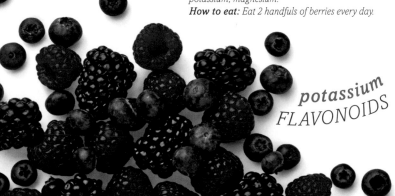

Carrots
These are high in antioxidant beta-carotene, which converts to vitamin A in the body. Vitamin A helps to promote strong bones and teeth. Carrots also provide vitamin C, which promotes healthy collagen production, in turn supporting the teeth and gum tissues. Other brightly colored vegetables such as sweet potatoes and squash are a source of beta-carotene.
Key nutrients: *Beta-carotene, vitamins B, C, E, and K, fiber, molybdenum, potassium.*
How to eat: *Eat ½ a medium-sized carrot daily as a snack or add to a salad or soup, or a juice or smoothie.*

Matcha
Drinking matcha (powdered green tea) is thought to help promote healthy, strong teeth and gums by reducing periodontal disease. The high levels of the antioxidant catechin in green tea are thought to help reduce inflammation of the gums. This in turn hampers the growth of the bacteria that leads to periodontal diseases.
Key nutrients: *Polyphenols, vitamin A.*
How to drink: *Add 1 scant tsp of matcha powder daily to drinks.*

Coconut oil
The practice of "oil pulling," whereby a small quantity of coconut oil is swished around the mouth for a few minutes and then spat out, is thought to literally pull toxins from the oral cavity. The medium-chain triglyceride (MCT) lauric acid, which makes up around 50 percent of coconut oil, is known to attack harmful bacteria that lurk in cavities in the mouth. Pulling with coconut oil has been shown to reduce the bacterium Streptococcus mutans, *which results in tooth cavities and plaque-induced gingivitis, or gum disease.*
Key nutrients: *MCTs, caprylic acid.*
How to eat: *Swill 1 tsp coconut oil around the mouth after brushing teeth, then spit out.*

Egg yolk
This is one of the best dietary sources of vitamin D. Vitamin D is metabolized in the body into a substance called calcitriol, which then helps the body to absorb calcium, an essential mineral for maintaining strong teeth.
Key nutrients: *Protein, vitamins B2, B12, and D, phosphorus.*
How to eat: *Eat an egg daily, poached or boiled for breakfast, lunch, or as a snack.*

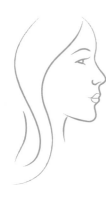

Coated tongue

The condition of our tongues can reveal our state of health, nutritional status, and even stress levels. For example, a whitish-yellow coating on the tongue may be a sign of dehydration. A healthy tongue should be pink in color, slightly moist, smooth with no spots, but layered with visible taste buds. Foods that are high in calcium and vitamins C and D can keep the mouth tissues healthy to boost oral health.

Superfood recipe suggestions...Overnight oats with superberry compote p168   Spiced apple oatmeal p170
Huevos rancheros p184   Summer asparagus salad p189   Greek vegetable mezze p198   Red berry smoothie p235

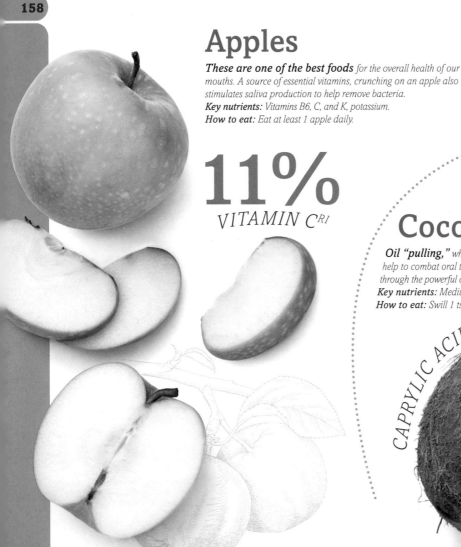

Apples

These are one of the best foods *for the overall health of our mouths. A source of essential vitamins, crunching on an apple also stimulates saliva production to help remove bacteria.*
Key nutrients: *Vitamins B6, C, and K, potassium.*
How to eat: *Eat at least 1 apple daily.*

11%
VITAMIN C[RI]

QUICK FIX

Cleanse the mouth with a crunchy salad. Core and slice 1 green apple. Peel and slice a shallot, then cook with 1 tsp coconut oil for five minutes. Mix with the apple and a squeeze of lemon juice.

Coconut oil

Oil "pulling," *where coconut oil is swished around the mouth, can help to combat oral thrush by collecting and trapping pathogens and through the powerful antifungal properties of caprylic acid in coconut oil.*
Key nutrients: *Medium-chain triglycerides (MCTs), caprylic acid.*
How to eat: *Swill 1 tsp around the mouth, then spit out.*

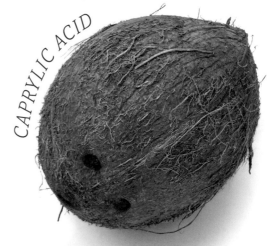

CAPRYLIC ACID

Berries

The high vitamin C content *in berries helps the body to fight off infections, and to combat yeasts such as candida that cause oral thrush. Bleeding gums are often the result of a lack of vitamin C, which helps maintain strong mouth tissue and capillaries.*
Key nutrients: *Vitamin C, potassium.*
How to eat: *Eat 2 handfuls of berries daily.*

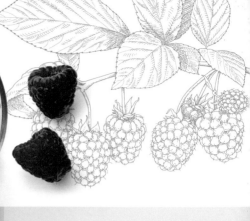

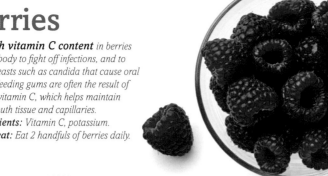

Eggs

The vitamin D *in egg yolk is essential for the absorption of calcium, which helps to keep our teeth strong and promotes good oral health.*
Key nutrients: *Protein, vitamins B2, B12 and D, phosphorus.*
How to eat: *Eat a poached or boiled egg daily for breakfast, lunch, or as a snack.*

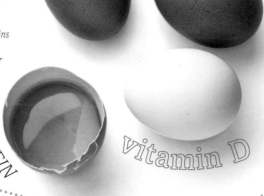

PROTEIN

vitamin D

Garlic

Fresh garlic, *known for its antifungal and antimicrobial action, can be effective in destroying the yeast candida in the body, which thrives in the mouth as oral thrush, forming a white, curdlike deposit on the tongue. Allicin, the active ingredient in garlic, helps to combat the yeast.*
Key nutrients: *Sulfur, selenium, vitamins B6 and C.*
How to eat: *Chew a clove of garlic or add 1–2 cloves crushed garlic to salads, dressings, and meals.*

vitamins B6 and C

SULFUR

21%
VITAMIN C RI

MORE SUPERFOODS

Green leafy vegetables
Leafy vegetables, such as kale, Swiss chard, and spinach, provide chlorophyll, which is thought to help combat the bad breath that can sometimes be an added symptom of a furry, unhealthy-looking tongue.
Key nutrients: *Chlorophyll, fiber, vitamins C and E, omega-3, beta-carotene, quercetin.*
How to eat: *Have a 3oz (85g) portion of green leafy vegetables daily with meals.*

Camu camu
The high vitamin C content of the camu camu fruit can help to combat the yeastlike fungus candida, which can cause a furry tongue. Camu camu also contains amino acids that help the body to absorb vitamin C, essential for healthy tissues.
Key nutrients: *Beta-carotene, vitamins B2, B3, and C, phosphorus, iron, potassium, calcium, amino acids.*
How to eat: *Have 1 tsp of fruit powder a day, added to oatmeal, meals, or smoothies.*

Natural live yogurt
Probiotics, the living microorganisms found in natural live yogurt, help to fight yeast infections. When the mouth environment has an imbalance of certain microorganisms, this is thought to result in a white tongue. Probiotic bacteria can help to control the growth of bacteria and fungi in the mouth.
Key nutrients: *Calcium, potassium, vitamin D.*
How to eat: *Eat a small pot daily for breakfast or mix into a smoothie.*

Spirulina
As with leafy greens, this microalgae contains chlorophyll, which can combat bad breath that may accompany a furry tongue.
Key nutrients: *Protein, antioxidants, fatty acids, B vitamins, calcium, chlorophyll.*
How to eat: *Start with ¼ tsp daily in a meal or drink and build up to 1 tsp.*

Meal planner
Healthy teeth and gums

Nutrient shortfalls or excesses quickly show up in mouth tissue. This meal plan, using recipes from the book and meal ideas, draws on whole foods, lean meats, and healthy fats to support teeth, gums, and oral health.

Your healthy mouth week Use this nutritionally balanced one-week meal plan to start you off on your healthy teeth and gums diet. For best results, continue for four weeks, using the alternatives, opposite, for variety. Start each day with a hot water and lemon drink to aid digestion.

Monday

Breakfast
Berry, seed, and nut granola (p.166)

Snacks
Sweet garden pea dip (p.190) with carrot sticks

Lunch
Broiled sardines on whole-wheat toast with green salad

Dinner
Baked stuffed squash (p.203)

Tuesday

Breakfast
Green smoothie (p.244)

Snacks
Slices of apple with nut butter with cup of green tea

Lunch
Spring veggie salad (p.183)

Dinner
Miso-glazed tofu with quinoa (p.218)

Wednesday

Breakfast
Poached egg on rye bread and an apple

Snacks
Handful of Hot nuts! (p.194) and a pear

Lunch
Crunchy apple, carrot, and radish salad

Dinner
Salmon with samphire (p.215)

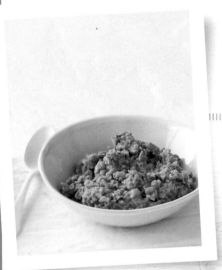

Sweet garden pea dip (p.190)

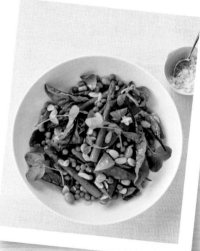

Spring veggie salad (p.183)

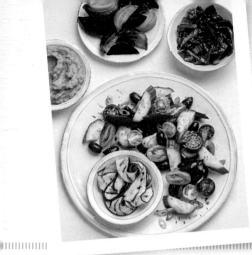

Greek vegetable mezze (p.198)

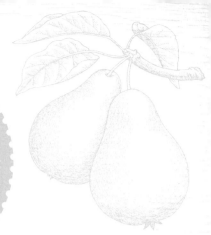

Thursday

Breakfast
Fruit salad with natural live yogurt

Snacks
Corn cakes with hummus and a pear

Lunch
Cannellini beans with bok choy, arugula, cherry tomatoes, and olives

Dinner
Greek vegetable mezze (p.198)

Friday

Breakfast
Fruity quinoa breakfast (p.169)

Snacks
Oat cakes with nut butter and apple slices

Lunch
Two-egg omelet with green salad

Dinner
Salmon with coconut rice (p.215, variation)

Saturday

Breakfast
Poached egg on rye bread

Snacks
Natural live yogurt with berries

Lunch
Cold chicken and raw veggie salad

Dinner
Black lentil and coconut curry (p.204)

Sunday

Breakfast
Blueberry and chia pancakes (p.171)

Snacks
Red berry smoothie (p.235)

Lunch
Winter veggie slaw (p.185)

Dinner
Rice salad (p.220, variation)

Sweet treat
Salted goldenberry chocolate cups (p.224)

Alternatives

To help you on your way, draw on these additional recipe suggestions to vary your meals over the course of four weeks.

Breakfast
Yogurt with apricots

Rye bread with nut butter

Snacks
Avocado on toast (p.180)

Lunch
Zucchini noodles with basil pesto (p.186)

Scrambled tofu (p.181)

Dinner
Japanese ocean soup (p.201)

Sweet potato, mackerel mash (p.219, variation)

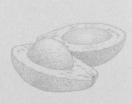

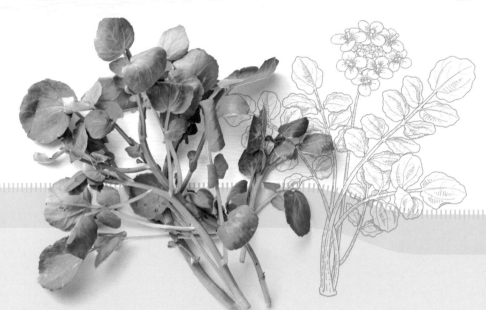

Recipes

for the whole day

Eat for beauty every day. These delicious, nutrient-packed recipes, each one targeting specific beauty concerns, will inspire you to include the top beauty foods in all your meals. Revitalizing breakfasts, nutrient-rich light bites and dinners, super-healthy sweet treats, and full-of-goodness drinks will all help you glow from the inside out.

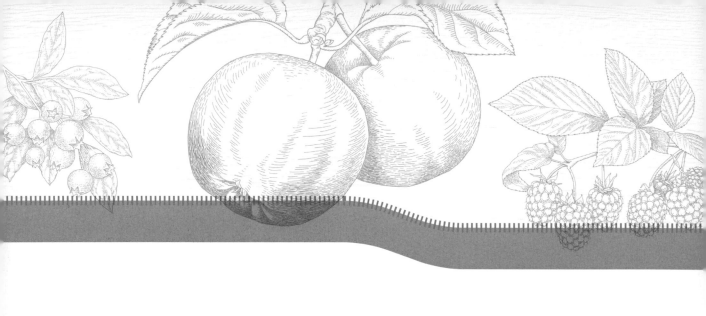

...for Breakfast

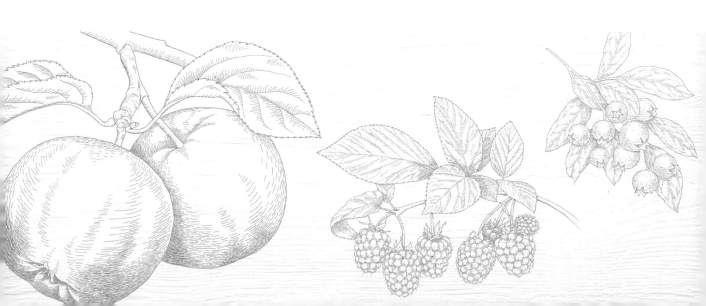

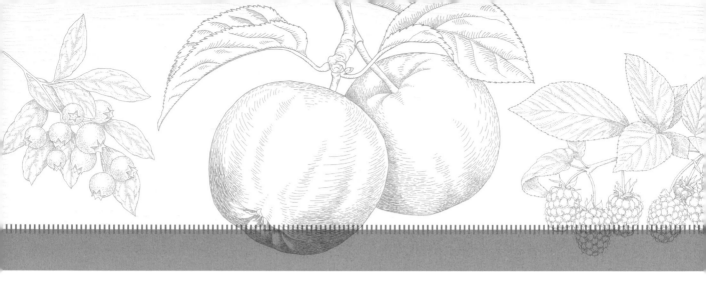

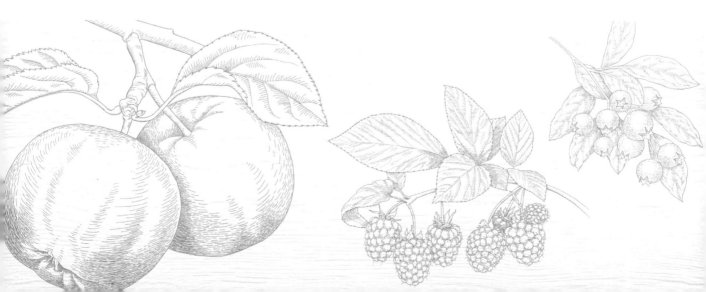

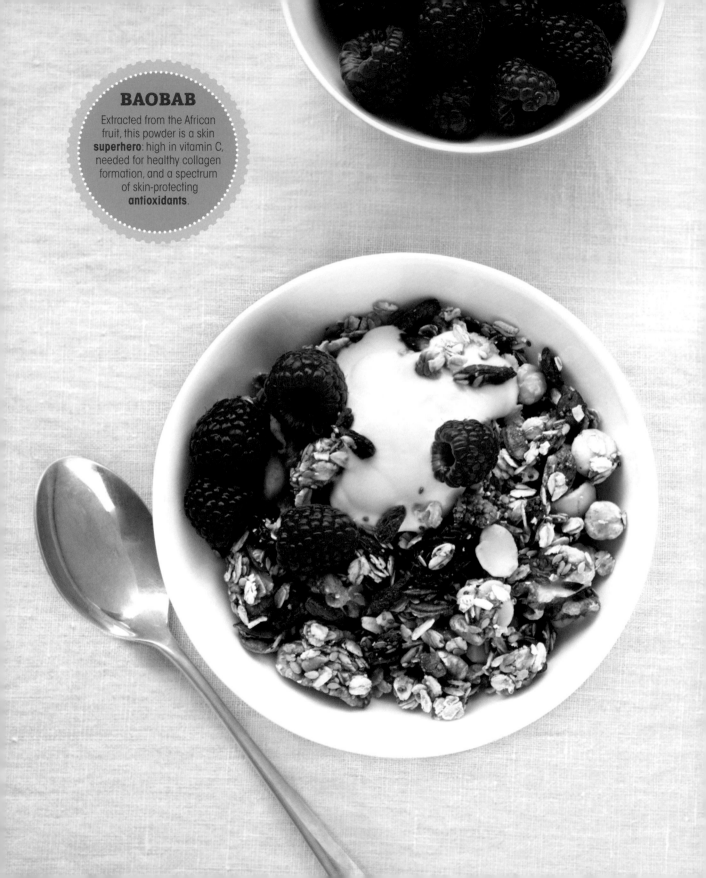

BAOBAB

Extracted from the African fruit, this powder is a skin **superhero**: high in vitamin C, needed for healthy collagen formation, and a spectrum of skin-protecting **antioxidants**.

ANTI-AGING   SKIN SMOOTHING   SKIN BALANCING   HAIR CONDITIONING   HEALTHY TEETH & GUMS   NAIL STRENGTHENING

Berry, seed, and nut granola

This heavenly granola is loaded with all the **essentials** for healthy skin—**restorative** fatty acids to keep fine lines at bay, **antioxidant-packed** berries, and vital minerals.

Makes 16 servings   Prep time: 10 mins   Cook time: 10–15 mins, plus cooling

Ingredients

⅔ cup honey (ideally raw or organic)

3 tsp lucuma powder

1 tsp ground turmeric

3 tsp baobab powder

3 cups rolled oats

⅓ cup sunflower seeds

¾ cup pumpkin seeds

½ cup walnuts

½ cup hazelnuts

¼ cup chia seeds

¼ cup flaxseeds

½ cup macadamia nuts

½ cup combined goji berries, mulberries, and chopped goldenberries

3 tbsp hemp seeds (shelled)

5 tsp bee pollen

natural live yogurt, raspberries (optional), and green tea (optional) to serve

How to make

1 Preheat the oven to 300°F (150°C). Gently heat the honey until it is a runnier consistency. Combine the honey, lucuma, turmeric, and baobab in a bowl, then transfer the mixture to a larger mixing bowl. Add all the other ingredients, except for the bee pollen and hemp seeds, and stir thoroughly.

2 Spread the granola mix evenly on a large baking sheet. Bake in the oven for 10–15 minutes, until golden brown, turning the mixture halfway through.

3 Remove the granola from the oven and sprinkle the hemp seeds and bee pollen over it.

4 Let the granola cool, then transfer to an airtight jar. Serve with natural live yogurt and, if you like, a few raspberries and a nice cup of green tea. The granola will keep for up to 3 weeks.

Nutritional information per serving:

Cals 230   Fat 13g   Saturated fat 1.5g   Carbohydrates 20g   Sugar 7g
Salt trace   Fiber 4.5g   Protein 6g   Cholesterol 0mg

ANTI-AGING

SKIN SMOOTHING

SKIN CALMING

HAIR CONDITIONING

NAIL STRENGTHENING

CHIA SEEDS

One of the top sources of **omega-3**, essential for nourishing skin, chia seeds are also high in **fiber**, promoting the healthy elimination of toxins.

Overnight oats with superberry compote

This soothing breakfast is a beauty treat. **Nutrient-rich** berries provide an **antioxidant boost** for radiant skin, while oats supply silica and calcium, both essential for healthy hair and strong nails.

Serves 2 **Prep time: 5 mins, plus soaking**

Ingredients

½ cup oat milk, plus a bit extra for serving (optional)

¼ cup coconut milk

1 cup organic jumbo oats

1½ cups mixed berries (fresh or frozen)

4 tsp omega-3, -6, -9 oil supplement (optional)

1 tbsp pumpkin seeds per serving

2 tsp chia seeds per serving

generous tbsp natural live yogurt, to serve

How to make

1 Combine the oat milk and coconut milk in a bowl. Place the oats in the bowl with the blended milks and soak overnight.

2 Make a compote of the berries by roughly blending them in a processor. Add the omega oil, if using.

3 In a bowl or lidded pot, layer the soaked oats, pumpkin and chia seeds, yogurt, and the berry compote. If the oats are too thick, add a little more oat milk to reach the desired consistency.

Variation

For a sweet-spicy and nutty twist, in step 3 replace the pumpkin and chia seeds with ¼ tsp cinnamon, a handful of mixed nuts, and 1 tbsp shredded coconut. Coconut is deeply hydrating, helping to refresh and rejuvenate skin.

Nutritional information per serving:

Cals 521   Fat 23g   Saturated fat 8g   Carbohydrates 56g   Sugar 15g
Sodium 60mg   Fiber 13g   Protein 16g   Cholesterol 6mg

SKIN
SMOOTHING

SKIN
BALANCING

SKIN
FIRMING

HAIR
CONDITIONING

HEALTHY
TEETH & GUMS

NAIL
STRENGTHENING

Fruity quinoa breakfast

Tasty quinoa is packed with **protein**. Adding **vitamin C–rich apricots** promotes collagen formation, helping to firm and strengthen skin and tackle stubborn areas of cellulite.

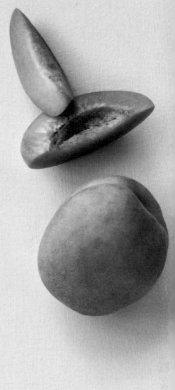

Serves 2   **Prep time: 5 mins**   **Cook time: 20 mins**

Ingredients

1½ cups almond milk

¼ cup quinoa, rinsed
   and drained

¾ cup fresh apricots, organic,
   if possible, pitted and sliced
   (or 6 dried apricots, sliced)

2 tbsp raisins

¼ tsp pure vanilla extract

How to make

1 Place the milk and quinoa in a pan, stir, and bring
   to a gentle simmer. Cover and cook for about
15 minutes, until the quinoa is tender.

2 Stir in the apricots, raisins, and vanilla extract.
   Cover and cook for another 2 minutes. Serve
warm or chilled. If eating chilled, once cooled store
in an airtight container in the fridge for up to 3 days.

Nutritional information per serving:

Cals 120   Fat 2g   Saturated fat 0.2g   Carbohydrates 21g   Sugar 14g
Sodium 76mg   Fiber 2.5g   Protein 3.5g   Cholesterol 0mg

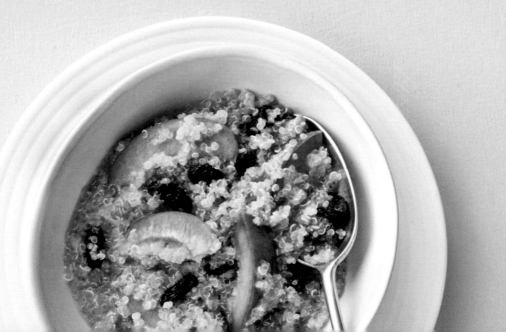

SKIN SMOOTHING

SKIN CALMING

SKIN FIRMING

HAIR CONDITIONING

Spiced apple oatmeal

This **warming** oatmeal provides a **nutrient-dense** start to the day. Nuts and seeds are a rich source of **healing** zinc, which can help to reduce the appearance of scars.

Serves 2   **Prep time: 5 mins**   **Cook time: 20 mins**

Ingredients

1 cup organic jumbo rolled oats

3 cups water

pinch of Himalayan pink salt

2 tsp coconut oil

¼ cup cashews

1 apple, cored and sliced

¼ tsp cinnamon

¼ tsp ground ginger

¼ tsp freshly grated nutmeg

2 tbsp maple syrup or honey, ideally raw

1 tbsp sunflower seeds

1 tbsp sesame seeds

handful of sliced almonds

How to make

1 Put the oats, water, salt, and oil in a pan. Bring to a simmer, then cook over low heat for 15 minutes, stirring occasionally. Add the cashews while cooking.

2 Serve the oatmeal in a bowl. Put the apple slices and spices on top, drizzle with the maple syrup, and sprinkle with the seeds and almonds.

Nutritional information per serving:

Cals 546   Fat 26g   Saturated fat 6g   Carbohydrates 59g   Sugar 21g   Sodium 209mg   Fiber 7g   Protein 15g   Cholesterol 0.1mg

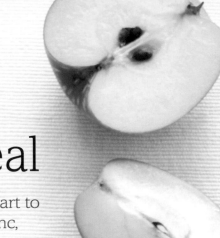

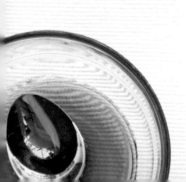

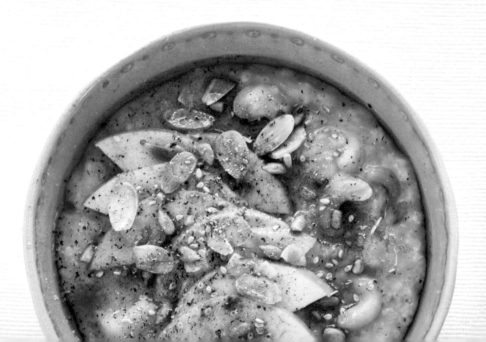

ANTI-AGING

SKIN
SMOOTHING

SKIN
CALMING

HAIR
CONDITIONING

Blueberry and chia pancakes

A breakfast treat, these pancakes have a **beauty kick**. The antioxidant rutin in buckwheat strengthens tiny blood vessels, **supporting** circulation to the fragile skin around the eyes.

CINNAMON
This sweet spice has stimulating properties that help to **boost** circulation, making it useful for tackling cellulite and for bringing a healthy **glow** to dull complexions.

Makes 6 pancakes   **Prep time: 10 mins**   **Cook time: 20–25 mins**

Ingredients

¾ cup buckwheat flour

1 tsp vanilla powder

½ tsp baking powder

½ tsp salt

1 tsp chia seeds, ground into a fine powder

a pinch of ground cinnamon

2–3 dates, pitted

¾ cup almond milk

squeeze of lemon juice

seeds from 1 vanilla bean

2 tsp whole chia seeds, to garnish

For the blueberry sauce

1 cup blueberries (fresh or frozen), plus extra to garnish

3 tbsp water

How to make

1 Combine all the dry ingredients, except the dates, in a mixing bowl. Place the dates, almond milk, lemon juice, and vanilla seeds in a food processor and blend until they form a smooth paste. Combine with the dry ingredients to form a not-too-thick batter.

2 Heat a nonstick frying pan and pour in about ¼ cup of batter at a time for each pancake. Cook slowly over low heat to keep the pancakes from burning or being undercooked, for about 2 minutes, until the pancake is firm on top with little bubbles in the center; flip and cook on the other side for another 2 minutes, or until a deep golden color.

3 To make the sauce, blend the blueberries and water with an immersion blender or in a food processor. Pour over the pancakes and garnish with extra blueberries and the chia seeds. Enjoy!

Nutritional information per serving:

Cals 85   Fat 1.2g   Saturated fat 0.1g   Carbohydrates 16g   Sugar 5g
Sodium 190mg   Fiber 2g   Protein 2g   Cholesterol 0mg

SKIN
SMOOTHING

SKIN
CALMING

SKIN
BALANCING

HAIR
CONDITIONING

Tasty toast toppings

Boost your essential fats with hemp seed butter, try **antioxidant-packed** chia jam, or enjoy guilt-free spread with skin-nourishing coconut oil. Enjoy on a slice of spelt or whole-wheat toast.

Hemp seed butter

Makes 3½oz (100g) jar   **Prep time: 5 mins**

Place ⅔ cup shelled **hemp seeds**, 1 tsp **coconut oil**, and ¼ tsp pink Himalayan **salt** in a blender and process until smooth, pausing the blender to push down any seeds from the side. Store in a jar in the fridge for up to 2 weeks.

Nutritional information per tbsp serving:
Cals 52   Fat 4.3g   Saturated fat 0.7g   Carbohydrates 0g   Sugar 0g
Sodium 39mg   Fiber 2g   Protein 2.5g   Cholesterol 0mg

LUCUMA

Full of minerals, lucuma powder, extracted from the South American fruit, has skin-healing properties that help to restore a smooth complexion.

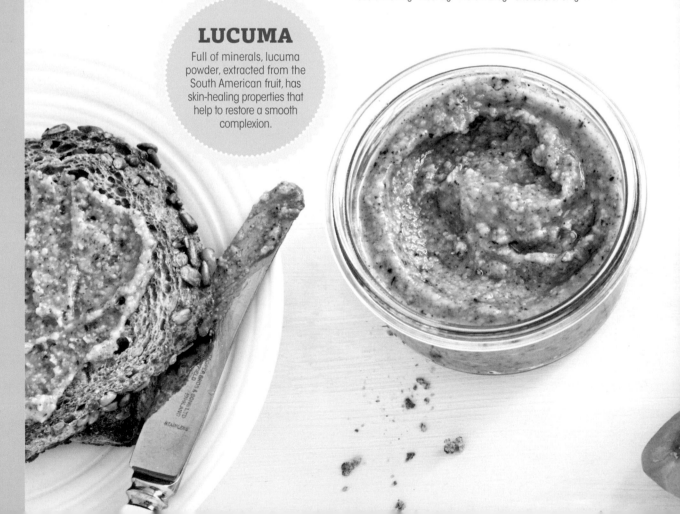

ANTI-AGING

SKIN SMOOTHING

SKIN BALANCING

NAIL STRENGTHENING

ANTI-AGING

SKIN SMOOTHING

SKIN FIRMING

NAIL STRENGTHENING

Fruity chia jam

Makes 9oz (250g) jar   Prep time: 10 mins, plus setting time

Pit 3 **apricots** and 2 **peaches** and coarsely chop the fruit. Place the chopped fruit in a blender with 2 tbsp **chia seeds** (grind first if you want a smooth jam), and blend until smooth. Place in the fridge until set—for at least 2 hours. Use within 3 days, freezing any surplus.

Nutritional information per 50g serving:

Cals 112   Fat 3.2g   Saturated fat 0.3g   Carbohydrates 14.5g   Sugar 10g
Sodium 4mg   Fiber 7g   Protein 3g   Cholesterol 0mg

Superfood spread

Makes 7oz (200g) jar   Prep time: 5 mins   Cook time: 10 mins

Preheat the oven to 350°F (180°C). Bake 1 cup **hazelnuts** for 10 minutes, then blend. Add ¼ cup **maple syrup**, 1 tsp **lucuma powder**, 1 tsp **coconut oil**, ¼ tsp pink Himalayan **salt**, and 3 tbsp **cacao**. Blend again. Add **water** until you get a smooth texture.

Nutritional information per 20g serving:

Cals 96   Fat 7.5g   Saturated fat 1.2g   Carbohydrates 4.5g   Sugar 3.5g
Sodium 27mg   Fiber 1.2g   Protein 2.4g   Cholesterol 0mg

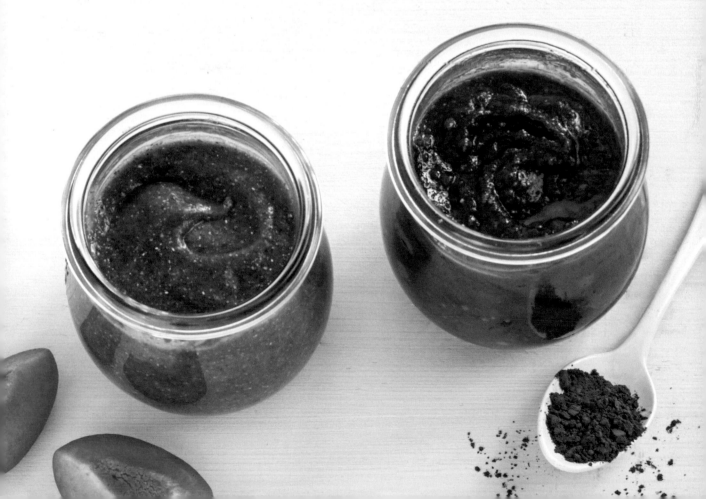

SKIN SMOOTHING

SKIN BALANCING

SKIN FIRMING

HAIR CONDITIONING

Cacao and chia chocolate "pudding"

This combo of fruits, chia seeds, and **creamy** oat milk makes a **deliciously nutritious** breakfast. High in **omega-3**, chia seeds moisturize from the **inside**, conditioning brittle hair and dry skin.

174

Serves 2   **Prep time: 10 mins, plus standing and chilling**

Ingredients

½ cup oat milk

1½ tbsp chia seeds

½ tsp maca powder

1 tsp raw cacao powder

1 tbsp maple syrup or honey

½ tsp vanilla paste, or seeds of ½ vanilla bean

2 tsp shredded coconut

2 tbsp coconut cream

handful of blueberries, or other berry, handful of pomegranate seeds, and 1 tbsp pumpkin seeds, to serve

How to make

1 Combine all the ingredients, except for the berries and pomegranate and pumpkin seeds, in a bowl, whisking to keep the chia seeds from sticking together. Cover and leave for 15 minutes, then whisk again.

2 Refrigerate overnight, or for at least 5–6 hours. Stir to check the consistency, adding more milk if the mix is too thick, or extra chia seeds if it's too runny.

3 Serve with the blueberries, or another berry, and the pomegranate and pumpkin seeds.

Variation

For a nonchocolate chia treat, mix 2½ tbsp chia seeds with ¾ cup coconut milk and refrigerate overnight. Serve with a sprinkle of cinnamon, 1½ tbsp shredded coconut, and 2 tsp sliced almonds. High in vitamin B2, almonds help regulate sebum levels to balance skin.

MACA POWDER

This **superfood** from the Andes is a natural **adaptogen**, which means it helps the body adapt to stress, so reducing the impact of stress on the complexion.

Nutritional information per serving:

Cals 187   Fat 12g   Saturated fat 5g   Carbohydrates 11g
Sugar 5g   Sodium 40mg   Fiber 6g   Protein 5g   Cholesterol 0mg

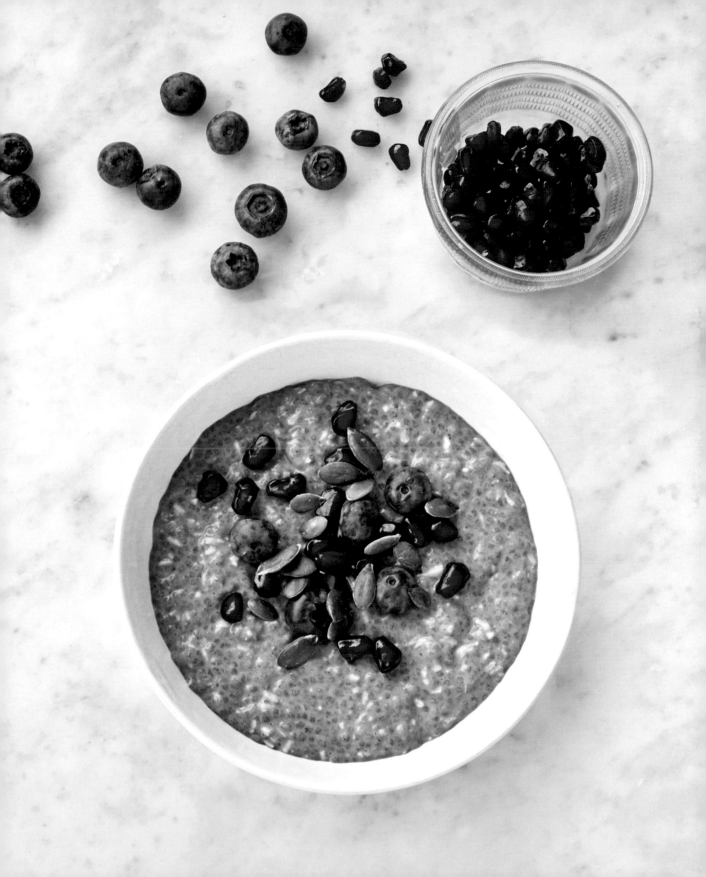

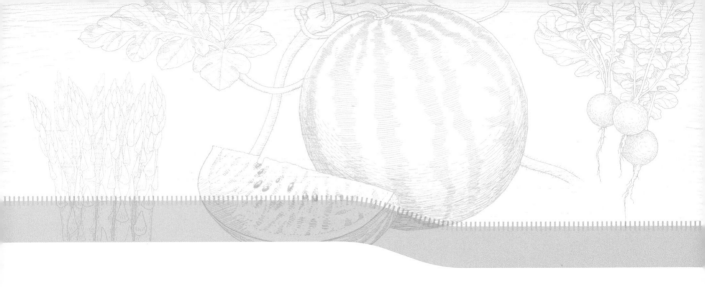

...for Snacks
and light bites

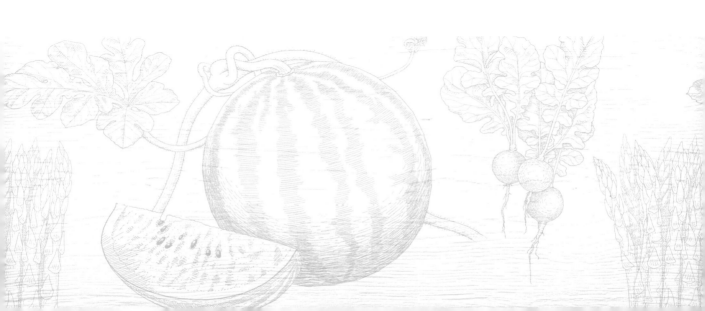

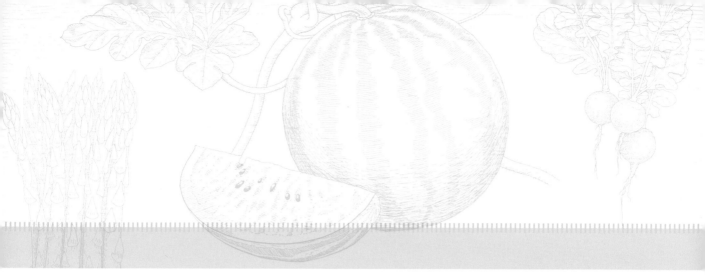

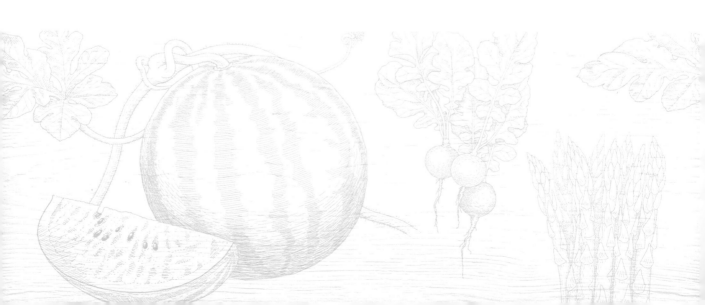

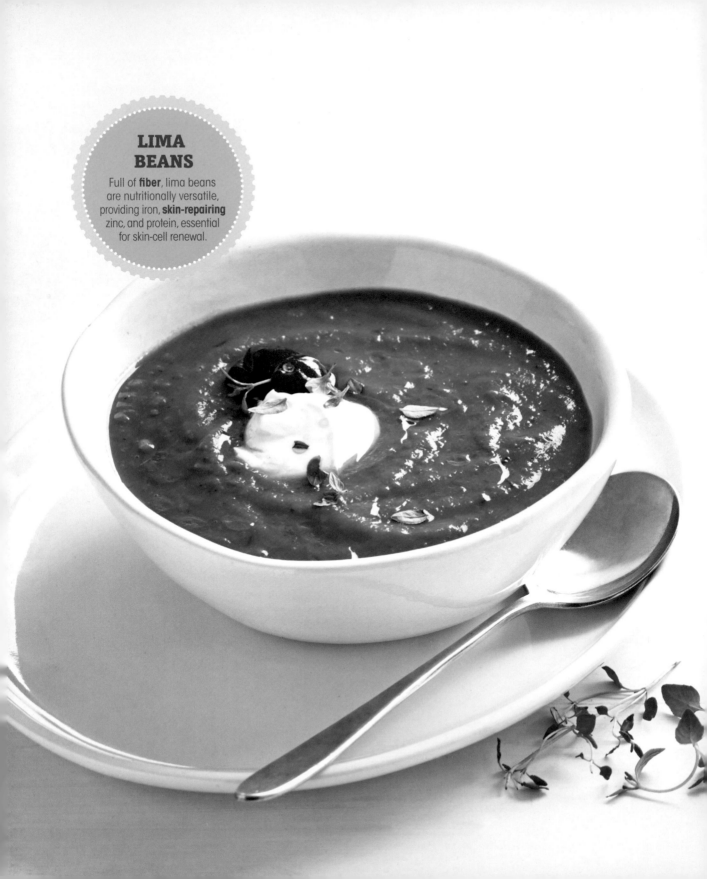

LIMA BEANS

Full of **fiber**, lima beans are nutritionally versatile, providing iron, **skin-repairing** zinc, and protein, essential for skin-cell renewal.

ANTI-AGING

SKIN SMOOTHING

SKIN BALANCING

SKIN FIRMING

NAIL STRENGTHENING

Fall flavors soup

This **nourishing** soup hydrates hair and skin. Protein-rich lima beans help keep skin **firm**, while a medley of vegetables provides **antioxidants** to protect skin from damaging UV rays.

Serves 2   Prep time: 10 mins   Cook time: 40 mins

Ingredients

- 2 sweet potatoes, or ¼ squash or butternut squash, peeled and cut into small cubes
- 2 carrots, peeled and cut into small cubes
- 2 red bell peppers, seeded and thickly sliced
- 4 sprigs thyme, leaves only, plus some for garnishing
- 1 tbsp olive oil, plus extra to drizzle
- 12 whole cherry tomatoes
- 2 red onions, finely diced
- handful of basil leaves, stems torn off
- 4 cups vegetable stock
- 6 garlic cloves, peeled
- Himalayan pink salt and freshly ground black pepper
- 14oz (400g) can lima beans
- dollop of natural live yogurt (optional), to serve

How to make

1 Preheat the oven to 400°F (200°C). Place all the vegetables, except the tomatoes and onions, and the thyme on a large baking sheet, drizzle with olive oil, and bake for 40 minutes. Bake the tomatoes with a drizzle of oil on a separate dish over lower rack.

2 Meanwhile, heat 1 tablespoon olive oil in a large pan, add the onions, and cook over low heat for about 15 minutes, or until soft and golden. Add the roasted vegetables to the pan, along with the basil, stock, and garlic, season, and simmer for 15 minutes.

3 Process with an immersion blender until smooth, add the beans, and blend again. Reheat the soup if needed.

4 Serve in bowls with a drizzle of olive oil, an optional dollop of yogurt, and a sprinkle of thyme leaves.

Nutritional information per serving:

Cals 669   Fat 20g   Saturated fat 3g   Carbohydrates 93g   Sugar 39g
Sodium 1354mg   Fiber 27g   Protein 17g   Cholesterol 0mg

**SKIN
SMOOTHING**

**SKIN
BALANCING**

**HAIR
CONDITIONING**

**HEALTHY
TEETH & GUMS**

**NAIL
STRENGTHENING**

Avocado on toast with mixed-herb pesto

Avocado is a fantastic source of healthy fats and oils, providing **vital moisture** for conditions such as eczema, and also supplying an important B vitamin, biotin, which **encourages hair growth**.

Serves 2   Prep time: 10–15 mins

Ingredients

portion Chile guacamole (see p.190)

slice of whole-wheat or spelt toast

handful of alfalfa seeds

For the herb pesto

2 cloves of garlic, peeled

pinch of Himalayan pink salt

1 cup mixed fresh basil, parsley, and mint, leaves only

¼ cup pine nuts

½ cup Parmesan, finely grated (use 1 tbsp nutritional yeast flakes if vegan)

¼ cup extra-virgin olive oil

freshly ground black pepper

squeeze of lemon juice

How to make

1 For the pesto, pulse the garlic, salt, and herbs in a food processor. Add the pine nuts and pulse again. Transfer to a bowl, stir in half the Parmesan, then add the olive oil. Season, adding more cheese to taste. Finish with a squeeze of lemon.

2 To serve, smooth a layer of the guacamole on a slice of whole-wheat toast, drizzle with the pesto, and sprinkle with the sprouted seeds. Herb pesto keeps in the fridge for up to 3 days.

Variations

For a nuttier pesto, you can use walnuts or hazelnuts in place of the pine nuts if you prefer. Instead of the classic guacamole, try mashing an avocado with 2 thinly sliced scallions, which have natural skin-healing properties, and 1 tbsp mixed ground sesame, sunflower, and flaxseeds for a zinc boost to help keep skin extra supple. If you wish, top the toast with cucumber and watercress instead of the sprouted seeds.

Nutritional information per serving:

Cals 747   Fat 65g   Saturated fat 14g   Carbohydrates 19g   Sugar 3g
Sodium 712mg   Fiber 7.3g   Protein 18.4g   Cholesterol 23mg

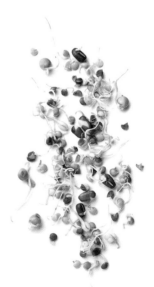

Fresh sprouted broccoli seeds have all essential vitamins and minerals.

ANTI-AGING

SKIN
BALANCING

SKIN
FIRMING

HEALTHY
TEETH & GUMS

NAIL
STRENGTHENING

TOFU

With omega-3 fats, zinc, calcium, selenium, and iron, this **protein-rich** soy curd is a top skin food, traditionally eaten to keep skin looking fresh and **youthful**.

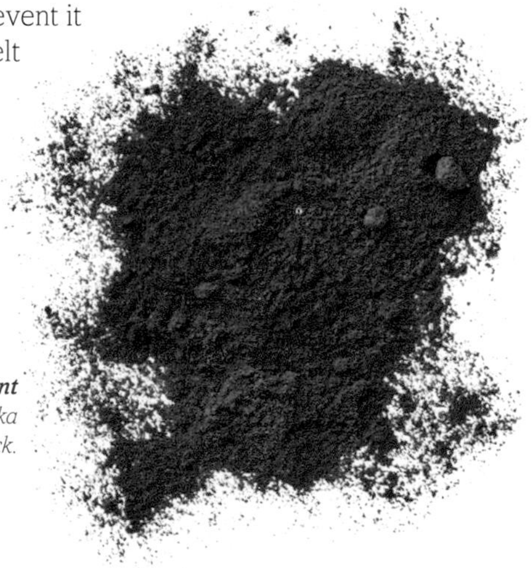

x

x

SKIN BALANCING

SKIN FIRMING

HAIR CONDITIONING

HEALTHY TEETH & GUMS

NAIL STRENGTHENING

Fava bean soup

This creamy soup is a boost for fragile hair and brittle nails. **Fiber-packed** beans and peas are a top source of vitamin A, essential for the production of **tissue-strengthening** collagen.

Serves 4 **Prep time: 10 mins** **Cook time: 30–35 mins**

Ingredients

1 onion, chopped

3 garlic cloves, crushed

4 cups vegetable stock

4 small potatoes, peeled and chopped into small pieces

2¼ cups fava beans, fresh or frozen

2 cups garden peas, fresh or frozen

½ cup oat cream, or soy or rice cream

2 tbsp olive oil, plus a drizzle, to serve

4 sprigs mint, minus stalks

2 scallions, finely chopped

toasted rye bread and butter, to serve

How to make

1 Cook the onion in a little oil in a saucepan over low heat for 10–15 minutes, until translucent. Add the garlic and cook for another minute.

2 Add the stock and bring to a simmer. Add the potatoes and simmer for about 10 minutes, until turning soft. Add the beans and peas, bring to a boil, and simmer for a couple of minutes.

3 Turn off the heat, add the oat cream, olive oil, and fresh mint. Pop in a blender and process until smooth and creamy. Serve with a sprinkle of scallions, a drizzle of olive oil, and with toasted spelt bread and melting butter.

Nutritional information per serving:

Cals 403   Fat 15g   Saturated fat 2.5g   Carbohydrates 45g   Sugar 7.5g
Sodium 606mg   Fiber 14g   Protein 15g   Cholesterol 0mg

SKIN CALMING

SKIN BALANCING

SKIN FIRMING

HEALTHY TEETH & GUMS

NAIL STRENGTHENING

Spring veggie salad

Light yet satisfying, this **protein-rich** salad is a tonic for irritated skin thanks to the **anti-inflammatory** effects of asparagus that help to soothe and calm.

PEAS

This sweet spring vegetable is packed with vital nutrients. In particular, peas contain the antioxidant saponin, which has strong **anti-inflammatory properties**.

Serves 2   **Prep time: 10 mins**   **Cook time: 5 mins**

Ingredients

10 asparagus spears

a generous handful of mixed salad leaves, torn into smaller pieces

¾ cup mange tout

¾ cup fava beans, fresh or frozen

¾ cup garden peas, fresh or frozen

¼ cup sliced almonds

2 tbsp olive oil

juice of ½ a lemon

freshly ground black pepper and Himalayan pink salt, to serve

How to make

1 Lightly steam the asparagus if you wish. Place the salad leaves, all the vegetables, and the almonds in a large serving bowl.

2 Pour over the oil and lemon juice, season, then mix together with your hands. Add the seasoning as needed and serve the salad immediately.

Nutritional information per serving:

Cals 319   Fat 20g   Saturated fat 2.5g   Carbohydrates 14.5g   Sugar 6.5g
Sodium 9mg   Fiber 11.5g   Protein 15g   Cholesterol 0mg

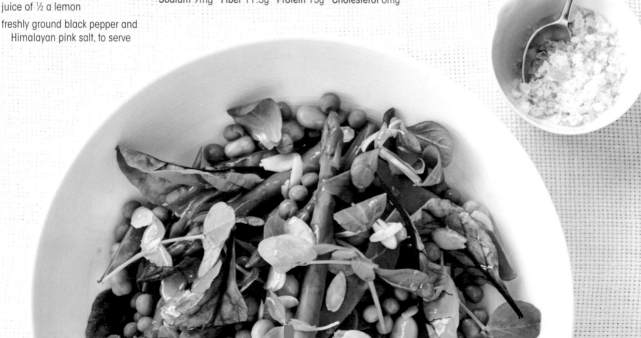

FLUID REBALANCING

SKIN CALMING

SKIN BALANCING

HAIR CONDITIONING

HEALTHY TEETH & GUMS

NAIL STRENGTHENING

Huevos rancheros

This traditional Mexican breakfast makes a winning brunch or light lunch. High in collagen-boosting **vitamin C**, it also contains the antioxidant lycopene, which helps to **protect** against sun damage.

Serves 2   Prep time: 10 mins   Cook time: 20 mins

Ingredients

2 kale leaves finely chopped

½ onion, finely chopped

½ green bell pepper, finely chopped

½ red bell pepper, finely chopped

½ bird's eye chile, chopped to taste

½ zucchini, finely chopped

½ clove garlic, finely chopped

⅓ cup tomato purée

freshly ground black pepper

2 tsp olive oil

pat of butter

4 organic eggs

fresh cilantro leaves, to serve

How to make

1 Place the kale, onion, bell peppers, chile, zucchini, garlic, and purée in a bowl. Season with pepper and mix well.

2 Heat the oil in a large lidded pan over medium heat. Add the vegetable mix, warm through for about 10 minutes, then make four holes in the mix. Quarter the butter and place in the holes, then break an egg into each one.

3 Put the lid on the pan and cook for 3–4 minutes. The dish is ready when the egg whites are firm. Slide the eggs and vegetables onto a large plate. Serve with cilantro leaves scattered on top.

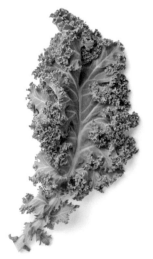

Steam or lightly sauté kale to maximize its nutritional benefits.

Nutritional information per serving:

Cals 241 Fat 15.5g Saturated fat 4.5g Carbohydrates 6.5g Sugar 6g
Sodium 279mg Fiber 3.5g Protein 18g Cholesterol 430mg

SKIN CALMING **SKIN BALANCING** **SKIN FIRMING** **HAIR CONDITIONING** **HEALTHY TEETH & GUMS** **NAIL STRENGTHENING**

CELERIAC

Similar in taste to celery, this root vegetable is seriously high in **skin-nourishing** nutrients, with magnesium, potassium, and vitamins B6, C, and K.

Winter veggie slaw

Here, sweet roots, fiery radishes, and a **warming** dressing make a delicious **skin-nurturing** combo. The tahini, made from calcium-rich sesame seeds, **strengthens** teeth, hair, and nails.

Serves 2   **Prep time: 15 mins**

Ingredients

¼ red cabbage, shredded

¼ savoy cabbage, shredded

¼ celeriac, peeled and grated

6 radishes, grated

2 carrots, grated

1 red onion, sliced as thinly as possible

For the dressing

½ clove garlic, crushed

2 tbsp light tahini

juice of ½ lemon

juice of ½ orange

½–1 tsp honey

2 tbsp olive oil

freshly ground black pepper and Himalayan pink salt

How to make

1 Place all the vegetables in a bowl and mix together well, using your hands.

2 For the dressing, combine all the ingredients in a small bowl, taste to check for seasoning, then mix into the vegetables, turning the slaw with your hands to make sure everything is well coated.

Variation

For an alternative winter salad with skin-nurturing benefits, preheat the oven to 400°F (200°C). Drizzle ⅓ cup coconut oil on 2 sweet potatoes and 3 beets, cut into wedges. Roast for 40–50 minutes, then cool. Place a handful each of arugula and kale in a bowl, a few chopped walnuts, and a 7oz (200g) can of lentils. Scatter with some finely sliced scallions and pomegranate seeds. Serve with the roasted veggies, 4–6 rehydrated figs, and drizzle with the dressing, opposite.

Nutritional information per serving:

Cals 417   Fat 21.5g   Saturated fat 3g   Carbohydrates 32g   Sugar 29.5g   Sodium 192mg   Fiber 23.5g   Protein 12g   Cholesterol 0mg

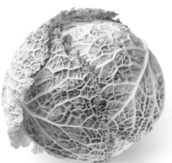

Raw cabbage *retains vitamin C often lost during cooking.*

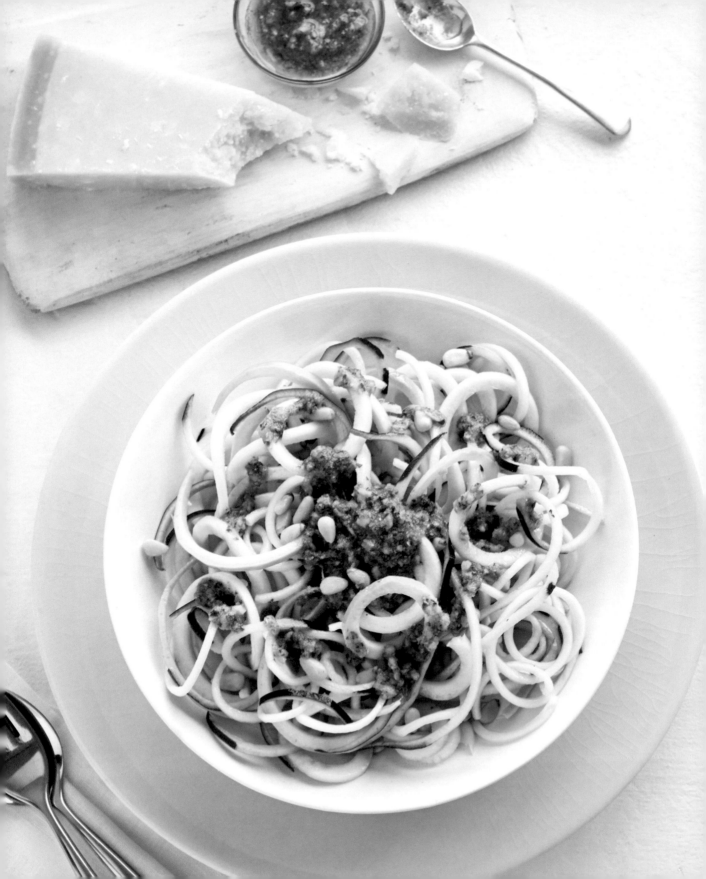

ANTI-AGING

SKIN SMOOTHING

SKIN CALMING

HEALTHY TEETH & GUMS

PINE NUTS

With **anti-inflammmatory** properties, pine nuts help **soothe** and calm sensitive skin, and their high vitamin E content adds **luster and shine** to dull hair.

Zucchini noodles
with basil pesto

Refreshing zucchini have an especially high water content that makes them **super-hydrating**, and are also naturally high in the anti-aging antioxidant **betacarotene**.

Serves 2 **Prep time: 20 mins**

Ingredients

1 green zucchini and 1 yellow squash, made into "noodle" ribbons with a spiralizer, or thin slices with a potato peeler

drizzle of olive oil

squeeze of lemon, and some lemon zest (optional)

For the pesto
1 garlic clove, peeled

pinch of Himalayan pink salt

freshly ground black pepper

1¼ cups basil, leaves only

¼ cup pine nuts, plus a few extra to garnish

¼ cup Parmesan cheese, finely grated (use 1 tbsp nutritional yeast flakes if vegan)

¼ cup extra-virgin olive oil

juice of ½ lemon

How to make

1 Place the zucchini and squash "noodles" in a bowl, add a drizzle of olive oil, a squeeze of lemon, and, if desired, a little lemon zest. Combine with your hands.

2 Prepare the pesto as shown on page 180. Put a dollop of the pesto on top of the noodles, add a sprinkle of pine nuts, and *voilà*!

Variation

Try this dairy-free pesto if you're cutting back on dairy, which is thought by some to exacerbate skin problems. (If you cut back on dairy, make sure you get sufficient calcium from other dietary sources.) Brown the pine nuts in a dry pan for about 3 minutes, being careful not to burn them—browning the nuts adds a deeper flavor, which you lose with the cheese. Then place all the ingredients, replacing the Parmesan with nutritional yeast flakes or a nondairy variety, in a blender and process.

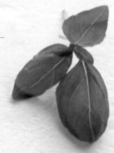

Nutritional information per serving:

Cals 429 Fat 41g Saturated fat 7g Carbohydrates 4g Sugar 3g Sodium 298mg Fiber 2g Protein 10.5g Cholesterol 14mg

ANTI-AGING

SKIN SMOOTHING

FLUID REBALANCING

SKIN FIRMING

HAIR CONDITIONING

NAIL STRENGTHENING

WATERMELON

Hydrating watermelon also supplies an amino acid, arginine that **boosts circulation** to the scalp, promoting healthy-looking hair.

Gazpacho with watermelon

Cooling and **hydrating**, this classic soup is full of raw goodness. The bright plant pigments contain **circulation-boosting** lycopene and sulfur, a vital mineral for strong and healthy nails.

Serves 4   **Prep time: 20 mins**

Ingredients

4–5 stems of basil

1 large tomato, coarsely chopped

2 cloves garlic, peeled and crushed

1 stalk of celery, chopped

½ chile, seeded and chopped (optional)

2½ cups watermelon, cut into cubes

½ small red onion, chopped

½ cucumber, sliced

¼ cup extra-virgin olive oil, plus a drizzle for the garnish

1 tsp red wine vinegar

freshly ground black pepper and Himalayan pink salt, to season

feta cheese (optional), to serve

How to make

1 Put a few of the basil leaves to one side for a garnish. Place all the ingredients, except for the olive oil, red wine vinegar, and seasoning, in a blender, and process to form a smooth and creamy purée.

2 Add the olive oil and red wine vinegar and pulse once more. Season to taste.

3 Pour the soup into chilled bowls and garnish with the remaining basil and a drizzle of olive oil. Crumble a little feta on top, if you wish. Refrigerate until ready to serve.

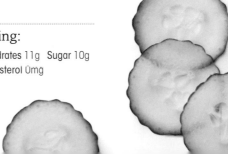

Most of a cucumber's nutrients, *such as vitamin C and copper, are in the skin.*

Nutritional information per serving:

Cals 181   Fat 14.5g   Saturated fat 2g   Carbohydrates 11g   Sugar 10g
Sodium 10mg   Fiber 1.5g   Protein 1.5g   Cholesterol 0mg

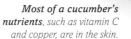

ANTI-AGING

FLUID
REBALANCING

SKIN
CALMING

SKIN
BALANCING

SKIN
FIRMING

NAIL
STRENGTHENING

Summer asparagus salad

This seasonal dish is loaded with antioxidants. A compound, saponin, in asparagus **calms** itchy skin, and **vitamin C–rich** fennel promotes collagen synthesis, helping to keep skin **taut** and prevent sagging.

Serves 2   **Prep time: 10 mins**   **Cook time: 5 mins**

Ingredients

10 asparagus spears

¼ cup olive oil

2 zucchini, cut into ribbons with a spiralizer or potato peeler

½ fennel bulb, thinly sliced across the whole head from bottom to top

2 handfuls of mixed salad leaves

handful of green olives, chopped or whole

4–5 stems dill, coarsely torn

juice and zest of 1 lemon

freshly ground black pepper and Himalayan pink salt

handful of pine nuts, to serve

How to make

1 Gently cook the asparagus spears for about 5 minutes in a little oil, until they are just soft and a little brown in places. Set aside to cool. Place the remaining vegetables, olives, setting aside a few to serve, and the dill in a bowl.

2 To make the dressing, add the lemon juice and zest to the olive oil. Pour the dressing over the salad, mixing it in well, and season to taste, mixing again.

3 Place the asparagus within the salad and sprinkle with the remaining olives and pine nuts to serve.

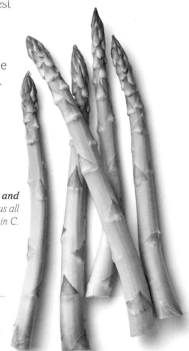

Green, purple, and **white** *asparagus all provide vitamin C.*

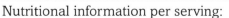

Nutritional information per serving:

Cals 292   Fat 25g   Saturated fat 3.5g   Carbohydrates 6.5g   Sugar 3.5g
Sodium 181mg   Fiber 7.5g   Protein 7g   Cholesterol 0mg

ANTI-AGING   SKIN SMOOTHING   SKIN CALMING   HAIR CONDITIONING

Skin-beautiful quick dips

These delicious dips provide a beauty boost. Opt for **moisture-replenishing** guacamole, **protein-packed** peas, or **antioxidant-rich** bell pepper and tomato, served with crunchy vegetable sticks.

Chile guacamole

Serves 2   Prep time: 5 mins

Peel and pit 1 medium ripe **avocado** and place both halves in a bowl. Add 2 tsp **olive oil**. Mash with a fork to your preferred texture. Season with freshly ground **black pepper** and Himalayan pink **salt**. Add ½–1 tsp **red chile flakes** and stir through. Squeeze over ½ **lemon** and mix to prevent it from turning brown. Keep any left over in an airtight container in the fridge for 2–3 days.

Nutritional information per serving:
Cals 177   Fat 17.5g   Saturated fat 3.5g   Carbohydrates 1.5g   Sugar 0.5g
Sodium 5mg   Fiber 3.5g   Protein 1.5g   Cholesterol 0mg

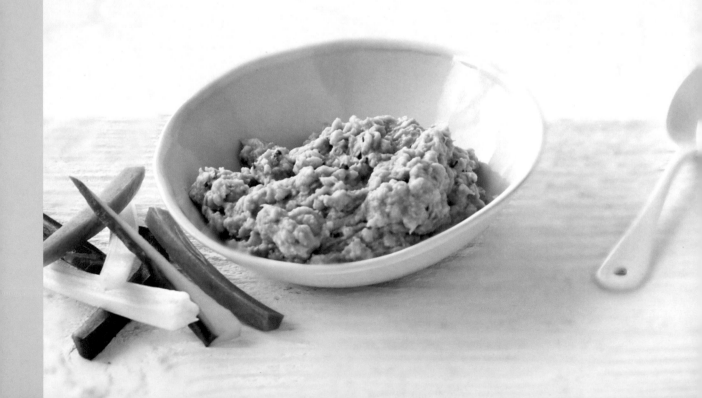

**SKIN
SMOOTHING**

**SKIN
BALANCING**

**HEALTHY
TEETH & GUMS**

**NAIL
STRENGTHENING**

ANTI-AGING

**SKIN
SMOOTHING**

**SKIN
CALMING**

**SKIN
BALANCING**

Sweet garden pea dip

Serves 2   **Prep time: 10 mins**

Place 1½ cups cooled cooked fresh or frozen garden **peas**, juice of ½ **lemon**, 2 stems **mint leaves**, ¼ cup olive oil, 1 tbsp natural live **yogurt** (optional), a pinch of Himalayan pink **salt**, and freshly ground **black pepper** in a food processor. Pulse until smooth, then put in a small bowl. Keep any leftover dip in an airtight container in the fridge for 2–3 days.

Nutritional information per serving:
Cals 299   Fat 24g   Saturated fat 4g   Carbohydrates 12g   Sugar 3g
Sodium 204mg   Fiber 6g   Protein 8g   Cholesterol 0.8mg

Bell pepper & tomato dip

Serves 2   **Prep time: 15 mins**   **Cook time: 40 mins**

Preheat the oven to 400°F (200°C). Wash, core, and seed 3 red **bell peppers**, brush with **olive oil**, and roast for 40 minutes, or until the skin is slightly charred. Let cool, then remove the skin. Place the peppers in a food processor with ½ tsp **paprika**, 4 **sundried tomatoes**, juice of ½ **lemon**, ½ cup **sunflower seeds**, 3 stems **basil** leaves, ¼ cup olive oil, 1 tbsp natural live **yogurt** (optional), a pinch of Himalayan pink **salt**, and freshly ground **black pepper**. Pulse until smooth. Put in a small bowl. Keep any left over in an airtight container in the fridge for 2–3 days.

Nutritional information per serving:
Cals 640   Fat 56g   Saturated fat 8g   Carbohydrates 18g   Sugar 11g
Sodium 308mg   Fiber 8g   Protein 12g   Cholesterol 0.8mg

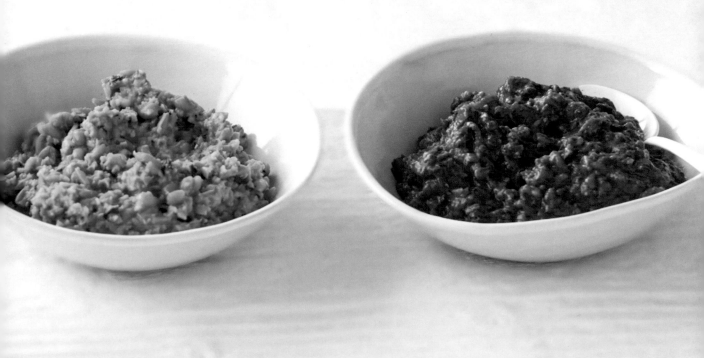

ANTI-AGING

SKIN SMOOTHING

FLUID REBALANCING

SKIN CALMING

HAIR CONDITIONING

NAIL STRENGTHENING

Beet and chickpea soup

Iron-rich beets provide the antioxidant **betacarotene**, which nourishes dry skin on the face and scalp, while chickpeas are high in **zinc**, which can help to deactivate the virus that leads to cold sores.

CHICKPEAS

High in **zinc**, essential for skin repair, chickpeas are also **full of fiber** and act as a prebiotic, promoting healthy gut bacteria and the elimination of toxins.

Serves 4   Prep time: 15 mins   Cook time: 40 mins

Ingredients

1 garlic clove, finely chopped

2 red onions, coarsely chopped

3 tbsp olive oil

1 tbsp ground cumin

4 sweet potatoes, sliced

4 cooked beets, chopped into chunks

5 cups chicken or vegetable stock

½ cup red lentils

Himalayan pink salt and freshly ground black pepper

14oz (400g) can chickpeas

juice of 1 lemon

handful of finely chopped chives (optional) and natural live yogurt (optional), to serve

How to make

1 In a medium pan, sauté the garlic and onions in the olive oil for about 10 minutes, until translucent. Add the cumin, sweet potatoes, and beets. Cook for another 5 minutes, stirring occasionally.

2 Add the stock and the lentils, bring to a boil, then reduce the heat and simmer for 15 minutes. Season to taste. Transfer to a food processor and blend until smooth.

3 Return to the pan. Add the chickpeas and the lemon juice and heat through once more.

4 Serve immediately, adding chives and a swirl of yogurt, if you wish.

Nutritional information per serving:

Cals 521   Fat 13g   Saturated fat 2g   Carbohydrates 73g   Sugar 20g
Sodium 131mg   Fiber 15g   Protein 21g   Cholesterol 0mg

ANTI-AGING **SKIN SMOOTHING** **SKIN CALMING** **HAIR CONDITIONING**

Salmon pâté

Easy to whip up, this delicious pâté delivers key beauty benefits. Rich in healthy omega-3 fats, salmon **hydrates** and **nourishes** skin cells, helping to delay the outward signs of aging, such as age spots.

Serves 2   **Prep time: 5 mins**

Ingredients

⅔ cup natural live yogurt or
   coconut yogurt

squeeze of lime juice

4oz (115g) cooked fresh salmon

freshly ground black pepper

rye bread and wedge of lemon,
   to serve, and sprig of thyme,
   to garnish

How to make

1 Place all ingredients in a blender and pulse to reach your preferred texture.

2 Serve with a slice of rye bread and a lemon wedge to squeeze on top, and garnish with a sprig of thyme.

Nutritional information per serving:

Cals 290   Fat 16g   Saturated fat 4.5g   Carbohydrates 8g   Sugar 8g
Sodium 132mg   Fiber 0g   Protein 28g   Cholesterol 70mg

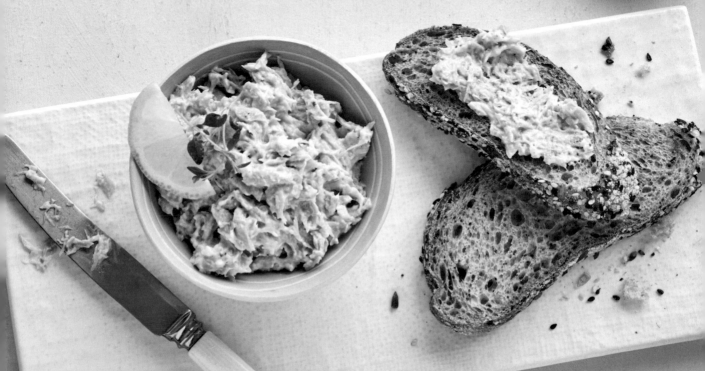

SKIN
CALMING

SKIN
BALANCING

HAIR
CONDITIONING

HEALTHY
TEETH & GUMS

NAIL
STRENGTHENING

Hot nuts!

Nuts and seeds are bursting with **rejuvenating** nutrients, including **omega fats**, which help to calm flushing, and essential **zinc**, which accelerates skin healing.

Serves 2   Prep time: 6–8 mins

Ingredients

1 tsp sesame seeds

1 tsp pumpkin seeds

1 tsp sunflower seeds

¼ cup whole almonds

¼ cup cashews

1 tsp red pepper flakes

1 tbsp tamari sauce

juice of 1 lemon

How to make

1 Heat a pan, then lightly toast the sesame seeds, just until they start to pop. Add the pumpkin and sunflower seeds and toast for another minute or so.

2 Add all the nuts to the pan and the red pepper flakes—adding a few extra if you want to increase the heat—and cook for another 3 minutes, stirring frequently to prevent the nuts and seeds from burning.

3 When the nuts and seeds are hot, add the tamari and lemon juice, being careful as this will sizzle! Enjoy as a tasty snack, or alternatively sprinkle this mix over a salad.

Variation

For a gluten-free alternative, use wasabi paste instead of red pepper flakes. This provides a different kind of heat, but is just as tasty!

TAMARI

Richly flavored and less salty than traditional soy, gluten-frees tamari is **high in minerals** and antioxidants. It helps digest grains and vegetables, **optimizing** nutrient uptake.

Nutritional information per serving:

Cals 298   Fat 24.5g   Saturated fat 3.5g   Carbohydrates 7g   Sugar 3g
Sodium 419mg   Fiber 1.5g   Protein 11.5g   Cholesterol 0mg

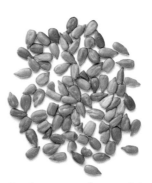

Snack on raw sunflower seeds to *get the maximum nutrient benefits.*

ANTI-AGING

SKIN
SMOOTHING

SKIN
BALANCING

SKIN
FIRMING

NAIL
STRENGTHENING

Protein power beauty bites

These **protein-rich** nutrient-packed balls are full of goodness. Almonds provide magnesium and potassium, which together help to balance fluids to **combat puffiness** and bloating.

Makes 20   **Prep time: 10 mins, plus soaking**

Ingredients

10 rehydrated figs or dates, coarsely chopped

1 cup blanched almonds

¼ cup chia seeds

¼ cup shredded coconut

¼ cup goji berries

2 tbsp maca powder

seeds from 1 vanilla bean

¼ cup cacao powder

How to make

1 Soak the figs, or dates if using, overnight in water to rehydrate them.

2 Place all the ingredients, apart from the cacao powder, in a food processor and blend until smooth and sticky. You may need to stop the processor several times to push the mixture down from the sides of the bowl.

3 Roll the mixture into 20 balls, then dust the balls with the cacao powder. These will keep for up to 1 week in the fridge.

Tip

Instead of using blanched almonds, you can presoak almonds in their skins overnight and then pop them out of their skins before using them. Soaking almonds in this way activates enyzmes that makes the nuts easier to digest.

Nutritional information per serving:

Cals 113   Fat 7.5g   Saturated fat 2.5g   Carbohydrates 7g   Sugar 5g
Sodium 7mg   Fiber 3g   Protein 3.5g   Cholesterol 0mg

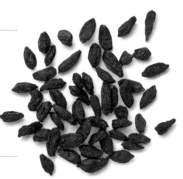

Presoaked goji berries
provide a hydrating snack.

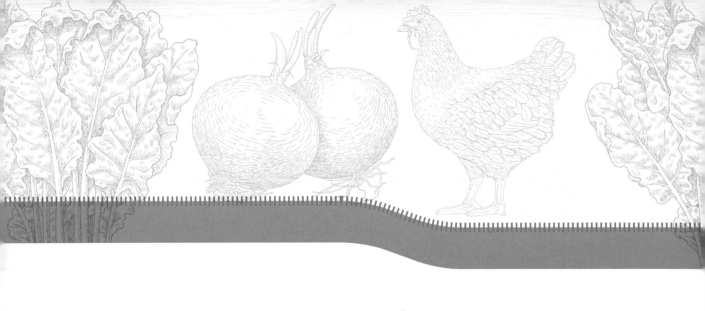

...for Dinner

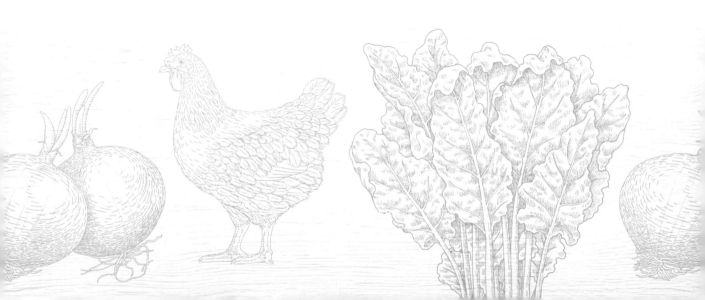

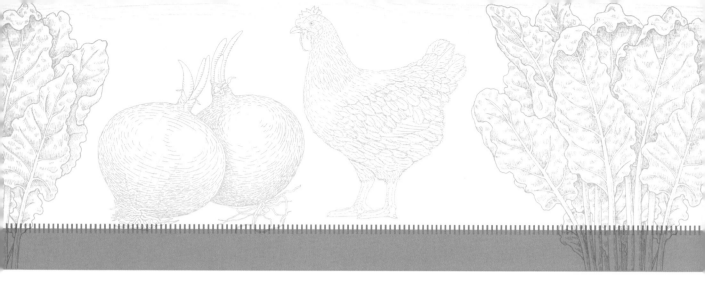

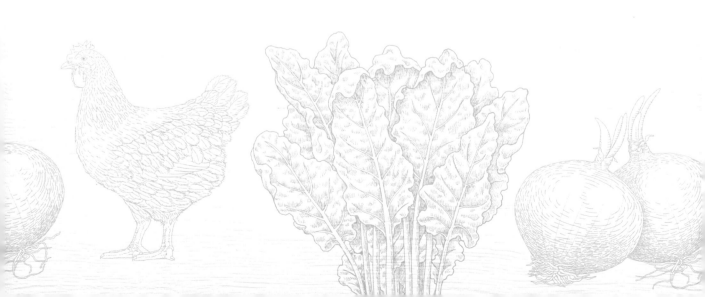

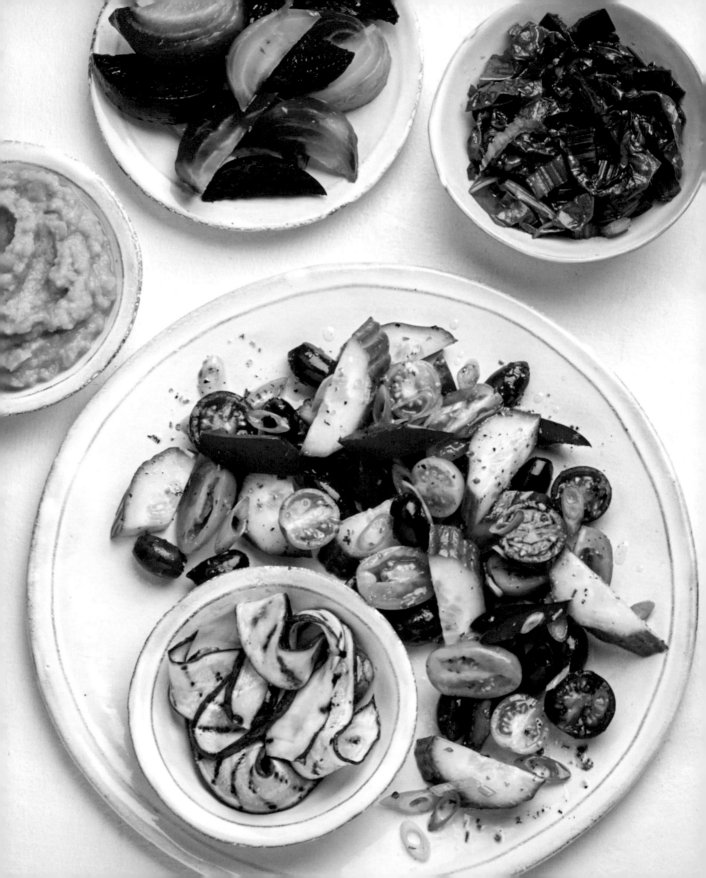

SKIN CALMING

SKIN BALANCING

HAIR CONDITIONING

HEALTHY TEETH & GUMS

NAIL STRENGTHENING

Greek vegetable mezze

This **colorful** dish is high in skin-protecting **antioxidants**. The split peas provide protein, B vitamins, iron, and zinc, all of which help to lift sallow complexions and add **luster** to dull hair.

Serves 4   **Prep time: 30 mins**   **Cook time: 50–55 mins**

Ingredients

1½ cups beets, cooked, peeled, and sliced

2 tbsp olive oil

freshly ground black pepper and Himalayan pink salt

12 cherry tomatoes, halved

½ cucumber, chopped

1 red bell pepper, seeded and chopped

3 scallions, finely sliced

handful of kalamata black olives, pitted

1 tsp dried oregano

2 zucchini, sliced lengthwise into ¼in (½cm) strips

2 handfuls mixed greens: bok choy, chard, spinach, spring greens

2 tsp lemon juice

For the *fava*

1 cup yellow split peas (soaked overnight in water)

1¾ cups vegetable stock

3 bay leaves

1 onion, chopped

1 whole garlic clove, peeled

How to make

1 To make the *fava*, put the split peas in a pan with the stock and bay leaves. Bring to a boil, then simmer for 40 minutes, or until soft. As the peas soften, add the onion and garlic and a little more water if too dry. Drain the peas, leaving a little water for blending. Remove the bay leaves. Blend the pea mixture until smooth, then place in a bowl and let cool and thicken.

2 Place the beets in a bowl and add a splash of olive oil and a little salt.

3 Place the tomatoes, cucumber, bell pepper, and scallions in a bowl. Add the olives, season, add the oregano and a generous amount of olive oil, stir, and set aside.

4 Heat a grill pan. Brush both sides of the zucchini with olive oil. Cook until soft and golden. Serve hot or cold.

5 Wilt the greens in a steamer. Place in a bowl, season, and add a splash of olive oil and lemon juice. Serve hot or cold.

6 Assemble the *fava*, beets, and mixed vegetables on a serving plate.

Nutritional information per serving:

Cals 589   Fat 13g   Saturated fat 2g   Carbohydrates 78g   Sugar 20g
Sodium 302mg   Fiber 18.5g   Protein 31g   Cholesterol 0mg

ANTI-AGING

SKIN SMOOTHING

SKIN CALMING

SKIN FIRMING

HAIR CONDITIONING

NAIL STRENGTHENING

DILL

This distinctive-tasting herb is high in **betacarotene**. This converts to vitamin A in the body, which is important for maintaining cell membranes and **promoting healthy skin**.

Barley vegetable risotto

A nutritionally versatile grain, barley has a range of beauty benefits. As well as boosting the body's **moisture quota**, it provides silica, which **promotes glossy hair** and strong, healthy-looking nails.

Serves 2   **Prep time: 10 mins**   **Cook time: 30–35 mins**

Ingredients

1 tbsp olive oil, plus extra to drizzle

1 large red onion, finely chopped

4 garlic cloves, crushed

8–10 stems of asparagus

1½ cups garden peas, fresh or frozen

1½ cups fava beans, fresh or frozen

1 cup whole or pearl barley, rinsed

2 cups vegetable stock

½ cup oat cream

4 stems dill, chopped, or 2 tsp dried dill

Himalayan pink salt and freshly ground black pepper

handful of pine nuts, arugula, and watercress, to serve

How to make

1 In a large heavy-bottomed pan, heat a little olive oil over medium heat, then cook the onion until soft, about 3 minutes. Add the garlic and cook for 1–2 minutes, being careful not to burn the onion or garlic. Remove from the pan and set aside. Add a little water to the pan and steam-fry the vegetables for 2 minutes, until firm but tender. Set to one side.

2 Place the barley in the pan over medium heat, add the stock, bring to a good simmer, then simmer gently until the barley is soft. Stir regularly to prevent the barley from sticking to the pan, adding extra water if the barley dries out. As the barley starts to soften, add the oat cream and dill and stir. Once the barley is soft to the taste, at around 25 minutes, turn off the heat and stir in all the other ingredients.

3 Season to taste. Serve sprinkled with pine nuts, a drizzle of oil, and an arugula and watercress salad.

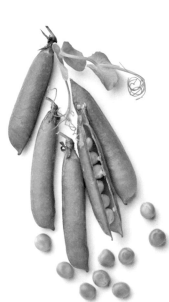

Freshly shelled peas are most flavorful and sweet when cooked within hours of picking.

Nutritional information per serving:

Cals 799   Fat 23g   Saturated fat 4g   Carbohydrates 113g   Sugar 13g   Sodium 34mg   Fiber 18g   Protein 27g   Cholesterol 0mg

ANTI-AGING

SKIN
SMOOTHING

FLUID
REBALANCING

HAIR
CONDITIONING

HEALTHY
TEETH & GUMS

NAIL
STRENGTHENING

Japanese ocean soup

With hydrating vegetables and **mineral-rich** seaweed, this **cooling** soup helps rebalance fluids to reduce bloating. Iron and B vitamins in the seaweed **strengthen** the hair shaft, helping prevent hair loss.

Serves 2   **Prep time: 10 mins, plus soaking**   **Cook time: 20 mins**

Ingredients

1 tbsp dried seaweed

7oz (200g) rice noodles

drizzle coconut oil (optional)

1 onion, sliced

1 garlic head, all cloves peeled

1 leek, sliced

8 stems broccolini

2 zucchini, sliced

3½oz (100g) French green beans, trimmed

1in (2.5cm) piece of ginger, peeled and cut into thin strips

2½ cups vegetable stock

2 tsp red pepper flakes (optional)

¼ savoy cabbage, cut into chunky ribbons

8 asparagus stems (if in season), chopped into 2in (5cm) pieces

1 heaped tbsp barley miso paste

10oz (300g) tofu, chopped into chunks

1 tsp raw sesame oil

sprouted seeds, and pumpkin and sesame seeds, to serve

How to make

1 Prepare the seaweed by soaking as per the instructions, rinse well, and, if you wish, cut into smaller pieces. Cook the noodles as per the instructions, strain, and let cool. If you wish, drizzle a little coconut oil on them to keep them from sticking together.

2 Place the onion, garlic, vegetables except the cabbage and asparagus, and ginger in a large pan with the stock and red pepper flakes, if using. Bring to a simmer, reduce the heat, and cook for about 5 minutes. Add the cabbage and asparagus and cook for 2 minutes more.

3 Now add the miso, mixing in well, the tofu, and the seaweed. Place the noodles in a bowl, pour the soup on top, drizzle with sesame oil, and scatter with the sprouted seeds and the pumpkin and sesame seeds.

Tip

A small amount of dried seaweed becomes a large amount when rehydrated; it keeps for several days in the fridge. Try adding to salads and stir-fries.

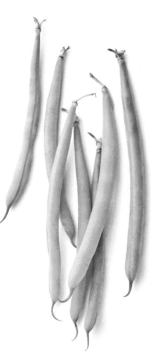

Green beans *lose a lot of their nutrients when overcooked. Steam for just a few minutes until tender.*

Nutritional information per serving:

Cals 866   Fat 16g   Saturated fat 3g   Carbohydrates 114g   Sugar 21g
Sodium 279mg   Fiber 28g   Protein 52g   Cholesterol 0mg

ANTI-AGING SKIN SMOOTHING SKIN CALMING SKIN BALANCING NAIL STRENGTHENING

Summer salad with pomegranate and pistachio

This Mediterranean salad is given a beauty kick with pomegranates, a key **rejuvenator** for tired-looking complexions, and pistachios, which provide **fluid-rebalancing** potassium to help reduce bloating.

Serves 2   **Prep time: 10 mins**   **Cook time: 20–30 mins**

Ingredients

1 eggplant, sliced lengthwise

2 red bell peppers, seeded and sliced lengthwise

2 zucchini, sliced lengthwise

Himalayan pink salt and freshly ground black pepper

1 tbsp of olive oil, plus a drizzle

handful of pistachios (unroasted and unsalted)

2¼oz (70g) arugula or watercress leaves

3 stems each of parsley, mint, and dill, finely chopped

squeeze of lemon juice

½ cup barley couscous

¾ cup hot vegetable stock

1 pomegranate, seeded

herb pesto (optional) see p.186

How to make

1 Preheat the broiler. Brush the eggplant, bell peppers, and zucchini on both sides with ½ tablespoon of oil. Put under the broiler for 15 minutes, or until soft and golden, turning to cook both sides. You may need to do several batches. Season, drizzle with oil, and set aside.

2 Smash the pistachios in a mortar and pestle and set to one side. Place the salad leaves and herbs in a bowl, season, and add the remaining oil and a squeeze of lemon juice.

3 Place the couscous in a bowl and add the vegetable stock. Cover, leave for 5 minutes, then fluff up with a fork. Once cool, stir in the pistachios and pomegranate seeds, leaving a few to decorate. Arrange all the elements on the plate, drizzle with herb pesto, if using, and the pomegranate seeds and pistachios, to serve.

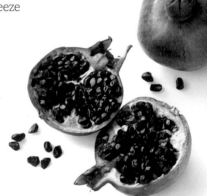

Nutritional information per serving:

Cals 513   Fat 21g   Saturated fat 3g   Carbohydrates 57g   Sugar 19g
Sodium 30mg   Fiber 14.5g   Protein 17g   Cholesterol 0mg

Ripe pomegranates are firm with a shiny, deep red skin.

SKIN CALMING

SKIN BALANCING

HEALTHY TEETH & GUMS

NAIL STRENGTHENING

Baked stuffed squash

Sweetly delicious, this divine squash supper is a nutrient powerhouse, high in **skin-firming** vitamins A, C, and E, and fiber to promote healthy digestion and **eliminate toxins**.

Serves 2   **Prep time: 10 mins**   **Cook time: 50 mins, plus standing**

Ingredients

1 squash (of choice), halved lengthwise, and seeded

Himalayan pink salt and freshly ground black pepper

6 garlic cloves, crushed

1 tbsp olive oil

½ cup quinoa

¾ cup hot vegetable stock

½ tsp ground turmeric

1 large onion, finely chopped

generous handful of chopped dill, sage, and chives

⅓ cup hazelnuts, chopped

3 tbsp pine nuts

grated cheese (optional) and green salad leaves, to serve

How to make

1 Preheat the oven to 400°F (200°C). Place the squash halves on a baking sheet, season, place the garlic in the hollows, and add a good splash of olive oil. Bake for 40 minutes, or until the flesh is soft. Remove from the oven to cool.

2 Meanwhile, rinse the quinoa. Place in a pan with the stock and turmeric, bring to a boil, cover, and simmer for 10 minutes. Remove from the heat, keeping the lid on. Let stand for 10 minutes, then fluff with a fork.

3 Cook the onion in a pan with a little oil. As the onion softens, add the chopped herbs, then remove from the heat. Scoop out the squash flesh and place in a bowl, preserving the squash halves. Roughly mash the flesh, then mix in the other ingredients. Spoon the mixture back into the squash halves. Return to the oven to bake for another 10 minutes, adding a sprinkle of cheese if you wish. Serve with green salad leaves.

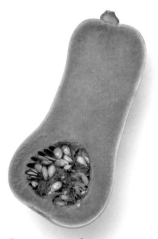
***Butternut squash** is one of the most nutrient-dense winter squashes.*

Nutritional information per serving:

Cals 709   Fat 33g   Saturated fat 3g   Carbohydrates 76g   Sugar 31g
Sodium 64mg   Fiber 18g   Protein 20g   Cholesterol 0mg

**SKIN
SMOOTHING**

**SKIN
CALMING**

**SKIN
BALANCING**

**HEALTHY
TEETH & GUMS**

**NAIL
STRENGTHENING**

Black lentil and coconut curry

Fiber-rich lentils are an abundant source of protein, vital for healthy collagen production, and of **zinc**, which has anti-inflammatory properties that can help to soothe inflamed, irritated skin.

Serves 4   **Prep time: 15 mins**   **Cook time: 1 hr**

Ingredients

1 cauliflower, divided into heads, large ones halved

2 tsp coconut oil solid

2 onions, finely chopped

5 garlic cloves, mashed

1in (2.5cm) piece ginger, grated

spices: ¼ tsp turmeric, pinch grated nutmeg, 8 cardamom pods, 4 cloves, ½ tsp red chile flakes, ¼ tsp ground coriander, ¼ tsp ground cinnamon, ½ tsp garam masala, ½ tsp paprika, and 1 tsp black mustard seeds

14oz (400g) can plum tomatoes, chopped

2½ cups hot vegetable stock

½ cup black lentils

2 large sweet potatoes, chopped into medium-sized chunks

14oz (400ml) can coconut milk

1 cup short-grain brown rice, or brown basmati

For the yogurt dressing

¾ cup natural live yogurt or coconut yogurt

¼ cucumber, grated

10 mint leaves, finely chopped (add more to taste)

pinch of Himalayan pink salt

How to make

1 Preheat the oven to 400°F (200°C). Place the cauliflower in a baking dish, drizzle with coconut oil, and roast for about 30 minutes, or until golden. Do this while the curry is cooking, then set to one side.

2 In a large pan, cook the onions, garlic, and ginger in 2 teaspoons coconut oil for about 10 minutes, then add all the spices and cook over low heat for a few minutes more.

3 Add the tomatoes, stock, lentils, and sweet potatoes, cover, and reduce the heat to a low simmer. Cook for about 30 minutes, stirring occasionally to make sure the bottom doesn't burn and that you have enough liquid. Top off with water if needed. Add the coconut milk and continue to cook until the lentils and sweet potatoes are very soft. Add the cauliflower to the sauce in the pan.

4 Let the curry stand while you cook the rice. Rinse the rice and add to a pot with 1¾ cups hot water, bring to a boil, then reduce to a simmer for about 20 minutes.

5 To make the dressing, place all the ingredients in a bowl and mix together well. Cover and keep in the fridge until needed. Serve the curry with the rice and the yogurt dressing.

Nutritional information per serving:

Cals 758   Fat 24g   Saturated fat 17.5g   Carbohydrates 105g   Sugar 28g
Sodium 238mg   Fiber 16g   Protein 24g   Cholesterol 6mg

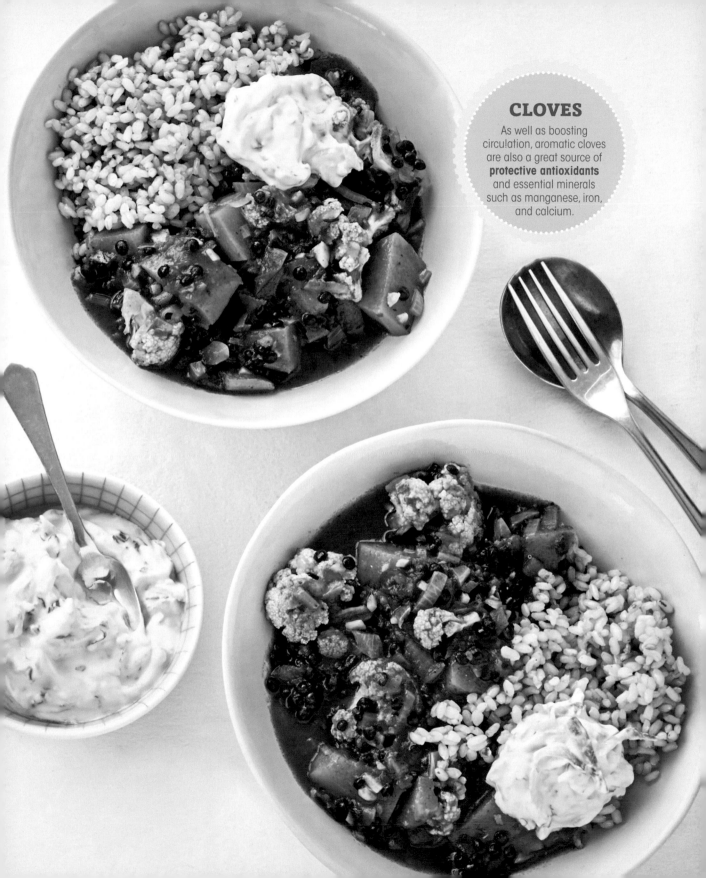

ANTI-AGING

FLUID REBALANCING

SKIN CALMING

SKIN BALANCING

HAIR CONDITIONING

HEALTHY TEETH & GUMS

Roasted broccoli and cauliflower with couscous

This **comforting** dish helps to hydrate both skin and hair. Broccoli is especially rich in anti-inflammatory **antioxidants**, making this an ideal dinner for those with skin sensitivities.

Serves 4   **Prep time: 20 mins**   **Cook time: 30–40 mins**

Ingredients

1 tsp coconut oil

½ head broccoli florets

½ head cauliflower segments

1 zucchini, sliced

¾ cup garden peas

1½ cups snow or sugar snap peas

1½ cups fava beans, fresh or frozen

Himalayan pink salt and freshly ground black pepper

1½ cups cherry tomatoes

drizzle of olive oil

½ cup barley couscous

15 saffron strands (optional)

¾ cup hot vegetable stock

generous handful of kale, chopped into ribbons

20 olives, pitted and halved

½ pomegranate, seeded

handful of walnuts, chopped

2 tsp red pepper flakes

How to make

1 Preheat the oven to 400°F (200°C). Melt the coconut oil in a roasting pan in the oven. Place the vegetables, except the tomatoes and kale, in a dish, season, and turn them so they are coated in the oil. Bake for 30–40 minutes, until golden brown.

2 Place the tomatoes in a separate dish, drizzle with olive oil, season, and bake for 20–30 minutes. Meanwhile, place the couscous in a heatproof bowl with the saffron, if using. Add the stock. Stir, cover, and steam for about 5 minutes, until you're ready to serve, then lightly fluff up the couscous with a fork.

3 Steam the kale for 5 minutes. Place in a large bowl, add the olives, pomegranate seeds, walnuts, red pepper flakes, and all the other ingredients, mix well, and serve.

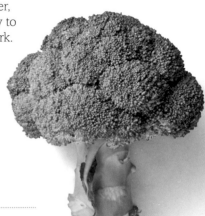

Eat broccoli stalks and florets to get the full nutrient quota.

Nutritional information per serving:

Cals 341   Fat 9g   Saturated fat 3g   Carbohydrates 39g   Sugar 12g
Sodium 233mg   Fiber 16g   Protein 18g   Cholesterol 0mg

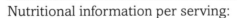

ANTI-AGING

SKIN
SMOOTHING

SKIN
BALANCING

HEALTHY
TEETH & GUMS

NAIL
STRENGTHENING

Ratatouille

Full of color, this classic dish is bursting with **protective** antioxidants. Red onions are an excellent source of sulfur, key for **healthy collagen** production and strong nails.

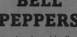

BELL PEPPERS

Try different-colored bell peppers for a variety of nutrients. Sweet red, yellow, and orange peppers are especially high in **vitamin C,** while green peppers are a good source of **vitamin A.**

Serves 4   Prep time: 15 mins   Cook time: 50 mins

Ingredients

2 tbsp olive oil, plus extra for drizzling

1 eggplant, chopped

3 zucchini, chopped

3 red, orange, or yellow bell peppers, seeded and chopped into wedges

2 red onions, peeled and cut into wedges

4 garlic cloves, peeled and coarsely chopped

3–4 sprigs of fresh oregano or thyme

6 ripe tomatoes, chopped

1 x 14oz (400g) can plum tomatoes, chopped

handful of black olives

1 tbsp balsamic vinegar

Himalayan pink salt and freshly ground black pepper

bunch of fresh basil, leaves only

zest of ¼ lemon

¼ cup feta or Parmesan (optional)

½ tsp red pepper flakes (optional)

rice or barley couscous, plus a poached egg (optional), to serve

How to make

1 Heat the 2 tablespoons of oil in a heavy-bottomed pan or casserole dish over medium heat. Add the eggplant, zucchini, and bell peppers and cook for around 5 minutes, or until golden and softened, but not cooked through. Put these vegetables in a large bowl and set aside.

2 Add the onions, garlic, and oregano or thyme leaves to the pan with a drizzle of oil. Cook over medium heat for 10 minutes, until soft and golden. Return the cooked vegetables to the pan then stir in the fresh and canned tomatoes, olives, and vinegar and season to taste, combining the ingredients together well.

3 Cover the pan and simmer over low heat for 30–35 minutes, or until reduced, sticky, and sweet. Tear in the basil leaves and add the lemon zest, then season to taste.

4 Drizzle with a little olive oil and, if you like, scatter some feta or Parmesan on top. Serve with the rice or couscous. You can also add a poached egg on top if you wish.

Nutritional information per serving:

Cals 176   Fat 4g   Saturated fat 1g   Carbohydrates 23g   Sugar 22g
Sodium 143mg   Fiber 10g   Protein 7g   Cholesterol 4.5mg

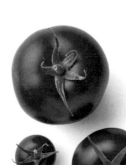
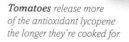

Tomatoes release more of the antioxidant lycopene the longer they're cooked for.

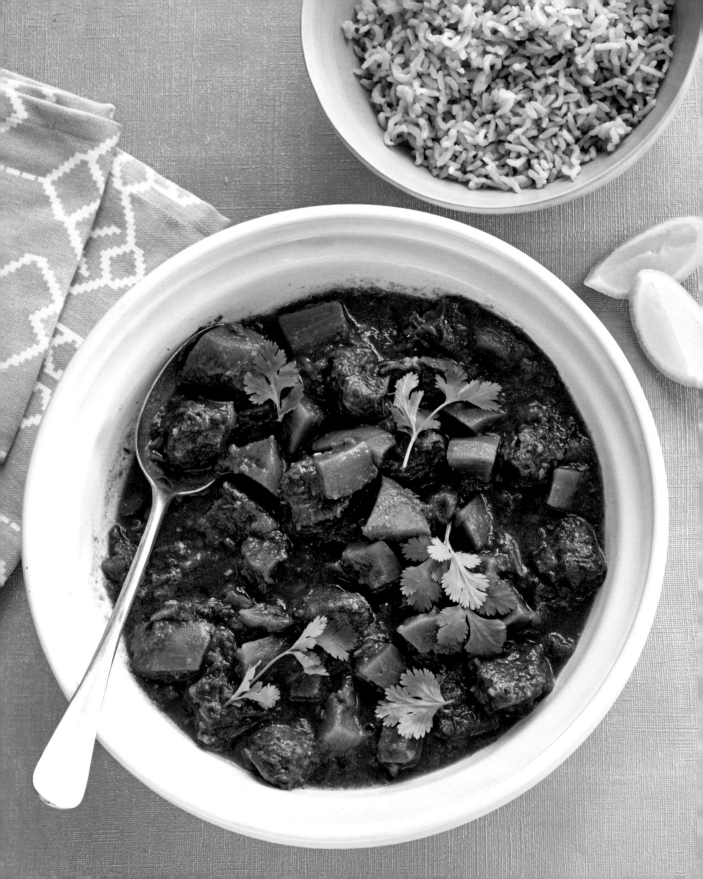

SKIN SMOOTHING

SKIN CALMING

SKIN FIRMING

HAIR CONDITIONING

Lamb tagine

High in **iron** and **B-complex vitamins**, lamb stands out among red meats for its **nutritional** value. B vitamins promote scalp health, helping to control conditions such as dandruff.

GINGER

As well as adding a spicy kick, pungent ginger has top beauty credentials. A natural anti-inflammatory, it **boosts circulation**, lending skin a healthy glow.

Serves 4   **Prep time: 10 mins**   **Cook time: 2 hrs 15 mins**

Ingredients

2 tbsp olive oil

1 onion, diced

2 carrots, peeled and diced

1lb 2oz (500g) leg of lamb, diced

2 garlic cloves, crushed

½ tsp ground cumin

½ tsp ground ginger

¼ tsp ground saffron

1 tsp ground cinnamon

1 tbsp honey

¾ cup soft dried apricots, quartered

2 cups hot vegetable stock

1 small butternut squash, peeled, seeded, and cut into ½in (1cm) cubes

cilantro sprigs, lemon wedges, and brown rice, to serve

How to make

1 Heat the olive oil over medium heat in a heavy-bottomed pan and add the onion and carrots. Cook for 3–4 minutes, until softened.

2 Add the lamb and brown all over. Stir in the garlic, cumin, ginger, saffron, and cinnamon and cook for another 2 minutes, or until the aromas are released.

3 Add the honey and apricots and pour in the vegetable stock, adding more to cover, if necessary. Give it a good stir and bring to a boil. Turn down to a simmer, put the lid on, and cook for 1 hour.

4 Remove the lid and cook for another 30 minutes, then stir in the squash. Cook for 20–30 minutes more, until the squash is soft and the lamb is tender.

5 Serve garnished with cilantro sprigs and with lemon wedges on the side. Accompany with brown rice.

Nutritional information per serving:

Cals 423   Fat 16g   Saturated fat 5g   Carbohydrates 35g   Sugar 27g
Sodium 145mg   Fiber 9g   Protein 29.5g   Cholesterol 92.5mg

SKIN SMOOTHING

FLUID REBALANCING

SKIN CALMING

SKIN FIRMING

HAIR CONDITIONING

OREGANO

This Mediterranean herb has **skin-healing** properties and also contains the **antimicrobial** compound thymol, which can help to stop cold sores in their tracks.

Lemon and herb-roasted chicken

Succulent chicken is a top source of healthy **protein**, vital for **skin-cell renewal**, and its anti-inflammatory properties make it especially beneficial for conditions such as rosacea.

Serves 2   Prep time: 10 mins   Cook time: 45 mins

Ingredients

zest of 1½ lemons

2 tbsp olive oil

1 tsp coarsely chopped oregano, plus 2 sprigs

1 tsp coarsely chopped thyme, plus 2 sprigs

1 tsp coarsely chopped rosemary, plus 2 sprigs

2 garlic cloves, crushed

freshly ground black pepper

2 x 5oz (140g) skin-on chicken breasts

8 small roasting potatoes, cut in half

2 carrots, peeled and cut into batons

2 small red bell peppers, seeded and sliced

2 small red onions, cut in wedges

1¼ cups vegetable stock or water

How to make

1 Preheat the oven to 400°F (200°C). Place the lemon zest, oil, oregano, thyme, rosemary, and garlic in a bowl, season with pepper to taste, and stir together well.

2 Spread the lemon-herb mixture onto the chicken breasts. Place the chicken breasts in a roasting pan and arrange the potatoes, carrots, bell peppers, onions, and sprigs of herbs around them. Add the stock or water, and roast the chicken for about 45 minutes, until the juice from the chicken runs clear when pricked and the vegetables have browned at the edges.

3 Remove the chicken from the oven. Take off the skin, discard the herb sprigs, and serve with the vegetables.

Nutritional information per serving:

Cals 383   Fat 13.5g   Saturated fat 2g   Carbohydrates 22g   Sugar 15.5g   Sodium 150mg   Fiber 8g   Protein 39g   Cholesterol 105mg

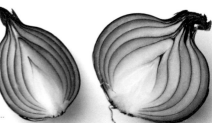

Resist overpeeling onions as antioxidants such as flavanoids are concentrated in the outer layers.

SKIN SMOOTHING   **SKIN BALANCING**   **HAIR CONDITIONING**

Potato and veggie bake

This quick-to-prepare vegetable bake is a twist on the traditional Greek "briam." **Nutrient-dense** spinach provides chlorophyll, a natural detoxer that helps to cleanse the liver.

Serves 2   Prep time: 10 mins   Cook time: 1hr 30 mins, plus cooling

Ingredients

3 zucchini, chopped into ½in (1cm) slices

1 eggplant, thinly sliced

2 red onions, sliced

3 bell peppers: 1 red, 1 orange, and 1 yellow, seeded and cut into chunky wedges

4–6 potatoes, chopped into ¼in (½cm) slices

1 head of garlic, peeled but left as whole cloves

Himalayan pink salt and freshly ground black pepper

3½ tbsp olive oil

7oz (200g) spinach

handful of olives

8–10 sundried tomatoes

handful each of dill and basil, very coarsely chopped

a little feta (optional), to serve

How to make

1 Preheat the oven to 375°F (190°C). Place all the vegetables, except the spinach and sun-dried tomatoes, and garlic in a large baking dish, season, mix together with your hands, add the olive oil, and mix again.

2 Bake in the oven for 1 hour, then add the spinach, olives, sundried tomatoes, plus the dill and basil. Bake for another 30 minutes, or until the top is slightly crispy and the eggplant is soft and gooey.

3 Let stand for 5 minutes, then serve. If you wish, a little feta crumbled on top is delicious.

Variations

If you wish, substitute the onions for a chopped leek. Leeks are high in the skin-protecting vitamins A, C, and E, which help prevent skin damage caused by harmful UV rays. You can also swap the potatoes for sweet potatoes if you prefer.

Nutritional information per serving:

Cals 896   Fat 35g   Saturated fat 5g   Carbohydrates 109g   Sugar 30g
Sodium 467mg   Fiber 28g   Protein 22g   Cholesterol 0mg

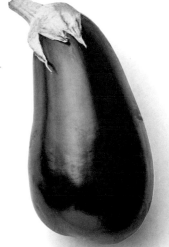

To ensure freshness, *look for shiny-fleshed eggplants, free from discoloration or marks.*

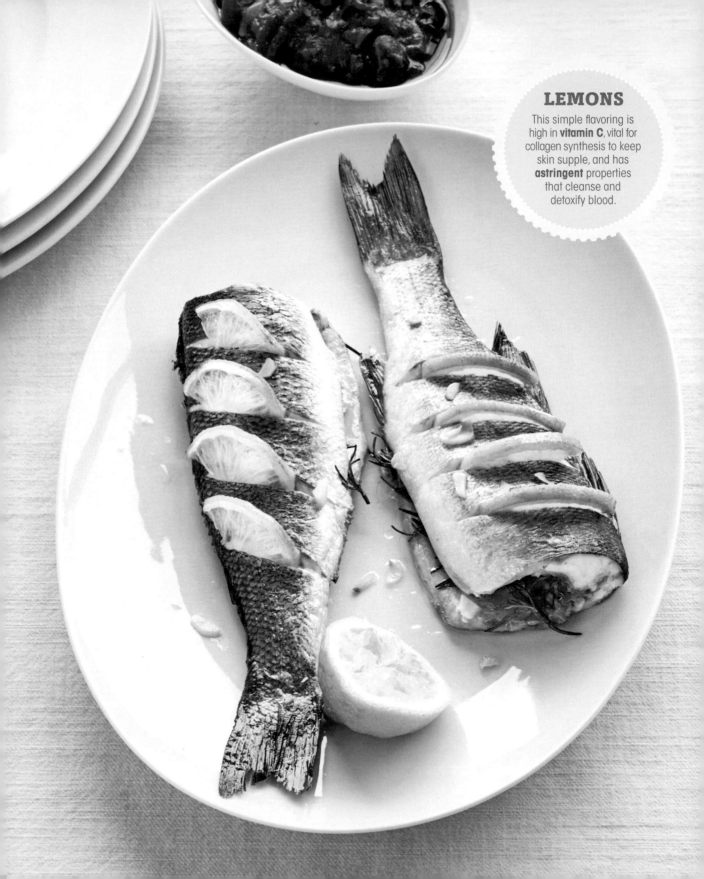

ANTI-AGING   FLUID REBALANCING   SKIN CALMING   SKIN FIRMING   HAIR CONDITIONING   NAIL STRENGTHENING

Roasted sea bass
with tomato salsa

Flavorful sea bass provides **omega-3** oils, which promote cell repair. The **antioxidant** lycopene in the tomato salsa strengthens delicate blood vessels, supporting fine skin on the neck and hands.

Serves 2   **Prep time: 30 mins**   **Cook time: 15 mins**

Ingredients

1 tbsp sea salt

2 x 1lb 2oz (500g) sea bass, scaled, cleaned, and heads removed

1 lemon, sliced, plus the juice of 1 lemon

2 sprigs of rosemary

¼ cup coconut oil

2 garlic cloves, coarsely chopped

For the tomato salsa

1 red onion, finely chopped

2 garlic cloves, finely chopped

1 red chile, seeded and finely chopped

1 tbsp olive oil

14oz (400g) can tomatoes

7oz (210g) can kidney beans, drained and rinsed

2 tbsp cilantro leaves

juice and zest of 1 lime

Himalayan pink salt and freshly ground black pepper

How to make

1 Preheat the oven to 425°F (220°C). Salt the inside of the fish, then set aside for 20 minutes. Rinse and pat dry. Slash the fish skin in 3–4 places and insert the lemon slices. Place the rosemary in the fish, then transfer to a lightly oiled baking sheet.

2 For the salsa, cook the onion, garlic, and chile in the oil over low heat for 10 minutes. Add the tomatoes and simmer for 10–15 minutes. Add the kidney beans, cilantro, and lime juice and zest, then season to taste.

3 Heat the coconut oil in a small pan over medium heat. Cook the garlic for 1–2 minutes. Pour the oil and garlic on top of the fish. Bake for about 15 minutes, basting frequently with the oil, until the fish flakes easily and the skin is slightly crisp. Pour the lemon juice over the fish and serve with the tomato salsa on the side.

Nutritional information per serving:

Cals 411   Fat 26g   Saturated fat 10g   Carbohydrates 7.5g   Sugar 4g
Sodium 386mg   Fiber 3g   Protein 36g   Cholesterol 118mg

SKIN BALANCING

SKIN FIRMING

HAIR CONDITIONING

NAIL STRENGTHENING

GARLIC

A pantry essential, garlic is a potent source of **skin-supporting nutrients**, providing manganese, vitamin B6, and vitamin C, essential for boosting collagen production.

Thai chicken and noodle soup

Simple but delicious, this aromatic soup provides cell-renewing **protein** and is a good source of **selenium**, an essential mineral that promotes a healthy scalp, nourishing dry, brittle hair.

Serves 4   **Prep time: 15 mins**   **Cook time: 20 mins**

Ingredients

4oz (115g) egg noodles

8oz (225g) chicken tenderloins

1 tbsp coconut oil

2in (5cm) piece ginger, peeled and finely chopped

2 garlic cloves, crushed

1 green chile, seeded and chopped

1 stalk lemongrass

½ tsp ground turmeric

1 x 14oz (400ml) can of coconut milk

2½ cups chicken stock

½ cup green beans

1 carrot, peeled and cut into matchsticks

3 scallions, trimmed and finely diced

¾ cup bean sprouts

2 tbsp tamari sauce

cilantro leaves, to garnish

How to make

1 Cook the noodles according to the package instructions. Cut the chicken into bite-sized pieces. Heat the oil over medium heat in a large saucepan and add the chicken, ginger, garlic, chile, lemongrass, and turmeric. Cook for 2 minutes, stirring well.

2 Pour in the coconut milk and stock, then bring to a boil, stirring. Simmer for 10 minutes. Stir in the green beans and the carrot and cook for another 5 minutes.

3 Add the scallions and bean sprouts and heat for 1–2 minutes, or until tender. Stir in the noodles and tamari sauce. Garnish with cilantro leaves.

Nutritional information per serving:

Cals 409   Fat 21g   Saturated fat 17.5g   Carbohydrates 28g   Sugar 6.5g   Sodium 707mg   Fiber 4g   Protein 25g   Cholesterol 40mg

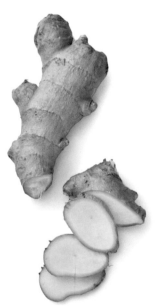

Just a small amount of freshly grated ginger supports digestion, helping to remove toxins.

FLUID REBALANCING

HAIR CONDITIONING

HEALTHY TEETH & GUMS
NAIL STRENGTHENING

Salmon with samphire

Rich in essential **omega-3** fats, salmon **nourishes** hard, rough skin. The sea vegetable samphire is rich in vitamins, silica, iron, zinc, and maganese, all of which **support skin**, hair, and nails.

Serves 2   Prep time: 10 mins   Cook time: 20 mins

Ingredients

½ cup short-grain brown rice

2 x 5oz (140g) salmon fillets

juice of 1 lemon and 1 lime

2 garlic cloves, finely chopped

2 tsp coconut oil

3½oz (100g) samphire

How to make

1 Preheat the oven to 400°C (200°C). Cook the rice according to the package instructions.

2 Place each salmon fillet on a piece of parchment paper, enough to cover each one, then place this on a piece of foil, large enough to wrap around it.

3 Pour the lemon and lime juice over the salmon. Mix the garlic and coconut oil and spread this over. Wrap the foil at the top to make a loose package.

4 Bake in the oven for 18–20 minutes, until the salmon flakes easily with a fork. Steam the samphire for 2–3 minutes, until tender. Serve the salmon on a bed of rice with the samphire on the side.

Variations

For a creamier version using skin-hydrating coconut, cook the rice in a combination of water and coconut milk. Use ¼ cup basmati rice and cook in ¼ cup each of coconut milk and water, according to the package instructions. If samphire is hard to find, replace this with broccoli and sugar snap peas.

Nutritional information per serving:

Cals 523   Fat 27g   Saturated fat 7g   Carbohydrates 32.5g   Sugar 1.5g
Sodium 65mg   Fiber 3g   Protein 36g   Cholesterol 101mg

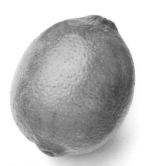

Both the tangy zest and the juice of limes contain vitamin C and betacarotene.

SKIN SMOOTHING

HEALTHY TEETH & GUMS

NAIL STRENGTHENING

Polenta with grilled vegetables

This rainbow of vegetables is abundant in antioxidants, including the flavonoid quercetin, in red bell peppers, which **rejuvenates** skin cells, promoting a smooth complexion.

Serves 4   Prep time: 10 mins, plus setting   Cook time: 20 mins

Ingredients

3 cups vegetable stock

1 cup polenta (quick cook)

1 cup fresh basil, leaves only and roughly torn

¼ cup Parmesan cheese (optional)

1 tbsp olive oil

2 zucchini, sliced into ribbons ⅛in (3mm) thick

1 eggplant, sliced into strips ⅛in (3mm) thick

2 red bell peppers, seeded and cut into strips

10 cherry tomatoes

freshly ground black pepper and Himalayan pink salt

arugula leaves and a drizzle of olive oil or herb pesto (p.180), to serve

How to make

1 Bring the stock to a boil, add the polenta, and cook for about 5 minutes, stirring constantly, until all the liquid has been absorbed and the mixture is thick. Add the basil and, if using, the Parmesan, stir for 30 seconds, then pour the mixture onto a large baking sheet lightly wiped with oil. Preheat the broiler.

2 Use a palette knife to spread out the polenta to about ½in (1.25cm) thick. Let set for about 20 minutes. Flip the baking sheet upside down onto a cutting board. Cut polenta into a rectangle, lightly brush with olive oil, then grill until golden and crispy. Set aside.

3 Brush the vegetables with olive oil, season, and lightly grill for about 15 minutes, until tender. Stack the vegetables on top of the polenta, scatter over the arugula leaves on top, and serve with a drizzle of olive oil or herb pesto.

BASIL

Fragrant basil is a delicious source of anti-aging antioxidants. Its oil also has **antibacterial** properties that help to clear acne and balance your complexion.

Nutritional information per serving:

Cals 472   Fat 8.5g   Saturated fat 3g   Carbohydrates 73.5g   Sugar 14g   Sodium 128mg   Fiber 13g   Protein 19g   Cholesterol 12mg

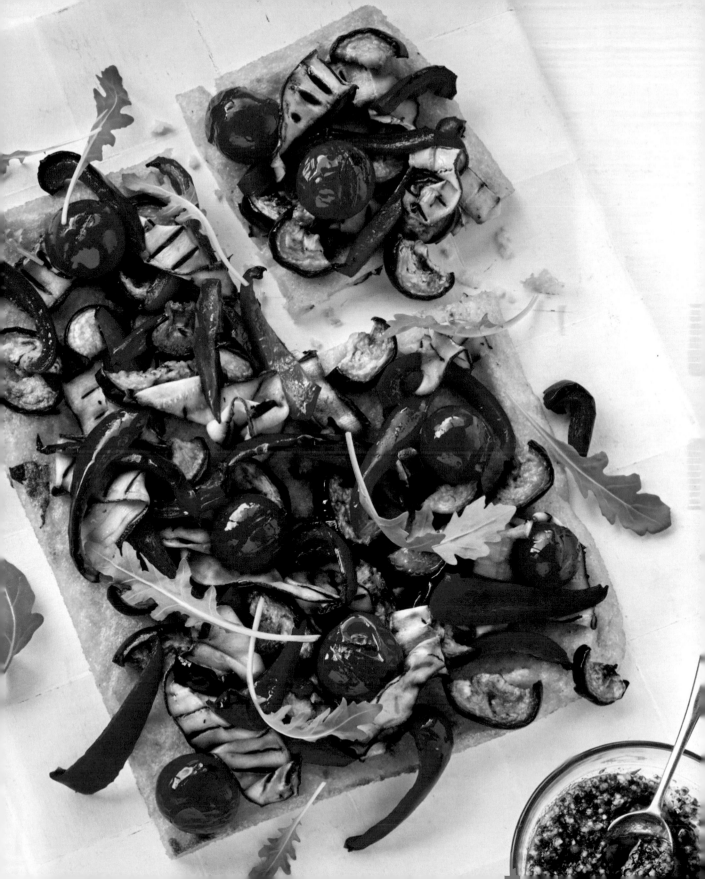

ANTI-AGING

SKIN BALANCING

SKIN FIRMING

HEALTHY TEETH & GUMS

NAIL STRENGTHENING

Miso-glazed tofu with quinoa

Sesame seeds and oil provide essential omega fats that help to **moisturize** skin, keeping it **supple** and soft, while tamari contains the B vitamin niacin, which boosts circulation to the skin.

MISO PASTE

This antioxidant-rich savory paste helps to support **good gut bacteria**, in turn promoting the body's uptake of skin-essential nutrients.

Serves 4   **Prep time: 10 mins, plus marinating**   **Cook time: 15 mins, plus standing**

Ingredients

1 tbsp miso paste

juice of 1 orange, plus some zest

1 tsp sesame oil

1 tsp tamari sauce

2 tsp light tahini

½ tsp maple syrup

¼ tsp red pepper flakes (optional)

2 cloves garlic, peeled and crushed

Himalayan pink salt and freshly ground black pepper

9oz (250g) firm tofu, cut into triangles about ½in (1cm) thick

drizzle of olive oil

½ cup quinoa, rinsed

¾ cup hot vegetable stock

2 tbsp sesame seeds

How to make

1 Mix the miso and orange juice and zest in a small bowl, smoothing out all lumps. Add the sesame oil, tamari, tahini, maple syrup, red pepper flakes if using, garlic, and seasoning, and mix well. Place the tofu in a dish, pour the marinade over the top, making sure the tofu is completely covered, and marinate for 1–2 hours.

2 Heat a little oil in a pan and cook the tofu for a few minutes on either side. Add any remaining marinade to the pan, lower the heat, and reduce down until slightly sticky. Keep warm.

3 Place the quinoa and stock in a lidded pan and bring to a boil. Reduce the heat to a low simmer for approximately 10 minutes, or until the water has been absorbed. Turn off the heat, but keep the lid on, and let stand for another 10 minutes.

4 Fluff up the quinoa with a fork and serve with the glazed tofu and sprinkled sesame seeds on top.

Nutritional information per serving:

Cals 241   Fat 12.5g   Saturated fat 2g   Carbohydrates 17g   Sugar 4.5g
Sodium 170mg   Fiber 4g   Protein 14g   Cholesterol 0mg

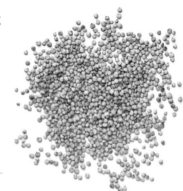

The three types of quinoa, black, red, and white, have similar nutrients.

ANTI-AGING

SKIN SMOOTHING

SKIN CALMING

SKIN BALANCING

NAIL STRENGTHENING

Potato mash with veggie mix

The orange pigment in sweet potatoes is rich in the antioxidant **betacarotene**. This converts to **vitamin A** in the body, an essential skin nutrient that helps to accelerate scar healing.

Serves 4   **Prep time: 10 mins**   **Cook time: 15–20 mins**

Ingredients

2 large sweet potatoes, peeled and chopped into chunks

2 large parsnips, peeled and sliced

2 large carrots, peeled and sliced

1 tbsp olive oil, plus a drizzle

freshly ground black pepper and Himalayan pink salt

handful of mixed sprouted seeds, 1 tbsp pumpkin, sunflower, and sesame seeds, to serve

For the steamed veggies

Choose from the following veggies:

¾ cup peas

1 onion, chopped

1 leek, chopped

1 cup green beans, trimmed

4–5 small cauliflower florets

handful Brussels sprouts, halved

4–5 stems broccoli, broccolini, or purple sprouting, chopped

handful of chard, spinach, or kale, chopped

How to make

1 Layer the vegetables to steam with the harder ones, such as cauliflower, in the bottom of the steamer. Steam the vegetables for 7–10 minutes, until still slightly firm. Add the leafy greens for a few minutes at the end of the steaming time.

2 Meanwhile, boil the potatoes, parsnips, and carrots for 15–20 minutes, until soft. Drain, mash with the olive oil, season, and cover to keep warm.

3 Serve the vegetables on top of the mash, season again, sprinkle with the sprouted seeds, other seeds, and a drizzle of olive oil.

Variation

For a boost of healthy omega fats, replace the carrots and parsnips in the mash with mackerel. Preheat the oven to 400°F (200°C). Wrap 2 mackerel fillets in parchment paper, then wrap loosely in foil. Cook for 16–18 minutes. Add to the sweet potato with finely chopped cilantro, and 1 or 2 tbsp of olive oil. Season and mash everything together.

Nutritional information per serving:

Cals 483   Fat 13g   Saturated fat 2g   Carbohydrates 67.5g   Sugar 27g   Sodium 146mg   Fiber 22g   Protein 12.5g   Cholesterol 0mg

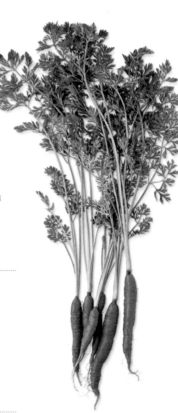

The leafy greens *of carrots are full of nutrients, too. Sauté them in olive oil and garlic for a tasty side dish.*

**FLUID
REBALANCING**

**SKIN
CALMING**

**SKIN
BALANCING**

**SKIN
FIRMING**

**HEALTHY
TEETH & GUMS**

**NAIL
STRENGTHENING**

...for Dinner

Nutty rice salad

With **hydrating** peppers and salad leaves, and high in essential **omega-3** oils from the avocado, this rice salad is a **nourishing** and conditioning treat for damaged, brittle nails.

220

Serves 4   Prep time: 10 mins   Cook time: 20 mins

Ingredients

1 cup brown rice

1¼ cups chicken or vegetable stock

1 onion, finely chopped

1 garlic clove, crushed

1 avocado, sliced

handful of roasted cashews or almonds

handful of golden raisins (optional)

1 red or green bell pepper, seeded and diced

handful of watercress or arugula,

handful of spinach

1 cup button mushrooms, sliced

1 tbsp olive, macadamia, or walnut oil and basil leaves, to serve

How to make

1 Cook the rice in the stock according to the package instructions, until cooked, but still with a little bite. Set aside to cool.

2 Meanwhile, gently cook the onion until soft and translucent, for about 10 minutes. Add the garlic and cook for another minute.

3 Place the cooled rice in a serving bowl. Add the onion and the remaining ingredients, then thoroughly combine. To serve, drizzle with the oil and scatter a few basil leaves over the top.

Variation

For an extra-hydrating rice salad, cook the rice as above, let cool, then add 1 tbsp each of pumpkin seeds, sunflower seeds, flaxseeds, hemp seeds, and toasted pine nuts; ½ tsp chopped garlic; 2 thinly sliced scallions; ¼ cucumber and ½ zucchini, sliced into matchsticks; and 2 tbsp chopped fresh herbs, such as basil, mint, rosemary, cilantro, or marjoram. Make a dressing by combining ⅓ cup olive oil, 2 tbsp lemon juice, and 1 tbsp soy sauce. Pour over the rice salad and serve.

Nutritional information per serving:

Cals 354   Fat 14g   Saturated fat 3g   Carbohydrates 44g   Sugar 9g
Sodium 18mg   Fiber 5.5g   Protein 9g   Cholesterol 0mg

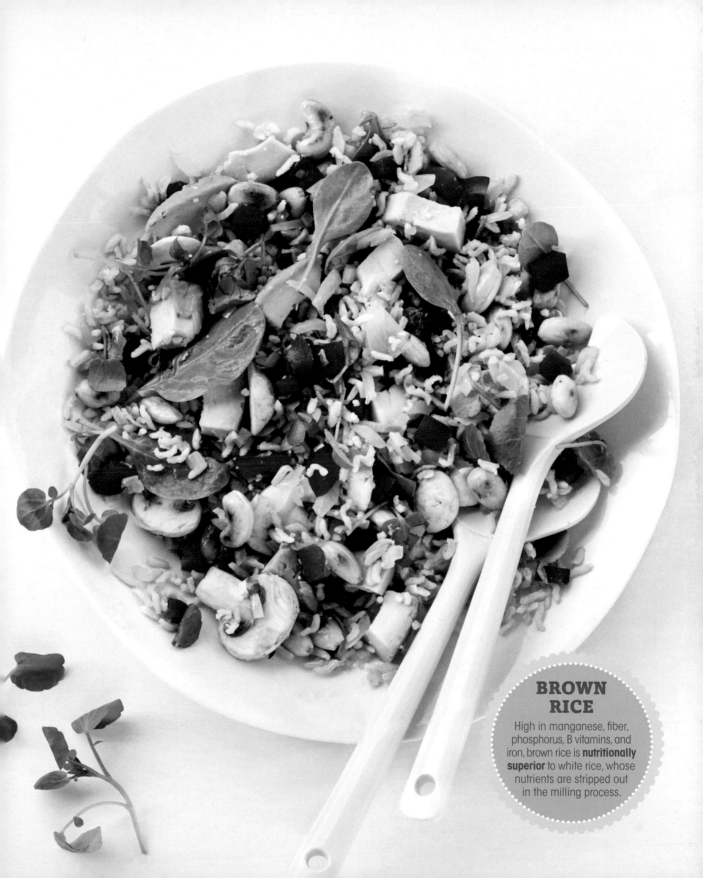

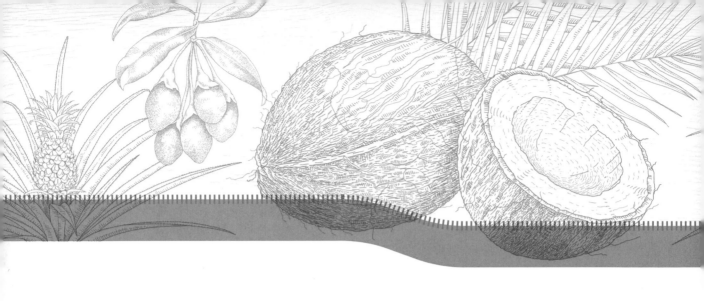

...for Sweet treats

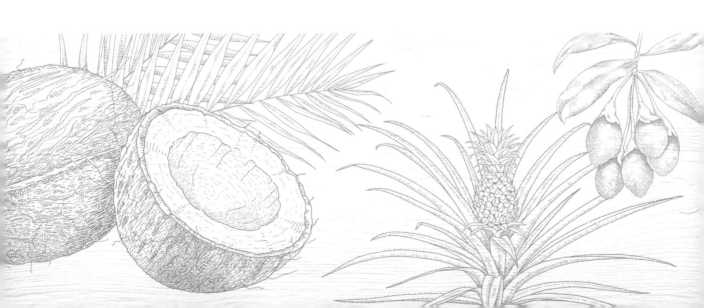

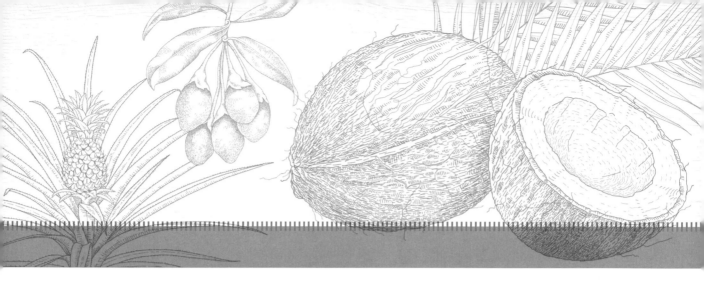

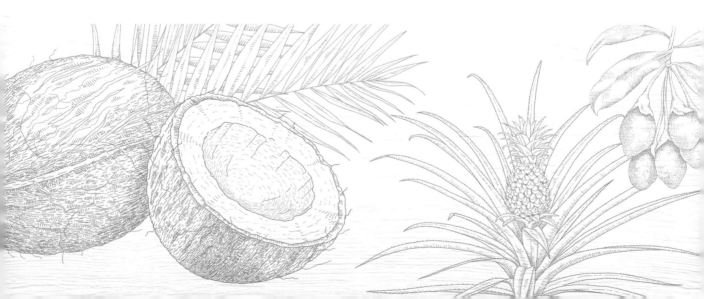

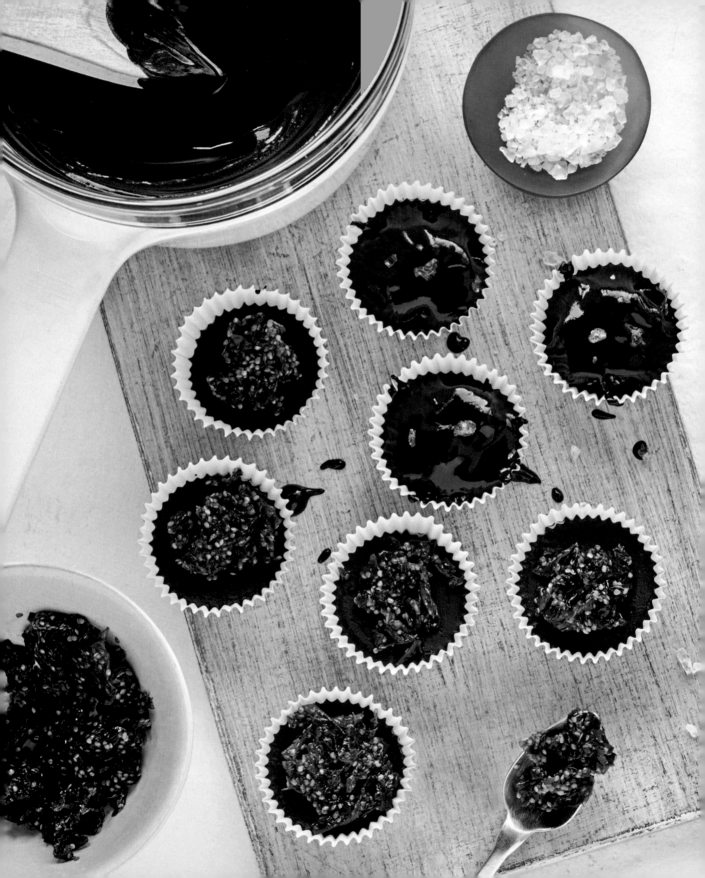

ANTI-AGING

SKIN
SMOOTHING

SKIN
FIRMING

HEALTHY
TEETH & GUMS

NAIL
STRENGTHENING

Salted goldenberry chocolate cups

These guilt-free sweet treats are full of **nourishing** coconut oil, which not only **hydrates** skin, but also has antifungal properties that help control perspiration and promote good oral hygiene.

VANILLA

This super-sweet spice is a source of **magnesium**, which helps the body assimilate nutrients, and **B vitamins**, which help to delay signs of aging such as age spots.

Makes 12 mini cupcakes   **Prep time: 10–15 mins, plus soaking and freezing**

Ingredients

For the salted goldenberry crush

¼ cup goldenberries (cape gooseberries), soaked for 2–4 hours

¼ tsp Himalayan pink salt

2 tsp goldenberry water

For the homemade chocolate

3½oz (100g) coconut oil

1 cup raw cacao powder

¼ cup maple syrup

1 vanilla bean, seeds only

¼ tsp Himalayan pink salt, to garnish

How to make

1 For the goldenberry crush, drain the goldenberries, reserving 2 teaspoons of the water, then blend the goldenberries and the reserved water with the salt in a food processor to form a paste.

2 For the chocolate, place the coconut oil in a bowl over a saucepan of hot water until it becomes liquid. Add the other ingredients to the bowl, except the salt, and mix thoroughly, keeping the bowl over the hot water to keep the coconut oil from resetting. Spoon a little of the chocolate mix into mini paper cups to form a base for the crush, and place in the freezer for about 15 minutes, until solid. Keep the rest of the chocolate mix warm, but set aside.

3 Place a little of the goldenberry paste on top of each set chocolate cup, then fill the cups with the remaining chocolate mix, sprinkle with the salt, and refreeze until solid. Enjoy!

Nutritional information per serving:

Cals 124   Fat 8.5g   Saturated fat 7g   Carbohydrates 9g   Sugar 7g
Sodium 75mg   Fiber 1.5g   Protein 2.2g   Cholesterol 0mg

ANTI-AGING

SKIN
SMOOTHING

SKIN
CALMING

SKIN
BALANCING

HAIR
CONDITIONING

NAIL
STRENGTHENING

Coconut yogurt with baobab and goldenberries

Bursting with minerals and antioxidants from goldenberry and baobab "superfruits," this creamy treat **aids** collagen synthesis, helping to **tackle cellulite** and promote healthy-looking hair and nails.

Serves 2   **Prep time: 5 mins, plus soaking**   **Cook time: 6 mins**

Ingredients

4 apricots, or 2 peaches, halved
  and pits removed

2 tsp coconut oil

zest of 1 orange

2 tsp baobab powder

½ cup coconut yogurt, or natural
  live yogurt

1 tsp bee pollen

2 tsp chia seeds

2 tsp raw honey

10 soaked goldenberries, or
  fresh physalis, quartered

How to make

1 Preheat the broiler. Place the apricot or peach halves flat sides up in a snug-fitting, heatproof dish. Drizzle some coconut oil over the fruit and scatter the orange zest over them. Place under the broiler for about 6 minutes, or until soft and golden.

2 Meanwhile, mix the baobab and yogurt in a bowl. When the fruit is ready, remove and let cool a little. Place the fruit in another bowl, flat sides up.

3 Spoon the yogurt mix inside the fruit hollows. Sprinkle the bee pollen and chia seeds on top, drizzle with a little honey, and serve with the goldenberries on the side.

RAW HONEY

Raw, unpasteurized honey retains the **health-giving properties** that are often destroyed in the heating process that pasteurized honey undergoes.

Nutritional information per serving:

Cals 276   Fat 17g   Saturated fat 13.5g   Carbohydrates 24.5g
Sugar 22g   Sodium 29mg   Fiber 4g   Protein 5g   Cholesterol 0mg

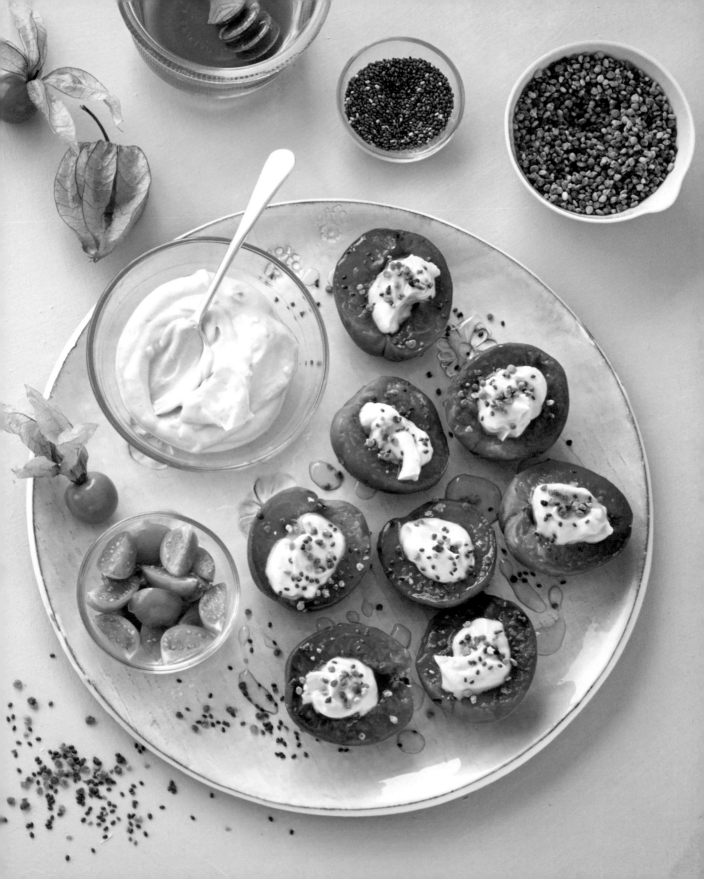

ANTI-AGING

SKIN SMOOTHING

SKIN CALMING

SKIN BALANCING

HAIR CONDITIONING

NAIL STRENGTHENING

MACADAMIA

Macadamia nuts are a beauty-food must. High in selenium, zinc, antioxidants, and fatty acids, they **nourish from within**, bolstering skin, hair, and nails.

Pineapple with cacao and coconut sauce

Sweet, delicious, and an excellent source of **skin-repairing** vitamin C, pineapple is always a hit. Coconut oil is **deeply nourishing**, helping to soften areas of hard, cracked skin.

Serves 4   **Prep time: 20 mins**   **Cook time: 20 mins, plus cooling**

Ingredients

1 pineapple, peeled and cut into ½in (1cm) slices

1 tbsp coconut oil

pinch of ground cardamom

For the macadamia cream

¾ cup macadamia nuts

1 tbsp maple syrup (or more for a sweeter taste)

1 tsp coconut oil

pinch of Himalayan pink salt

¾ cup water

For the sauce

¼ cup raw cacao powder

¼ cup melted coconut oil (stand in a bowl of hot water if solid), plus a little extra for brushing

1 tsp maple syrup

How to make

1 To make the macadamia cream, put all the ingredients except for the water in a blender, then pulse, adding the water a little at a time until the mixture is smooth. Store in the fridge. For the pineapple, preheat the broiler. Place the pineapple slices on a baking sheet and brush the tops with the coconut oil. Sprinkle the slices with the cardamom and broil for about 20 minutes, until the tops are golden.

2 To make the sauce, place a heatproof bowl over a pan of boiled water. Place all the ingredients in the bowl and combine until there are no lumps of cacao powder. The sauce will set as it cools, so keep it over the bowl of hot water until you're ready to use it.

3 Place the pineapple slices on a plate and let cool for a couple of minutes. Drizzle with the cacao and coconut sauce and serve with the macadamia cream.

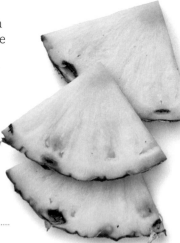

The soft innner flesh of the pineapple is nutrient-rich.

Nutritional information per serving:

Cals 419   Fat 36g   Saturated fat 17g   Carbohydrates 18g   Sugar 17g   Sodium 126mg   Fiber 4g   Protein 4g   Cholesterol 0mg

ANTI-AGING

SKIN
SMOOTHING

SKIN
CALMING

HAIR
CONDITIONING

Sweet green ice cream

With **hydrating** cucumber, **moisture-replenishing** coconut milk, and vitamin C–rich pineapple, this healthy ice cream is a treat for dry skin and helps to **condition** and strengthen fragile, thinning hair.

Serves 8   **Prep time: 15–20 mins, plus setting**

Ingredients

- 1 x 14oz (400ml) can coconut milk
- large handful of spinach
- 1 x 14oz (400g) can pineapple chunks, including the core
- 4 tsp baobab powder
- 1 avocado
- ¼ cucumber
- juice of ½ lemon
- ½ tsp guar or xanthan gum
- 1 cup cashews

How to make

1 Mix all the ingredients together in a food processor until thoroughly combined. Pour the ice cream mixture into a freezerproof container with a lid, or cover in plastic wrap.

2 Remove the ice cream from the freezer every 30 minutes and stir the mixture well. Do this until the ice cream is frozen (you will need to do this about 4–5 times) to prevent crystal build-up. Store the ice cream in the freezer.

3 Remove from the freezer and allow to sit for 10 minutes at room temperature to soften before serving.

Variation

Try adding 2 teaspoons of matcha powder to the mixture for extra antioxidant support for the skin.

Nutritional information per serving:

Cals 135   Fat 12g   Saturated fat 8g   Carbohydrates 4g   Sugar 3g
Sodium 11mg   Fiber 1.8g   Protein 1.5g   Cholesterol 0mg

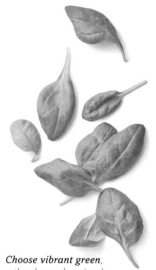

Choose vibrant green, *rather than pale, spinach leaves, as these have higher levels of vitamin C.*

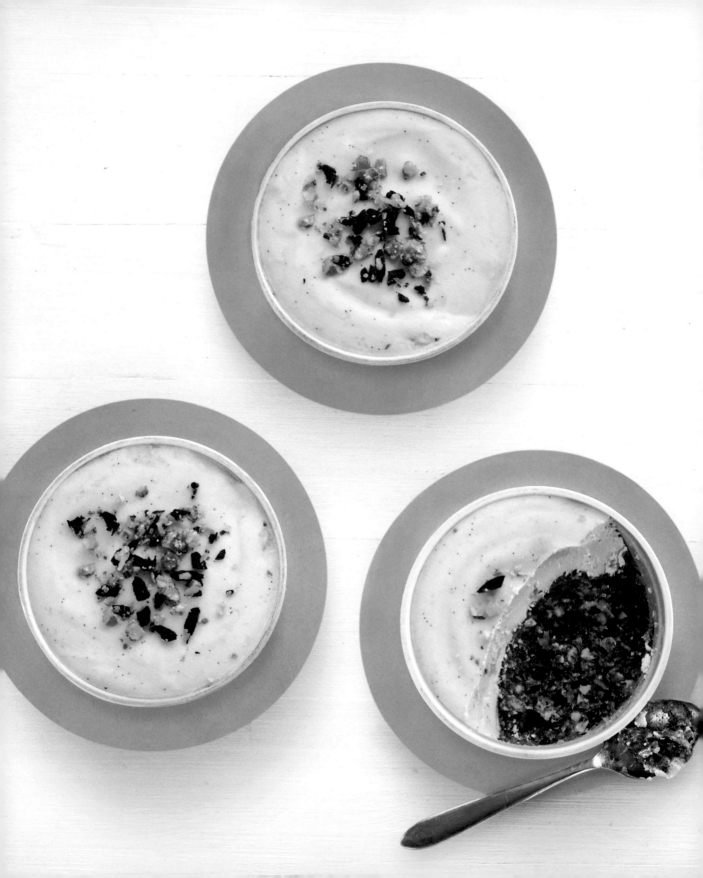

ANTI-AGING

SKIN
SMOOTHING

HAIR
CONDITIONING

HEALTHY
TEETH & GUMS

NAIL
STRENGTHENING

Cashew and goji berry cheesecake

Perfect for celebrations, this dessert uses **sugar-free** cacao. The cashews provide copper, which **boosts melanin production**, helping delay the onset of gray hairs.

Serves 8   **Prep time: 10–15 mins, plus soaking, setting, and chilling**

Ingredients

For the crumble base

2 tbsp goji berries, plus 1 tsp chopped dried goji berries for the topping

handful each of walnuts, almonds, pumpkin seeds, and hulled hemp seeds

2 tsp coconut oil

8 dates, ideally Medjool, chopped

For the topping

2 cups cashews, soaked for at least 4 hours

¾ cup coconut oil

½ cup lemon, lime, or orange juice

seeds of 1 vanilla bean

4–6 tbsp maple syrup

How to make

1 Soak the 2 tablespoons goji berries in a little water until plump. Set aside 3–4 walnuts, then place all the ingredients for the cheesecake base in a food processor and process until the mixture sticks together, stopping to push the mixture back down in the bowl if needed until the texture is sufficiently fine.

2 Press the crumble base into small ramekins and place in the freezer for 30 minutes, until set.

3 To make the topping, place all the ingredients in a food processor and blend until smooth and creamy. Spoon over the crumble base. Chop 1 teaspoon goji berries and the reserved walnuts and sprinkle over the cheesecake tops. Chill in the fridge for a minimum of 3 hours, until set, then serve. The cheesecakes will keep for up to 2 days.

DATES
These natural sweeteners are full of beauty benefits. High in the **essential skin vitamins** B and C, dates also top off our calcium levels to **strengthen teeth and hair**.

Nutritional information per serving:

Cals 490   Fat 41g   Saturated fat 20g   Carbohydrates 19g   Sugar 14g
Sodium 12mg   Fiber 2.5g   Protein 10g   Cholesterol 0mg

...for Drinks

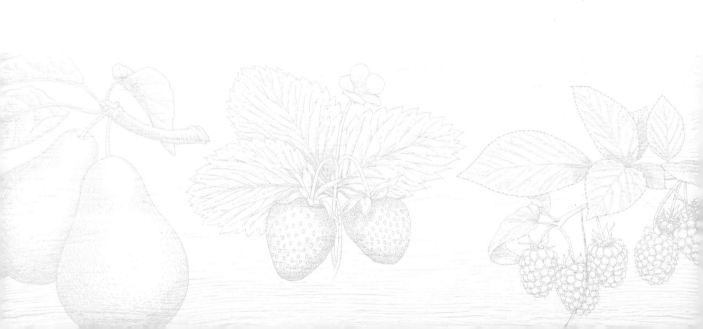

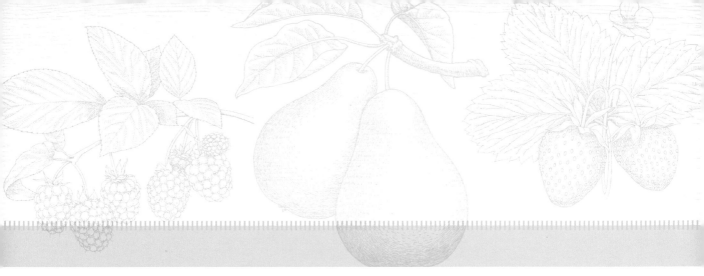

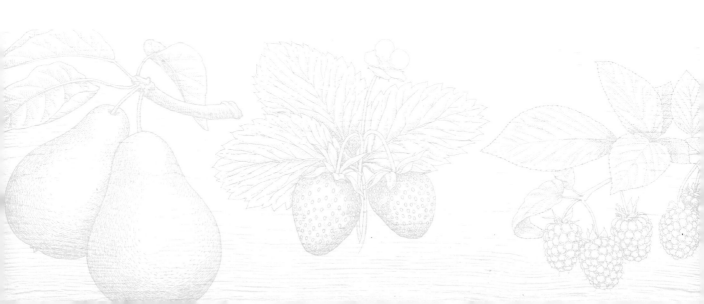

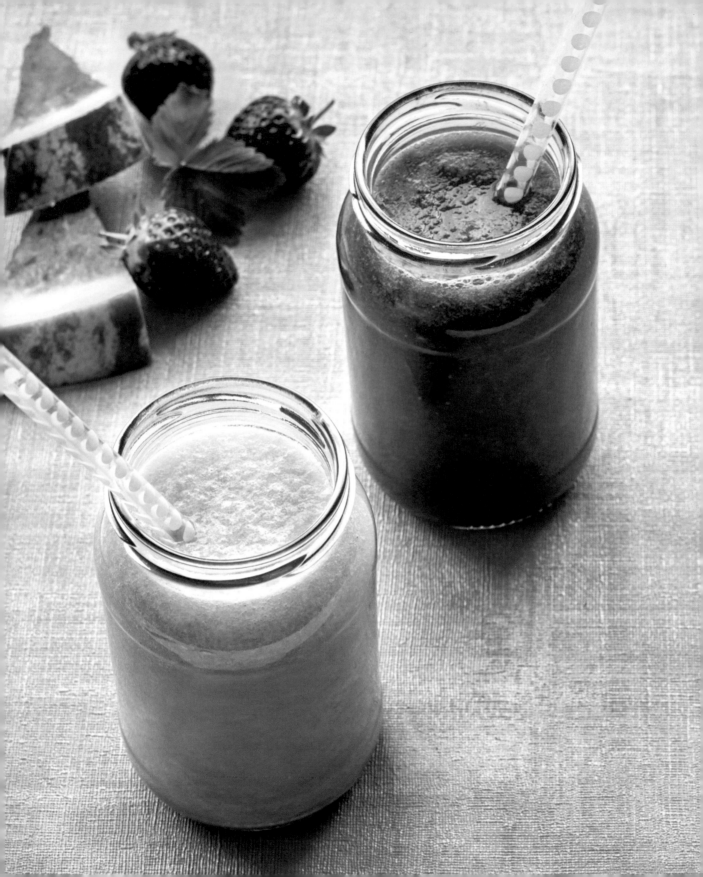

ANTI-AGING   FLUID REBALANCING   SKIN CALMING   SKIN FIRMING   HEALTHY TEETH & GUMS

Red berry smoothie

Full of **beta-carotene**, this skin-protecting smoothie helps ward off tell-tale signs of aging, such as age spots.

Serves 2   **Prep time: 5 mins, plus infusing**

Ingredients

2 tsp pink rose buds or petals

¼ chilled watermelon, chopped and seeds removed

5 strawberries (optional)

6 tsp goji berries, rehydrated and puréed

How to make

1 First, make a rose infusion by placing the pink rose buds in a cup of boiling water. Infuse for 5–10 minutes, let cool, then drain.

2 Put all the ingredients in a blender, together with at least 12 ice cubes. Blend the mixture, then serve immediately.

Nutritional information per serving:

Cals 181   Fat 1.5g   Saturated fat 0.5g   Carbohydrates 39g   Sugar 39g   Sodium 17mg   Fiber 2g   Protein 2g   Cholesterol 0mg

ANTI-AGING   FLUID REBALANCING   SKIN CALMING   SKIN BALANCING   SKIN FIRMING

Coconut smoothie

This coconut water smoothie is the ultimate **thirst quencher**, helping to **hydrate** dry skin and hair and regulate perspiration.

Serves 2   **Prep time: 5 mins**

Ingredients

2½ cups coconut water

juice of 1 grapefruit

3 tsp baobab powder

flesh of ½ honeydew melon

How to make

Put all the ingredients in a blender and process for 1 minute. Serve immediately.

Nutritional information per serving:

Cals 184   Fat 1.5g   Saturated fat 0.5g   Carbohydrates 37g   Sugar 37g   Sodium 400mg   Fiber 5g   Protein 3.5g   Cholesterol 0mg

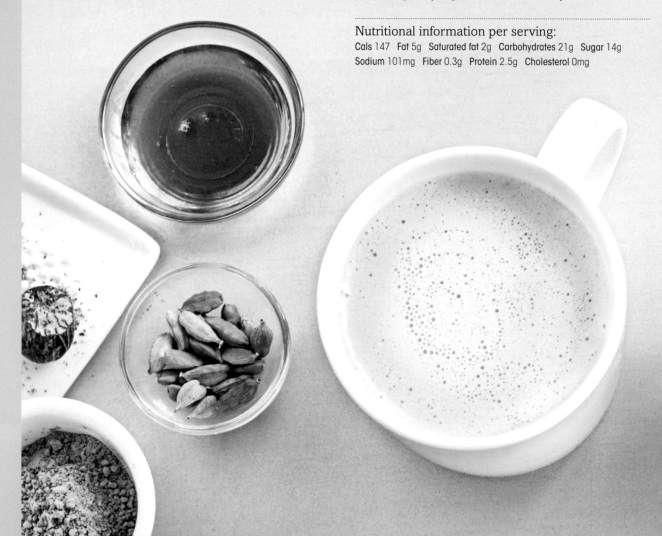

Winter warmers

Start the day with one of these warming beverages. **Calming** matcha provides powerful **antioxidants**, while cacao makes a circulation-boosting hot chocolate that leaves skin **glowing**.

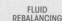

ANTI-AGING   SKIN SMOOTHING   FLUID REBALANCING   SKIN BALANCING

Matcha latte

Serves 2   **Prep time: 5 mins**   **Cook time: 10 mins**

Make a paste with 1 tsp **matcha powder** and a little **hot water**. Top off with ½ cup hot water. Gently heat 2 cups **oat milk** in a pan with a pinch each of grated **nutmeg** and **cardamom** and 1 tsp **coconut oil** for 10 minutes. Be sure not to overheat the oat milk as it may split. Whisk in the matcha water (ideally with a bamboo matcha whisk), or mix in a blender. Add 2 tsp **maple syrup**. Serve immediately.

Nutritional information per serving:
Cals 147   Fat 5g   Saturated fat 2g   Carbohydrates 21g   Sugar 14g
Sodium 101mg   Fiber 0.3g   Protein 2.5g   Cholesterol 0mg

ANTI-AGING   SKIN SMOOTHING   SKIN FIRMING

ANTI-AGING   FLUID REBALANCING   SKIN BALANCING   SKIN FIRMING

Cacao comfort

Serves 2   **Prep time: 5 mins**   **Cook time: 5–10 mins**

In a saucepan, make a paste from 6 tsp **raw cacao powder**, 1 tsp **maca powder**, and a little of 1 cup **oat milk**. When smooth, whisk in the remaining oat milk. Add 2 tsp **lucuma powder**, the zest of an **orange,** the seeds of 1 **vanilla bean**, 1–2 tbsp **maple syrup**, and ½ cup **coconut milk**. Heat slowly without boiling. Serve immediately.

Nutritional information per serving:

Cals 222   Fat 13.5g   Saturated fat 9.5g   Carbohydrates 18g   Sugar 11.5g   Sodium 51mg   Fiber 3.5g   Protein 5.5g   Cholesterol 0mg

Matcha beauty shot

Serves 1   **Prep time: 5 mins**

Put ½ tsp **matcha powder** in a small bowl. Add ½ cup **hot water** and a generous squeeze of **fresh lemon juice**. Whisk until you get a beautiful green foam. Add a dash of **maple syrup**, if you wish, to sweeten. Enjoy!

Nutritional information per serving:

Cals 21   Fat 0g   Saturated fat 0g   Carbohydrates 5g   Sugar 4.5g   Sodium 1mg   Fiber 0g   Protein 0g   Cholesterol 0mg

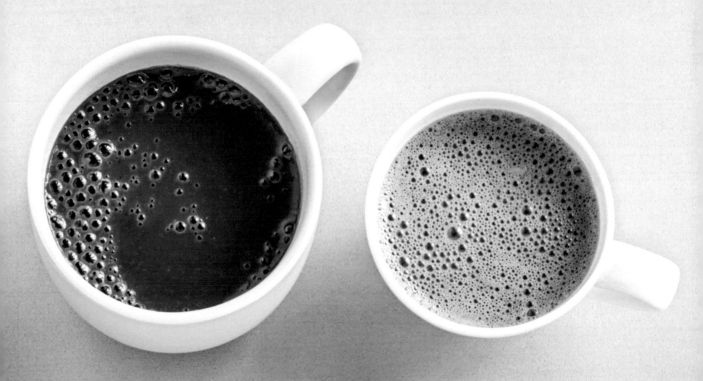

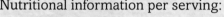

ANTI-AGING SKIN SMOOTHING SKIN CALMING SKIN FIRMING NAIL STRENGTHENING

Berry nice skin!

Naturally sweet, antioxidant-rich berries help to **support the micro-circulation** to the delicate skin around the eyes, lifting dark shadows and giving eyes a healthy sparkle.

Serves 2   **Prep time: 5 mins**

Ingredients

½ cup coconut yogurt
½ cup blueberries
½ cup raspberries or strawberries
1 banana
½ pineapple, peeled and sliced
1 heaping tsp coconut oil
2½ tbsp chia seeds
1¾ cups water

How to make

Place all the ingredients in a blender, setting aside a few berries and chia seeds. Process until smooth and creamy. Serve with a sprinkling of berries and chia seeds on top.

Nutritional information per serving:

Cals 401   **Fat** 17.5g   **Saturated fat** 10.5g   **Carbohydrates** 47g
Sugar 38g   **Sodium** 30mg   **Fiber** 13.5g   **Protein** 7g   **Cholesterol** 0mg

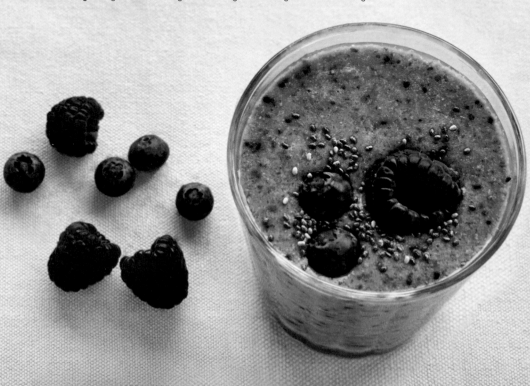

ANTI-AGING　　SKIN SMOOTHING　　SKIN CALMING　　SKIN BALANCING　　HAIR CONDITIONING

Pineapple smoothie

This smoothie take on the milky Indian drink "lassi" is full of **beneficial enzymes** from the pineapple, mango, and papaya that support digestion and the efficient **elimination** of toxins.

Serves 2　　**Prep time: 5 mins**

Ingredients

handful of mango pieces

handful of pineapple pieces

½ cup natural live yogurt, or coconut yogurt

12 strands of saffron (optional)

½ tsp ground turmeric

1 tsp ground ginger

4 tsp baobab powder

¼ tsp ground cardamom

1¼ cups water

pinch of Himalayan pink salt

sprinkle of bee pollen

How to make

Place all the ingredients, except for the bee pollen, in a blender and process until smooth. Serve the smoothie immediately, with a sprinkle of bee pollen over the top.

Variation

If you wish, you can try papaya instead of mango in this smoothie. Similarly sweet and delicious, papaya has a high water content to give skin a hydrating boost.

CARDAMOM

This aromatic spice has good beauty credentials. A source of **fiber**, cardamom aids the elimination of toxins and also provides **iron**, which helps oxygenate skin tissues.

Nutritional information per serving:

Cals 257　Fat 22g　Saturated fat 19g　Carbohydrates 10.5g　Sugar 9.5g
Sodium 244mg　Fiber 2.5g　Protein 4g　Cholesterol 0mg

ANTI-AGING

SKIN SMOOTHING

FLUID REBALANCING

SKIN CALMING

SKIN BALANCING

SKIN FIRMING

for Drinks

Matcha fruit shake

MANGO

A superfood among fruits, mango is a rich source of prebiotic dietary fiber, and is high in vitamins, including vitamin A for **eye health**, minerals, and antioxidant flavonoids.

Filled with **antioxidants**, matcha is a top **anti-aging** ingredient. Simple to make, this sweet smoothie supports the circulation, helping to **lift** sallow, dull-looking skin.

240

Serves 2   **Prep time: 5 mins**

Ingredients

1 tsp matcha

1¼ cups oat milk

1 tsp coconut oil

large handful of mango pieces

2 tsp baobab powder

1–2 tsp maple syrup

4 tsp shredded coconut

How to make

Process all of the ingredients together in a blender, along with a good handful of ice cubes. Sit back and enjoy!

Variations

You can easily use pineapple pieces in place of the mango here, if you prefer. High in vitamin C, pineapple boosts collagen production, helping to keep skin firm.

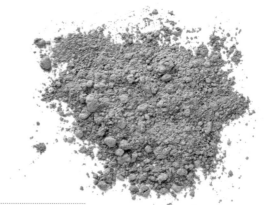

Matcha has a higher antioxidant count than standard green tea.

Nutritional information per serving:

Cals 178   Fat 10g   Saturated fat 7g   Carbohydrates 18g   Sugar 13.5g   Sodium64mg   Fiber 4g   Protein 2.3g   Cholesterol 0mg

SKIN CALMING

SKIN BALANCING

SKIN FIRMING

HAIR CONDITIONING

HEALTHY TEETH & GUMS

NAIL STRENGTHENING

Homemade oat milk

Soothing oats have myriad benefits for dry skin, providing **skin-repairing silica**, B vitamins, and **essential fats**. To get all their goodness, nothing beats homemade oat milk.

Serves 2   **Prep time: 10 mins, plus soaking**

Ingredients

1 cup jumbo rolled oats

2½ cups water

seeds of 1 vanilla bean

4 Medjool dates

¼ tsp ground cinnamon

How to make

1 Soak the oats in water for 20 minutes, then rinse through a strainer. Put the oats, fresh water, and other ingredients into a blender and process on a high setting until smooth.

2 Strain the oat milk by pouring it through a nut milk bag (or cheesecloth) into a jug or bowl. Use your hands to squeeze the milk out of the nut milk bag.

3 Store the oat milk in the fridge for 2–3 days. Shake thoroughly before using. Don't heat as this will make it thicken! Try composting the oat pulp.

Nutritional information per serving:

Cals 112   Fat 2g   Saturated fat 0.3g   Carbohydrates 19g   Sugar 2.5g
Sodium 1mg   Fiber 2.5g   Protein 3g   Cholesterol 0.1mg

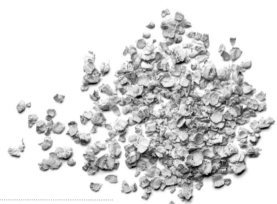

The process of rolling oats into flakes helps to stabilize the healthy oils.

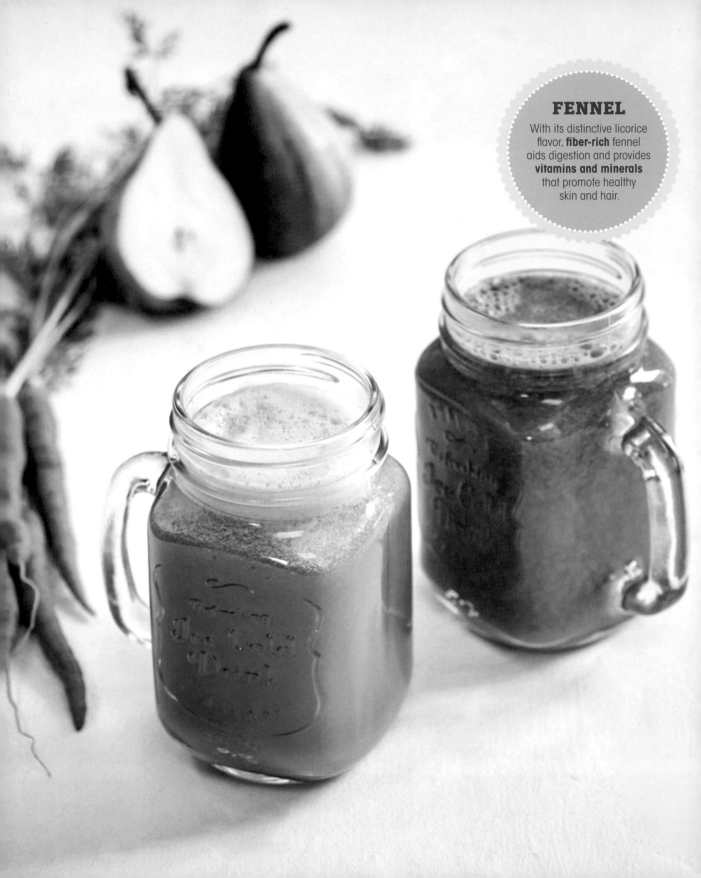

FENNEL

With its distinctive licorice flavor, **fiber-rich** fennel aids digestion and provides **vitamins and minerals** that promote healthy skin and hair.

ANTI-AGING FLUID REBALANCING SKIN BALANCING SKIN FIRMING NAIL STRENGTHENING

Grapefruit and pear juice

Revitalizing and refreshing, this clever mix of **cleansing** grapefruit and slightly aniseed fennel is guaranteed to quench your thirst.

Serves 1   **Prep time: 5 mins**

Ingredients

1 grapefruit, peeled

2 pears

½ fennel bulb

½ cucumber

3 carrots

½in (1cm) piece fresh turmeric (optional)

How to make

Put all the ingredients through a juicer or process in a blender. If you have a centrifugal juicer, you may need to squeeze the grapefruit separately and then add to the juice. Serve immediately.

Nutritional information per serving:

Cals 308 Fat 2.5g Saturated fat 0.5g Carbohydrates 53g Sugar 52g Sodium 147mg Fiber 23g Protein 6.5g Cholesterol 0mg

 SKIN SMOOTHING FLUID REBALANCING SKIN BALANCING SKIN FIRMING

Cucumber and kale juice

Sweet and tangy, this super healthy juice has **detoxifying** greens that help to **flush out** toxins and reduce bloating.

Serves 1   **Prep time: 5 mins**

Ingredients

½ large cucumber

½ bulb fennel

1 large handful kale

2 apples, peeled and cored

3 celery stalks

juice of ½ lemon or lime

½in (1cm) piece fresh ginger

How to make

Put all the ingredients through a juicer or process in a blender. Serve immediately.

Nutritional information per serving:

Cals 140 Fat 0g Saturated fat 0g Carbohydrates 29g Sugar 29g Sodium 40mg Fiber 1g Protein 3g Cholesterol 0mg

ANTI-AGING

SKIN
SMOOTHING

FLUID
REBALANCING

SKIN
BALANCING

HAIR
CONDITIONING

HEALTHY
TEETH & GUMS

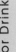

...for Drinks

244

Green smoothie

This **nourishing** smoothie, high in essential fats, vitamin C, and antioxidants, makes an all-in-one breakfast or healthy snack, giving skin, hair, and nails a **complete nutrient boost**.

Serves 1   **Prep time: 5 mins**

Ingredients

1 avocado, pitted and peeled

1 large handful spinach

¼ cucumber

handful of blueberries

6 strawberries

generous squeeze of lemon juice

1 cup coconut water

How to make

Process all the ingredients together in a blender until smooth. Enjoy immediately.

Variations

Instead of spinach, try adding kale or even lettuce—just keep it green. Leafy green vegetables have more nutrition per calorie than any other food. Kale is especially rich in calcium, helping to keep teeth strong and healthy.

BLUEBERRY

The succulent blueberry is renowned for promoting eye health. Blueberries contain the antioxidant **lutein**, which protects the delicate blood vessels around the eyes.

Nutritional information per serving:

Cals 419   Fat 31.5g   Saturated fat 7g   Carbohydrates 20.5g   Sugar 18.5g
Sodium 383mg   Fiber 12g   Protein 7g   Cholesterol 0mg

ANTI-AGING

SKIN SMOOTHING

SKIN CALMING

SKIN BALANCING

SKIN FIRMING

Vitamin C boost

Full of superfoods, this revitalizing smoothie delivers a **vitamin C** boost, providing all the **skin-healing** and **anti-inflammatory** benefits of this important skin vitamin.

Serves 2   Prep time: 5 mins

Ingredients

½ pineapple, peeled, de-eyed, cored, and chopped

juice of 1 pink grapefruit

½ tsp ground turmeric

1 heaping tsp camu camu powder

2 heaping tsp baobab powder

3 heaping tsp presoaked goldenberries

1 heaping tsp coconut oil

4 heaping tsp coconut cream

2 cups water

How to make

Place all the ingredients in a blender and process until smooth and creamy. Serve immediately.

Nutritional information per serving:

Cals 227   Fat 9g   Saturated fat 7g   Carbohydrates 31g   Sugar 31g
Sodium 8.5mg   Fiber 5.5g   Protein 2.5g   Cholesterol 0mg

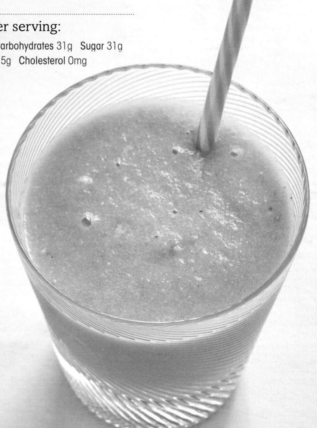

Nutrition reference charts

Eating a varied diet is the most important way to give your body the nutrients it needs to function healthfully and enhance your natural beauty. These pages show the nutritional information for each beauty food in this book, helping you to choose which foods are best for your needs.

Beauty food **nutrition**

Each of the foods in this book contains a cocktail of beauty-boosting ingredients. This chart details the key nutrients—vitamins, minerals, phytonutrients, and macronutrients—found in each beauty food.

Reference intakes (RIs)

Previously known as Guideline Daily Amounts (GDAs), reference intakes (RIs) are a guide to the approximate amount of each nutrient you should consume every day. RIs are based on official guidelines and are different for each individual, as factors such as age and gender affect energy and nutrient requirements.

Food	Nutrients
Alfalfa seeds	vitamin K, B vitamins, magnesium, silica
Almonds	vitamin E, B vitamins, biotin, calcium, copper, iron, magnesium, manganese, potassium, selenium, zinc, omega-6
Aloe vera juice	vitamins A, C, and E, calcium, chromium, magnesium, polysaccharides, potassium, selenium, zinc, beta-carotene, salicylic acid
Apple	vitamin C
Apple cider vinegar, raw	acetic acid
Asparagus, raw	vitamins B1, B3, B5, C, and K, calcium, choline, copper, fiber, folate, iron, potassium, phosphorus, manganese, selenium, zinc
Arugula	vitamin C, folate, calcium, iron, sulfur
Avocado	vitamins A, C, E, and K, B vitamins, folate, copper, iron, lutein, magnesium, potassium, beta-carotene, fatty acids, omega-3, -6, and -9
Banana	vitamins B6 and C, biotin, copper, manganese, potassium, fiber, lutein
Baobab	vitamins A, B1, B6, and C, calcium, potassium, magnesium, zinc, fiber, bioflavonoids
Barley	vitamins B1 and B3, chromium, magnesium, phosphorus, selenium, fiber
Bee pollen	B vitamins, amino acids, fatty acids, protein
Beets	vitamins A, B1, B6, and C, folate, magnesium, betalains
Black beans	vitamin B1, folate, iron, magnesium
Black-eyed peas	vitamin C, B vitamins, folate, iron, zinc

Food	Nutrients
Blueberries	vitamins C and K, manganese, anthocyanins, lutein, omega-3, quercetin
Broccoli	vitamins A, B5, C, E, and K, B vitamins, choline, folate, calcium, chromium, iron, manganese, phosphorus, potassium, selenium, zinc, omega-3, protein, sulforaphane
Brazil nuts	calcium, copper, iron, magnesium, manganese, potassium, phosphorus, selenium, zinc
Brown rice	B vitamins, zinc, fiber
Brussels sprouts	vitamins A, B1, B6, and C, folate, omega-3
Buckwheat	magnesium, quercetin, rutin, fiber, protein
Burdock root tea	vitamins C and E, potassium
Cacao, raw	vitamins B1 and B2, calcium, chromium, copper, iron, magnesium, sulfur, carotene, fatty acids, flavonoids, protein
Camu camu	vitamin C, copper, manganese, zinc, beta-carotene
Carrots	vitamins A, C, E, K, B vitamins, biotin, iron, magnesium, zinc, phosphorus, beta-carotene, carotenoids, fiber, lutein, molybdenum, potassium
Cayenne pepper	vitamins C and E, beta-carotene, capsaicin
Celery	vitamins A and C, magnesium, potassium, silica, sodium, fiber, quercetin
Chamomile tea	vitamin A, calcium, magnesium, zinc
Chia seeds	vitamins D and E, phosphorus, selenium, protein

Food	Nutrients
Chicken	vitamins B6 and B12, phosphorus, selenium, protein
Chickpeas	vitamin B6, folate, copper, iron, zinc, fiber, protein, quercetin
Chlorella	B vitamins, calcium, fatty acids, protein
Cilantro	vitamins A, B1, C, and E, zinc
Cinnamon	calcium, iron, manganese
Coconut	vitamin B6, manganese, potassium, fiber, medium-chain triglycerides
Coconut oil	vitamins E, D, and K, iron, fatty acids, medium-chain triglycerides, omega-3
Coconut water	B vitamins, potassium, sodium
Cucumber	vitamins A, B5, B6, C, E, and K, biotin, magnesium, phosphorus, potassium, silica, sulfur
Dandelion	vitamins A and C, calcium, iron, magnesium, manganese, potassium
Eggs	vitamins A, B2, B5, B12, and D, biotin, choline, iodine, phosphorus, selenium, sulfur, zinc, carotenes, lutein, omega-3, protein
Figs	vitamins A and E, B vitamins, copper, iron, magnesium, potassium, fiber
Flaxseeds	vitamins B1 and B6, copper, iron, magnesium, manganese, phosphorus, potassium, selenium, zinc, omega-3
Garlic	vitamins B6 and C, selenium, sulfur, allicin
Ginger	gingerols, volatile oils
Goji berries	vitamin C, B vitamins, calcium, copper, iron, selenium, zinc, amino acids, beta-carotene, polysaccharides, zeaxanthin
Gotu kola tea	vitamins B1, B2, and C, calcium, beta-carotene, saponins
Grapes	vitamins A, B6, C, and K, folate, copper, magnesium, selenium, resveratrol
Green beans	vitamin C and K, B vitamins, folate, iron, potassium, silica, zinc, beta-carotene, fiber, hyaluronic acid, protein
Green tea	vitamins A, B1, and B2, magnesium, potassium, catechins, epigallocatechin gallate, L-theanine
Hemp seeds	gamma linolenic acid, omega-3, -6, and -9
Kale	vitamins A, B3, C, and E, B vitamins, folate, calcium, iron, magnesium, phosphorus, potassium, omega-3

Food	Nutrients
Kefir	B vitamins, calcium, potassium, omega-3, protein
Kelp	folate, vitamins B2 and B5, iron, magnesium, zinc, L-lysine
Kidney beans	vitamin B1, iron, magnesium, manganese, phosphorus, potassium, protein
Kiwi	vitamins C, E, and K, folate, copper, manganese, potassium, fiber
Lemon	vitamin C, folate
Lentils	B vitamins, iron, potassium, zinc, fiber, protein
Lettuce	vitamins A, C, and K, biotin, folate, iron, potassium, fiber
Lima beans	vitamins B1 and B6, biotin, folate, iron, potassium, fiber
Macadamia nuts	calcium, iron, magnesium, manganese, selenium, zinc, fatty acids
Mango	vitamins A, B6, and C, folate, silica
Marigold herbal tea	lutein, lycopene, zeaxanthin
Matcha	vitamins A and K, catechins, epigallocatechin gallate, L-theanine, polyphenols
Milk thistle	vitamins C and E
Miso	vitamin K, phosphorus, zinc, fatty acids, kojic acid, omega-3, protein
Mulberries	vitamins A, B1, B2, and C, anthocyanins, protein, resveratrol
Nettles	vitamins A, D, and K, calcium, iron, potassium, silica
Nori	folate, vitamins B2 and B5, iodine, iron, magnesium, zinc
Oats	vitamin E, B vitamins, biotin, calcium, chromium, copper, iron, magnesium, silica, zinc, fiber, polysaccharides, protein
Olive leaf	elenolic acid, oleuropein

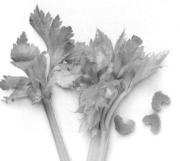

Celery is high in silica, which helps to renew the protein collagen.

Food	Nutrients
Olive oil	vitamins E and K, flavonoids, omega-9, quercetin
Onion	vitamins B1, B2, C, and E, biotin, folate, copper, magnesium, potassium, sulfur, fiber, flavonoids, inulin, quercetin
Oranges	vitamins B1 and C, folate, potassium
Papaya	vitamins A, C, E, and K, B vitamins, folate, copper, magnesium, potassium
Paprika	vitamins B2, B6, C, and E, beta-carotene
Parsley	vitamins A, C, and E, B vitamins, potassium, carotenoids, chlorophyll
Peas	B vitamins, folate, iron, potassium, zinc, fiber, protein
Pepper, orange	vitamin C, B vitamins, carotenoids, flavonoids
Pepper, red	vitamins B6 and C, folate, beta-carotene, lycopene
Pineapple	vitamins B1, B2, B5, B6, and C, folate, copper, manganese, potassium
Pink Himalayan salt	calcium, iron, magnesium, potassium
Pomegranate	vitamins B6, C, and E, folate, magnesium, zinc, folate, fiber, polyphenols
Pumpkin seeds	copper, iron, magnesium, manganese, phosphorus, zinc, fatty acids, fiber, phytosterols, protein
Quinoa	vitamins B1, B2, B6, and E, folate, copper, magnesium, manganese, phosphorus, silica, zinc, lysine, protein, quercetin
Radish	vitamins A, B3, B6, and C, folate, sulfur
Salmon	vitamins B12 and D, biotin, magnesium, potassium, selenium, omega-3, protein
Sardines	vitamins B12 and D, selenium, omega-3
Sauerkraut	vitamins C, and K, B vitamins, calcium, fiber
Sea buckthorn fruit oil	vitamins C, and E, beta-carotene, omega-7
Sesame seeds	vitamin B1, calcium, iron, magnesium, phosphorus, selenium, zinc
Snow peas	B vitamins, iron, potassium, zinc, fiber, protein
Soybeans	vitamins B2 and K, biotin, folate, iron, magnesium, potassium, omega-3
Spinach	vitamins A, B1, B2, B6, C, E, and K, folate, calcium, iron, magnesium, potassium
Spirulina	B vitamins, calcium, sulfur, beta-carotene, chlorophyll, fatty acids, gamma linolenic acids

Food	Nutrients
Sprouted seeds	vitamins A, C, E, and K, B vitamins, calcium, iron, selenium, sulfur, fiber, omega-3, protein
Strawberries	vitamins C and E, magnesium, potassium, anthocyanins, flavonoids, omega-3
Sunflower seeds	vitamins B1, B2, B3, B6, and E, folate, iron, magnesium, manganese, phosphorus, selenium, zinc, omega-3
Sweet potatoes	vitamins A, C, and K, B vitamins, biotin, folate, calcium, copper, manganese, potassium, beta-carotene, fiber, lutein, lycopene, polysaccharides
Swiss chard	vitamins A, C, E, and K, copper, iron, magnesium, manganese, potassium
Tempeh	vitamin B2, phosphorus, magnesium
Tofu	B vitamins, calcium, iron, magnesium, selenium, zinc, omega-3
Tomatoes	vitamins A, C, E, and K, B vitamins, biotin, folate, manganese, phosphorus, potassium, beta-carotene, lutein, lycopene, quercetin
Turmeric	vitamin B6, iron, manganese, potassium, beta-carotene, curcumin
Walnuts	vitamin E, B vitamins, folate, copper, iron, magnesium, potassium, alpha-linoleic acid
Watercress	vitamins A, C, and E, B vitamins, folate, calcium, iron, magnesium, manganese, phosphorus, potassium, sulfur
Watermelon	vitamins B1, B6, and C, magnesium, potassium, beta-carotene, fiber, lycopene
Wheatgrass	vitamins A, C, and E, B vitamins, iron, potassium, selenium, zinc, chlorophyll, fiber, protein
Whole-grain bread	vitamin E, B vitamins, folate, potassium, fiber, omega-9
Yogurt, natural live	B vitamins, calcium, potassium, protein
Zucchini	vitamins B6 and C, folate, magnesium, potassium, carotenoids, omega-3 and -9

Pomegranates have powerful antioxidants that help to firm and strengthen the skin.

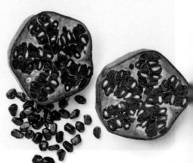

Supplement **boost**

Alongside beauty-enhancing meals, dietary supplements help tackle problem areas by boosting your nutrient intake. Choose good-quality, natural supplements, and follow recommended dosage instructions.

Area	Recommended supplement
Beauty detox kickstart	**Psyllium husks** encourage a gentle bowel movement while cleaning the bowel walls of impurities to help absorb nutrients. Add 1 tsp to 250ml (9fl oz) water, stir, then drink immediately.
	Cascara sagrada and yellow dock contain anthraquinones, which promote bowel movements. Take as teas or tinctures for 1–2 weeks if you are prone to constipation. Avoid cascara if you are taking prescribed drugs, or are pregnant or breastfeeding.
	Dandelion and burdock root help ease bowel movements, and can be taken as teas, tinctures, pills, or capsules. Follow dosage instructions.
	Milk thistle helps the liver to eliminate toxins that have been neutralized during a detox. Take as a tea, tincture, or capsule during your detox, or for a mini cleanse. Follow dosage instructions.
Oily skin	**Zinc complex** helps to balance sebum and aid repair. Take every day.
Anti-aging	**An antioxidant complex** containing grape seed, pycnogenol, and carotenoids boosts circulation to the skin. Follow dosage instructions.
	MSM, or organic sulfur, aids collagen synthesis. Take daily in water.
	Hyaluronic acid, boosts collagen and improves skin tone. Follow dosage instructions.
Sallow skin	**An antioxidant complex** containing grape seed, pycnogenol, and carotenoids, protects blood vessels which improves circulation to the skin. Take the recommended dosage.
Sensitive skin	**An antioxidant complex** containing grape seed, pycnogenol, and carotenoids, protects the skin and blood vessels. Follow dosage instructions.
	Quercetin helps alleviate skin sensitivities caused by allergies. Take the recommended dosage.
Acne	**MSM**, or organic sulfur, helps collagen synthesis, calms skin, and speeds repair. Take daily in water.
Rosacea	**An antioxidant complex** containing grape seed, pycnogenol, and carotenoids, strengthens the blood vessels. Take the recommended dosage.
Cold sores	**Olive leaf** has antiviral, antibacterial, and antifungal properties. It blocks virus-specific systems without affecting gut flora. Take once a day.

Area	Recommended supplement
	L-lysine is an amino acid that helps to prevent outbreaks of cold sores and reduces their severity. Take the recommended dosage.
Cellulite	**Glucosamine** builds and protects the connective tissues in the body, preventing the appearance of cellulite. Follow dosage instructions.
	Omega-3 fatty acids contain anti-inflammatory properties which help to control cellulite and protect collagen. Take every day.
	A multivitamin complex contains several vitamins that tackle cellulite. Vitamin B6 reduces the build up of fluid, while vitamin C boosts collagen levels, which promotes elasticity and keeps skin firm. Vitamin E improves circulation and encourages healthy skin. Take the recommended dosage.
Water retention	**A vitamin B complex** with a good balance of B vitamins can combat water retention. Vitamin B5 helps the body to excrete excess fluid, while vitamin B6 controls the level of the amino acid homocysteine, helping to reduce the risk of water retention caused by heart disease. Take for 4 weeks to see if symptoms subside.
Stretch marks	**Vitamin D** helps to stop skin thinning when it is overstretched, or during rapid growth. Take every day, especially when lacking sun exposure.
Dry body skin	**Biotin** is a B vitamin that helps enzymes to regulate fatty acid metabolism. This helps to promote healthy skin and protect skin cells against free-radical damage and water loss. Take a B-vitamin complex every day for 4 weeks.
Eczema	**MSM**, or organic sulfur, helps collagen synthesis and reduces redness. Take daily in water.
Scars	**Vitamin C** is important for collagen production and is believed to help heal wounds. Choose vitamin C as calcium ascorbate and follow dosage instructions.
	A vitamin B complex aids wound healing by boosting the repairing cells in a wound and the synthesis of protein. Follow dosage instructions.
Hair loss	**Biotin**, taken as part of a good-quality vitamin B complex, promotes healthy hair and prevents hair loss in men. Take the recommended dosage.
Greasy hair	**A vitamin B complex** helps to maintain healthy hair and prevents excess oil and grease. Take the recommended dosage.
Dandruff	**Lecithin** protects the scalp and strengthens the cell membranes of the scalp and hair. Take 1 tsp before eating fatty foods, such as oily fish, to aid fat digestion and help absorb the essential fats needed for a healthy scalp.

Index

Acknowledgments

The authors at Neal's Yard Remedies would like to thank:
our great editor, Claire Cross, from DK.

DK would like to thank: the great team at Neal's Yard Remedies for their
expertise and guidance throughout.

Photography William Reavell
Food styling Penny Stephens and Kate Wesson
Photoshoot prop styling and art direction Isabel de Cordova
Illustration stuart@kja-artists, mike@kja-artists, and Debbie Maizels
Editorial assistance Georgina Palffy and Alice Kewellhampton
Proofreading Nikki Sims
Indexing Vanessa Bird

Disclaimer

Every effort has been made to ensure that the information in this book is accurate.
However, the publisher is not responsible for your specific health or allergy needs that may
require medical supervision, nor for any adverse reactions to the recipes contained in this
book. Neither the authors nor the publisher will be liable for any loss or damage allegedly
arising from any information or suggestion in this book.

Do not give bee pollen to young children, or take it if you have an allergy to honey, honey
products, or bee stings, or if you're pregnant or if breastfeeding. Never exceed the dosage
recommended on the packaging.